P. SIDEBOTHAM

CW01080413

Physical Disability in Childhood

For Churchill Livingstone

Publisher: Georgina Bentliff
Editorial Co-ordination: Editorial Resources Unit
   Copy Editor: Neil Pakenham-Walsh
   Indexer: Joy Warren
Production Controller: Nancy Henry
Design: Design Resources Unit
Sales Promotion Executive: Hilary Brown

Physical Disability in Childhood

An Interdisciplinary Approach to Management

Edited by

Gillian T. McCarthy MB FRCP DCH

Medical Director, Chailey Heritage Rehabilitation and Development Centre;
Consultant Neuropaediatrician, Royal Alexandra Hospital for Sick Children, Brighton;
Visiting Consultant, Ingfield Manor School, Billingshurst, West Sussex

Foreword by

B. G. R. Neville FRCP

Professor of Paediatric Neurology, Institute of Child Health, London; Honorary Consultant
Paediatric Neurologist, The Hospitals for Sick Children, Great Ormond Street, London

CHURCHILL LIVINGSTONE
EDINBURGH LONDON MADRID MELBOURNE NEW YORK AND TOKYO 1992

CHURCHILL LIVINGSTONE
Medical Division of Longman Group UK Limited

Distributed in the United States of America by Churchill
Livingstone Inc., 650 Avenue of the Americas, New York,
N.Y. 10011, and by associated companies, branches and
representatives throughout the world.

First published 1992

ISBN 0-443-04288-8

British Library Cataloguing in Publication Data
A catalogue record for this book is available from the British
Library.

Library of Congress Cataloging in Publication Data
Physical disability in childhood: an interdisciplinary approach to
    management / edited by Gillian T. McCarthy.
        p.   cm.
    Rev. ed. of: The Physically handicapped child. 1984.
    Includes index.
    ISBN 0-443-04288-8
    1. Physically handicapped children.   I. McCarthy Gillian T.
II. Physically handicapped child.
    [DNLM: 1. Child, Exceptional.   2. Handicapped.   3. Rehabilitation-
–in infancy & childhood.   WS 368 P5765]
RJ138.P44   1992
618.92'003—dc20
DNLM/DLC
for Library of Congress   91-23089

Produced by Longman Singapore Publishers (Pte) Ltd
Printed in Singapore

Foreword

A comprehensive clinical textbook on physical disabilities in childhood is much needed and this book fills the gap. I believe it is a major achievement to have produced a cohesive account of such a disparate range of pathologies. The logic of putting them together is that the children and their families have common needs which should lead professionals to provide a multidisciplinary community service and to access tertiary expertise where necessary. It is the 'state of the art' on the subject which is meant as a compliment to the writers but not necessarily to the scientific status of the subject. However, many references to important research set the scene for the revolution which this subject is now ready to experience.

Despite having many authors, the approach holds together because the majority of the writers have worked together, particularly at Chailey Heritage, but also in the South East Thames Region. Chailey is a special place providing medical and educational services for some of the most disabled children in southern England. It has high quality neurology, orthopaedic, orthotic, therapy and engineering input. The writers are both very experienced and busy and their interests within the subject are much wider than the area which they have specifically addressed.

Each chapter is full of useful ideas and the reader is quite appropriately led to think of unanswered questions. A lack of dogmatism and openness is very welcome in a subject which has sometimes produced clashes of belief systems laced with irrelevant appeals to the emotions.

The chapters are free-standing which is particularly useful if this book is used as a course textbook. I believe that doctors, therapists, psychologists and teachers will all find this book a valuable resource and will use it very often as a starting point in developing their own ideas. David Taylor's excellent chapter on 'Mechanisms of Coping with Handicap' is an example of such an essay. Psychiatry is integral to the approach which is truly multidisciplinary. It represents UK practice but the approach is of general applicability. Philippa Russell's excellent analysis of services will be extremely useful for United Kingdom readers and may well be of considerable interest to people outside the UK.

The approach is both compassionate and professional. There are important contributions from two young people who are disabled and from two parents and I think it is a book that one can recommend to interested lay people.

The book represents the level of care for childhood disability which should be available in a developed country. It is a challenge to health and educational authorities to organise this quite ordinary level of provision. There is a need for good research into the effectiveness of intervention strategies in childhood disability but most of what is presented here is a suitable minimum structure which civilised society should be providing for the physically disabled. Many, however, look in vain within their community for a flexible and integrated service for children recovering from head trauma and for a tertiary service which can provide high quality assessment and advice on bladder and bowel care, augmentative communication, special seating and disability orientated orthopaedics. Both super-specialists within the subject and service planners should, I believe, read the whole book, see the big message that it contains as well as its undoubtedly valuable detail. I congratulate Gillian McCarthy on completing this major contribution to the subject.

Brian Neville

Preface

It is nearly a decade since the book out of which *Physical Disability in Childhood* developed—then called *The Physically Handicapped Child*—was published by Faber. In that time society has become more aware of the disabled people in its midst. Parents are asking for more to be done to help their children, however great their disability. Disabled people themselves are demanding to be heard. Politicians are making us aware of the high cost of medical care and education for children with special needs.

The Children Act 1989 lays specific duties upon social services departments, education and health authorities to work together more effectively in the best interests of children. The Act requires every local authority to provide 'services designed to minimise the effect on disabled children . . . of their disabilities and to give such children the opportunity to lead lives which are as normal as possible.'

It is important to look critically at services for disabled children and to ensure that all the people involved in their day-to-day management understand and carry out recommendations made by their therapists, teachers, nurses and doctors. In turn it is important that the therapists, teachers, nurses and doctors understand the complexity of each child and family. Communication is vital and is best achieved by regularly meeting and working together.

All of us who work closely with children and families want our efforts to be effective. Interdisciplinary working implies the merging of roles across disciplines, *enabling* the people closely and constantly in touch with the children—parents, care workers and teachers—to facilitate their development. It is a goal to be strived for and, since staff are constantly changing, one that may feel always just beyond reach! It is therefore essential to establish a teaching programme centred on individual children.

The authors are drawn from all the disciplines working at Chailey Heritage as well as our visiting consultants. We are also fortunate to have contributions from Malgozata Borzsykowski, Professor David Taylor, Philippa Russell, Stephen Dorner, Phil Madden, Judith Middleton and Mother Frances Dominica. Each of these has brought special experience and insight from their particular fields.

Inevitably some background knowledge has to be assumed. References and bibliography are provided at the end of each chapter to encourage pursuit of further information. There is also a glossary at the end of the book.

At Chailey Heritage we have established a 'Charter of Children's Rights' to enable us all to keep in mind that children are the centre of our work.

FOR EVERY CHILD WE CARE FOR, TEACH OR TREAT:
wherever I am, whoever I am with, whatever I am doing, I have these
fundamental rights:
to be valued as an individual,
to be treated with dignity and respect,
to be loved and cared for as a child first,
to be safe.

The aim of this book is to educate and enlighten people who care for children with disabilities. We hope to promote their best possible development and alleviate some of the problems they, and their families, will encounter as they grow up.

Chailey Heritage, East Sussex   G.T.McC.

Acknowledgements

A multi-author book is particularly difficult to draw together. If it is also attempting to be interdisciplinary the problems are multiplied! I would like to thank all the contributors for their hard work, co-operation and patience throughout the elephantine gestation period. The in-house multidisciplinary team of Mary Jones, Valerie Moffat, Sue Crane, Ruth Cartwright and Terri Fearn had a particularly difficult task combining writing with their full clinical workload.

I also wish to acknowledge the contribution of Paddy Downie FCSP, formerly Medical and Therapy Editor of Faber, who sadly died before the second edition was completed. Without her wit, wisdom and support the task would never have been started.

Thanks are also due to Neil Pakenham-Walsh, copy editor, who has been patient, enthusiastic and helpful.

Thanks also to Sam Higgins, Director of the Department of Clinical Photography and Illustration at the Royal Sussex County Hospital, who has taken many of the photographs.

Particular thanks go to the children and parents for allowing us to publish photographs which make the text come alive.

I would also like to thank Neurodevelopmental Paediatricians Dr Peter Rosenbaum, from McMaster University, Canada, and Dr Carolyn West, from Royal Alexandra Hospital for Children, Sydney, Australia, for providing the information for the Select List of useful addresses at the end of the book.

Finally my thanks to all the secretaries who have helped in typing the various chapters. Special thanks to my husband, Stephen, and foster-daughter, Sarah, for putting up with all the paper and my cloistered attachment to the word processor.

G.T.McC.

Contributors

Ulfur Agnarsson MB MRCP
Honorary Lecturer in Paediatrics, King's College Hospital, London and
Royal Alexandra Hospital for Sick Children, Brighton

Gillian Baird MB BChir FRCP
Consultant Developmental Paediatrician, Newcomen Centre, Guy's
Hospital, London

Malgorzata Borzyskowski MB MRCP
Consultant Developmental Paediatrician, Newcomen Centre, Guy's
Hospital, London

Andrew Brown MSc MBES
Deputy Technical Director, Rehabilitation Engineering Unit, Chailey
Heritage

Alistair C. Bruce BEd ADES
Deputy Principal–Head of School, Chailey Heritage

Ruth Cartwright MCSP
Superintendent Physiotherapist (Retired), Chailey Heritage

Jennifer Cattermole BSc Home Office Letter of Recognition in Child
Care, Social Worker, Chailey Heritage

Morwenna Cork SRN HVTutCert
Senior Lecturer in Health Studies, Brighton Polytechnic, Brighton

Sue Crane LCST
Specialist Speech Therapist, Chailey Heritage

R. Dominic Croft MB MRCP
Clinical Medical Officer, Chailey Heritage

Mother Frances Dominica SRN RSCN FRCN
Helen House, Oxford

Steven Dorner MA
Principal Clinical Psychologist, Wessex Unit for Children and Parents,
Middleton Ford, Portsmouth

Terri A. Fearn MCSP
Superintendent Physiotherapist, Chailey Heritage

John A. Fixsen MChir FRCS
Consultant Orthopaedic Surgeon, St Bartholomew's Hospital, London
and The Hospital for Sick Children, Great Ormond Street; Honorary
Consultant Chailey Heritage

Ian Fletcher MRCS LRCP
Senior Medical Officer (Retired), Limb Fitting Centre, Roehampton and
Chailey Heritage

John Florence FBIST
Director, John Florence Orthotic Workshop, Chailey Heritage

William Fuller RSCN
Charge Nurse, Chailey Heritage

Elizabeth M. Green MB ChB DCH
Locum Consultant in Paediatric Rehabilitation, Chailey Heritage;
Developmental Paediatrician, Royal Alexandra Hospital for Sick
Children, Brighton

Alec Harden FRCS FCOpth
Consultant Ophthalmologist, Sussex Eye Hospital, Brighton; Visiting
Consultant, Chailey Heritage

Mary Jones MBAOT SROT
Head Occupational Therapist, Chailey Heritage

Rosemary Land MA MPhil CPsychol
Senior Clinical Psychologist, Royal Alexandra Hospital for Sick Children,
Brighton

Phil Madden BA Diploma in Applied Social Studies
Service Manager, Avon Social Services, Bristol

Ruth Marchant BA (Hons) Developmental Psychology, Child Care
Services Manager, Chailey Heritage

M. Frances Martin MSCP
Superintendent Physiotherapist, Worthing Mental Handicap Team

Gillian T. McCarthy MB FRCP DCH
Medical Director, Chailey Heritage; Consultant Neuropaediatrician,
Royal Alexandra Hospital For Sick Children Brighton; Visiting
Consultant, Ingfield Manor School, Billingshurst, West Sussex

Judith A. Middleton PhD
Principal Clinical Psychologist, Director, Head Injury Unit, Tadworth
Court Children's Hospital, Tadworth, Surrey

Valerie Moffat LSCT
Senior Specialist Speech Therapist, Chailey Heritage

Timothy R. Morley MA MB BChir FRCS
Consultant Orthopaedic Surgeon, King's College Hospital and Royal
National Orthopaedic Hospital; Honorary Consultant Orthopaedic
Surgeon, Chailey Heritage

Catharine M. Mulcahy BScOT MBAOT SROT
Research Occupational Therapist, Chailey Heritage

Roy L. Nelham BEng CEng MIMechE MBES
Technical Director, Rehabilitation Engineering Unit, Chailey Heritage

Carolyn Shumway Nicholls BSc (Mass) RPT MCSP
Formerly Research Physiotherapist, Cheyne Walk, London

Diane Nurse MB ChB FRCS
Senior Registrar in Urology, Guy's Hospital, London

Hugh Parrott CertEd Dip Spec Ed
Principal, Chailey Heritage

Terry E. Pountney MCSP
Research Physiotherapist, Chailey Heritage

Valerie Raynar-Smith DBO(D)
Head Orthoptist, Sussex Eye Hospital, Brighton

Richard O. Robinson MA MB FRCP
Consultant Paediatric Neurologist, Guy's Hospital, London and Chailey
Heritage

Philippa Russell BA
Principal Officer, Voluntary Council for Handicapped Children, London

Martin Samuels MB MRCP
Respiratory Physician, The Brompton Hospital, London

David C. Taylor MD MSc FRCP FRCPsych
Professor of Child and Adolescent Psychiatry, University of Manchester,
Manchester

Carol Thornett BSc PhD
Senior Research Scientist, Chailey Heritage

Lisa Wintle MCSP
Senior Physiotherapist, Chailey Heritage

Alison Wisbeach SROT
Head Occupational Therapist, Department of Neurology and Developmental Paediatrics, The Wolfson Centre, London

Christine S. Young BSc MCSP
Superintendent Physiotherapist, Royal Alexandra Hospital for Sick Children, Brighton

Christina Zergaeng BSc MEd (Ed Psych)
Educational Psychologist, Chailey Heritage

Contents

Introduction: from the inside out

Ann Jones   Christine Howard   Sharon O'Leary
Sarah Thurgood

Much has been written about disability from the professional viewpoint: from the outside in. This chapter takes the personal view: from the inside out. Everyone contributing to this chapter lives with disability, either in themselves or their children.

After high tech intensive care it can be a cruel shock for parents to discover that their child is handicapped. Even if the diagnosis is not made at birth and parents suspect something may be wrong, they are often not prepared for the adjustments to expectations or lifestyle which may be necessary. It is important to recognise how variable responses will be.

A PARENT'S VIEW (1)
Ann Jones

We had only reached month seven in the childbirth guide when, as two very inexperienced parents, we were faced with the news of having given birth to triplet girls 2 months early, their chances of survival only fifty-fifty. We had seen how ill Joanna was; although the biggest and first born, she had jaundice, a stomach block, and had stopped breathing in the incubator. I remember calling a nurse and saying Jo was a funny colour and being told gently but firmly to go back to the ward and I would be called later. Even then we did not contemplate handicap in any of the three girls and optimistically just thought it was a matter of gaining weight.

At first all seemed fine with the three babies although Joanna cried much more than the others . . . but then they can't be all the same; and then Joanna did not focus on toys or pick them up . . . but of course they are bound to do things at a different rate; but then Joanna didn't try to crawl or sit up, and by the time she was showing signs of stiffness and slow development, we had stopped trying to justify her difference. This gradual awareness of problems was, we feel, easier to take than a dramatic announcement earlier on of possible handicap. The actual diagnosis—to have a name, a prognosis, something tangible—was in a way a relief.

The one stage at which we desperately needed help was when Joanna could not (although, having been a difficult baby all along, it looked more like 'would not') take solids. The other two just opened their mouths like little cuckoos and gulped it down. Joanna just seemed to let it slide out, even when I resorted to lying her on her back and tried pouring it down her throat. At this time a gentle word from the health visitor—that perhaps because of Jo's early problems she might not physically be able to eat— would have stopped me feeling literally murderous towards her. The suggestion of giving rice in her milk only delayed what needed to be said. When quadriplegic cerebral palsy was diagnosed at 11 months, weekly physio started. Regular visits and tests at the developmental clinic gave professional support and kindness to dazed parents in great need of reassurance.

We were lucky to live in an enlightened area of Kent where a Dr Barnado's play group could give Joanna, and me, the individual help that was needed. Having two sisters the same age helped us and Jo, in that she joined in everything they did, visiting their playgroup, going on physically active outings, even having ballet lessons with Mum trying to hold Jo and be invisible while tiptoeing like a fairy or stamping like a giant. Joanna loved every moment of this and I am sure would have been denied many such experiences without her sisters leading the way.

Joanna started at Chailey Heritage when she was 3 years 10 months. Physiotherapy started immediately and soon Jo was going to school two mornings a week. She could say very few words but soon began making sentences, and I can remember my joy when she had been on a school outing and could tell me about something she had experienced without me. With her first teacher, music was an important part of each day and I am sure that the repetitious songs helped Jo's speech amazingly. It soon became obvious that she had good comprehension and could handle elementary number work, which was very encouraging.

The difference between Jo and her sisters had not seemed so very great while they were under 5 but the gulf grew greater with the mobility and independence of the able girls. Activities they could whole-heartedly share became less, but still the benefits of three the same age outweighed the lack of time to devote completely to Jo. The worry we often have is not giving enough importance or time to other problems when there is one seemingly insurmountable one.

The next big frontier to cross was surgery. Jo was 'scissoring' badly and, knowing the specialist did not advise surgery until really necessary, we realised the time had come to have the adductor muscles released. There was no other path to be taken. Jo had an extremely successful operation carried out and wonderful postoperative care. She coped well with her 'A' frame plaster and the nights of interrupted sleep have lost their horror, now that they are in the past. With lots of physiotherapy Jo could walk well with a walking frame and was learning to use clumper sticks. Her walking was slow and tiring for her and not particularly useful except as necessary exercise. The extra walking gradually showed up a dragging foot so the specialist did a tendon transplant operation very successfully; we hoped this would be the last operation needed. How many other parents pray that the 'last' operation is the last, only to find more are needed? When Jo was 12 her left hip became critically dislocated. She could not sit or walk with any comfort; the time had come for another, and the most major operation yet. Again we were delighted that this could be done at Chailey and the amazing postoperative care, amongst all the nurses and friends Jo already had, made it less traumatic.

We can look back on the 13 years of Jo's life so far without any regrets and without too many wrong decisions. Maybe we have been rather too complacent but there is only so much energy and time in a day to be striving all the time.

As Jo gets older, correct body positioning wherever possible becomes obviously vital. Having accepted that for speed and independence within the school day she needs to be in a wheelchair, it becomes important that she is seated as perfectly as possible. This is where the Rehabilitation Engineering Unit at Chailey is so ideal, as it is truly multidisciplinary.

For Joanna to go into an Adapta seat seemed a huge decision. We had seen the physically less able children at school using this seating which enables them to be securely seated and increases their abilities when not having to concentrate on sitting. We realised that this seat would mean less independence for Jo initially as transferring in and out was not possible, and with all the necessary 'anchors' to hold her steady she needed help to undo everthing. She looked far more disabled in the Adapta seat but she was sitting beautifully—she said herself that she loved it because she felt safe and secure, comfortable for the first time in her life. We then found that when not using the Adapta at home she felt unsteady and worried in chairs she coped with before, but this has now ceased to be a problem. Cosmetically, and from the independence viewpoint, the chair leaves a lot to be desired, but we realised that the benefits of Jo's major hip operation would be lost if she went back to old habits of bad posture.

Decisions such as the seating are just another example of stress and pressure on us! Jo needs to be on a front-lying board at night to train her positioning. She can only tolerate it for 1½ hours until the onset of spasms, then goes into a night wedge lying on her back. She gets very tired with the unsettled nights, and we also get very fed up and tired, but while she is growing we all know how important this positioning is.

Time seems to be passing very quickly and more decisions will have to be made. Residential schooling may be desirable in the future; we know education up to 19 years and further is possible. Just as hopefully the other two girls will go away to college. After that we hope Jo will be able to find suitable accommodation with enough 'care' to make her independent from us. We will need to be free from the aspect of 'caring' and responsibility for Jo as we get older; we look forward to a life of our own with a relationship with Jo as with Nicky and Emma—background support and love without the burdens of physical caring which can lead to bitterness and boredom.

We want for Jo the same as for her sisters, a happy independent life with the ability to make her own decisions to give her the quality of life and fulfilment that we all seek.

All parents desire a good quality of life for their children , but the parents of handicapped children often feel that the onus is upon them to provide it. This feeling is often all the stronger because they are so aware of what their child is missing. The extra care and attention required by the disabled child can put much stress on the family, and many parents need to develop strategies for coping with it.

A PARENT'S VIEW (2)
Christine Howard

'You're no good', 'you're lazy', 'you're useless'. These are expressions we have all used, or heard others use when tempers are a bit frayed, perhaps at the end of a long and tiring day. All these feed into a child's negative feelings about himself. They might bring out feelings of rejection or low self worth, of being useless and unloved, even though such feelings may be momentary. These feelings are bad enough for a 'normal' child, but they are a hundred times worse for a child with special needs who already has to face the seemingly insurmountable problems ahead of him.

How much better it is to feed these children with positive encouragements. When a child is battling to control uncoordinated body movements it is far more constructive to say 'Come on, lean forward, that's it—good !' rather than a sharp 'No! That's naughty ! Don't throw yourself back.' Telling a child he is naughty when he is struggling to keep his body upright is no encouragement at all.

Experience has taught me as a parent how even a severely handicapped child will respond to a smile and an encouraging tone of voice, rather than a cross look and an irritable voice.

It is also important for professionals to take a positive attitude with children, and parents, in all situations: in preschool play groups and nurseries, in the physiotherapy or speech session, in the classroom, and at clinic appointments. I believe it should be possible to give parents information and advice about their children in a positive way, not 'doom and gloom' without an element of hope. Make them aware of the good points and tell them the many areas of help and support available.

Parents should be actively encouraged to take part in the work with their child—a partnership between parents and professionals. This is easier when the professionals work together with parents as a multidisciplinary team where there is regular discussion about the child's progress. It is also important to set realistic goals for the child, both short and long term so that achievement of a short-term goal is a step nearer the long-term goal.

There are some times where it may not be practical or possible for the parents to be involved, but in most cases parents want and need to be active in working with their children. The atmosphere of the classroom or centre is important. A bright, happy, busy atmosphere can be very stimulating despite the age of the building. On a recent visit to the Pető Institute in Budapest, I was impressed by just such a feeling of enthusiasm and I am aware of other schools and institutions where this is also the case.

An increasing number of parents are sacrificing a great deal to obtain this positive approach. Some are seeking help from abroad and working to raise vast sums of money to fund their trips. They endure long unspecified periods away from the rest of their families for the best of motives, because they feel it will help their children. Although not all parents feel the need to go to such great lengths, most will make frequent sacrifices on behalf of their handicapped child. They will willingly give up their own interests and hobbies to give the maximum amount of time working for and with their child.

There are frequent appointments to be kept with different specialists; there is the constant need to stimulate the child with exercises provided by the physiotherapist and portage worker, as well as working out their own scheme to stimulate the child. Often household chores go unheeded. There is a danger that brothers and sisters may feel left out, or that one parent may take on all the work with the child. It is good to involve all the family, including grandparents who often give much needed love and support, but they need to understand how to handle the child appropriately too.

A link family can be very supportive, giving a break for short or longer periods to allow recharging of batteries.

If the bonding process was difficult the mother may feel rejected by her baby and unable to cope with him in the early days. These feelings often return especially when she is tired. As the child gets older, feelings of guilt may recur because of lack of time or energy—there is always the feeling of not doing enough.

It is good to develop a routine to work to during the day, allowing time for relaxation as well as intensive work times. A child must learn to amuse himself for a short period of time and not always rely on adult company for amusement; this is part of growing up. If the day has a good all round structure involving physical exercises, times for books and games, as well as sociable meal times and toilet training where appropriate, and if there is plenty of conversation, looking, listening, and fun, then the child will progress. There should be flexibility allowing for treats and outings as well. All children feel safe and secure if they have a routine, and for the mothers of handicapped children the structure helps to give a plan to work around. It avoids the problem of feeling 'I'm not doing enough', and if other family members are included it helps to take some of the pressure off the mother and at the same time makes them feel valued and included.

As a parent of a severely handicapped boy I began to develop quite definite ideas about how I wanted my child handled, and what I needed to do in order to help him. I found the structured day worked well for us and it was easy to keep a routine going at home. I have also insisted on consistent handling of my child, although at times it has been difficult convincing people that this is important to Matthew's wellbeing. It is not always easy to give him choices as it is often easier and quicker to do it myself, but it is important to be allowed to make decisions.

On returning to work as a teacher, it seemed right to work with children with special needs. I realise that not all parents feel as I do about working with their children, but I hope I can encourage them to do so and show them the pleasure they can derive from it. It is also important to remember that there are many different approaches—no single path is correct for all children.

I would encourage any mother of a handicapped child to think deeply about her child's needs and formulate a working programme setting realistic short-term goals.

Professionals please continue to help and support the families in the work that they do with their children at home, taking note of what mothers say, as they have care of the children all the time and are the children's first and most important teacher.

It is only in the last 10 years or so that the institutionalised disabled have been considered to have valid opinions of their own. Thirty years ago it was not unusual for parents of severely disabled children to be advised to place them in an institution. This involved a very different way of living and did not prepare the young people for the 'mainstream world'.

British society prides itself on its open-minded attitude to the disabled in recent years. This view is particularly prevalent amongst the able-bodied. Not many ask the disabled what they think . . .

THE CONSUMER VIEW
Sharon O'Leary

I find it difficult to discuss the pros and cons of living in a special boarding school because I have nothing else in the way of family life to compare it with, but a major upheaval that we often faced was becoming emotionally attached to staff who left after a short time. This had emotional repercussions, especially later in life. I enjoyed the sense of camaraderie between the children and staff which I have not felt to such a degree since. Also my reaction on leaving school after 15 years was one of great sadness at being separated from all the people I had grown up with. Maybe it would have been an idea to set up an annual residential reunion to soften the blow a little.

Another concern I have about residential special schools is the alienation they bring. I feel that the Victorian philosophy of providing isolated institutions is largely responsible for many of the prejudices which still exist today. Now, however, this policy has been reappraised and care is slowly becoming more community orientated, particularly since the introduction of child development centres and integrated education.

A third major drawback was the standard of education. Life was definitely geared more towards learning independence skills and medical care. This was good, but education suffered as a result. I realise now that a balance is needed but I felt that the school did not play its part adequately.

Retrospectively, the concentrated specialisation of medical care, independence training and assistance on the premises was a great advantage. This has become more apparent since leaving school. Medical follow-up has sometimes been quite poor, often as a result of ignorance in the general medical world with regard to specialised problems and conditions.

Having left a school where my medical needs were met automatically, I was unsure what medical follow-up I required or what was available. It became apparent that there was a lack of communication between GPs, who seemed equally unsure about special needs, and the appropriate specialists. It was too easy to fall through the net. Had it not been for the consultant I worked for I don't know how long I might have been without the medical care that I required. The follow-up system for adults with multiple problems seems very fragmented, with a lack of liaison between involved professionals. It would make sense to establish adult assessment clinics for people with long-term needs—as far as I know, none exist.

Another thing that worries me is the priority status of the disabled as regards medical care, especially given the present state of the NHS. I have always had the medical treatment I need, but I know that some people have not. I wonder by what criteria people will be deemed worthy of treatment in the future.

I would also like to speculate about the extensive research into prenatal diagnosis. Why is there a need for such techniques in the first place? If they are used purely for the detection of abnormality in order to enable parents and support agencies to prepare for potential problems before birth, this is a reasonable use. But why do so many parents opt for an abortion after diagnosis? I feel this attitude can be attributed to a lack of communication and integration. Because, on the whole, inadequate provision is made, we are often considered a liability, which can only cultivate such a negative attitude. If we were generally considered as equal human beings, with spiritual, emotional, sexual and social drives, many parents might be spared such an agonising choice. 'Abnormality' should be accepted as a natural occurrence, a fact of life, certainly not something to be eliminated. All people should be allowed to 'be'. Who has the right to judge the quality of another's life?

After leaving school my first stop was a further education college for the disabled. I enjoyed much more freedom than previously. The college had good liaison with the technical college next door. Some courses were mixed and students were able to use the facilities of both. The sudden freedom proved too much; I was not used to working without supervision and consequently failed the 'O' levels. From there I was thrown onto a course at a local technical college to retake the examinations I had failed. I had to adjust to a completely new system. Life at college hit me as so fast—up and down stairs, carrying books. Often I felt indebted to other students for the help I constantly needed. If it hadn't been for the great support of a few people, my basic right to study could not have been fulfilled through the existing system. Basically this college, like so many others, was not geared to providing access, and thus opportunities, for the disabled.

Another major adjustment I had to make during this time was moving into a flat on my own. Having always lived with other people, being alone was very difficult. I felt very isolated, was unused to housework and was still only 17.

Independent living means being able to live in a home of your own choice without political, social or access restraints. This is possibly a very idealistic outlook for anybody, and for many disabled people quite unrealistic. Resources vary from area to area, some providing social and nursing services which enable people to have whatever assistance they require for independent living. Some areas also provide cheap transport which permits more journeys a week than the Mobility Allowance. Other areas are unable to provide such services. Consequently people are unable to live independently, and either return to, or cannot leave a residential institution. These services should respect people as individuals and provide for individual needs and freedom of choice.

Spiritual independence means being given the chance to make personal choices, and not being forced by circumstances to follow other people's decisions. It means being in control of your own life, and may sound impossibly altruistic for somebody who is severely disabled.

As for access to public buildings, there is still a disturbing lack of awareness of the needs of the disabled. We are often regarded as a fire hazard, which can only be seen as a measure of our low status in society. The 'fire hazard syndrome' has become an excuse to keep us out, to protect the image of some places. It is also used as a money saving tactic by those not wanting to afford necessary adaptions.

On leaving tech as a qualified medical secretary, I naively assumed that getting a job in the Health Authority would be no problem, but this employer, like many others, was unwilling to employ someone with a disability, not even offering me an interview after many applications. I am convinced that it is essential to present yourself at the employer's office, under the guise of collecting an application form, to conduct your own diplomatic interview. An employer is going to find any excuse to reduce the application forms to an interview list; the disabled applicants will be first in the bin.

I feel the law concerned with employing a percentage of the disabled is a farce. If we must resort to positive discrimination the Department of

Employment should monitor its effectiveness more carefully and support employers who need to make adaptions.

I did eventually get a job with a doctor I knew personally. I took my place on the other side of the desk with trepidation, for I had been affected by other people's blinkered attitude and my self-confidence had taken a beating. I felt I had a lot to prove and the feeling of being on trial was a great pressure, but as it turned out I spent four very happy, successful years in the job.

I then moved away and decided to 'temp' for a time. I haven't had much difficulty getting a foot in, but four wheels hasn't been so easy. I have again been faced with discrimination due to access problems. Unemployment is a major problem for the disabled. Why should people be deemed unemployable and be expected to live on non-contributory benefits when a desperate lack of opportunities oppresses our capabilities?

A PERSONAL VIEW OF DISABILITY
Sarah Thurgood

It's hard to pin-point a time when I didn't realise I was, if not handicapped, at least different. I had five able-bodied brothers who ran everywhere. It didn't take much deduction to realise most people didn't spend their days lying on the floor. But to me that wasn't disability, that was life—my brothers ran, I crawled.

Understanding of any situation changes with the growing up process. Children don't think about life, they just live it. During my childhood I think the only thing my disability really meant to me was physio. I hated it. Infamous battles raged when I was required to do anything at all. I don't believe I had any other understanding of what living with a disability could mean until I left Chailey. Perhaps that sounds impossibly naive, as if I went round with a bucket over my head; perhaps I did. The environment of my childhood was such that my disability hardly impinged on my life. It never prevented me from doing anything I wanted to; there were always care-staff to help, and my natural laziness insured sedentary hobbies anyway. I enjoyed anything I could do easily like reading, and fiction is a good source of insulation when life becomes difficult. I didn't need a bucket. I had an institution, and books.

I remember how I used to laugh when my teachers at Chailey talked about 'Life in the Big Wide World'. I was firmly convinced, aged 15, that I lived in it. That's how I thought of it, in inverted commas and capital letters. The school tried to prepare us for life outside Chailey, and the difficulties we could face, but like all lessons they seemed pleasantly abstract and unlikely. If only I'd known! I was shocked and terrified by the second school I attended. I had never heard such atrocious language! No one at Chailey swore with such monotonous regularity. Neither had I ever seen so many people in one place going so fast. I spent at least the first term wandering around in a daze, utterly panic-stricken and totally lost. Of course I have since discovered that at Chailey life moves in slow-motion and no one ever swears, but I thought that was normal then. I do not know whether it is usual for the long-term institutionalised to have such limited horizons. But I think so.

Leaving Chailey made me realise how facilities for and attitudes to disability vary. For instance the ethos of my second school emphasised independence to a great extent, more so than Chailey. I do not think this is a bad thing in itself, but the general atmosphere at this school seemed unhappy in consequence, and student self-esteem very low. It was my disabled friends who used the derogatory term 'veggie' to describe themselves. Some were convinced they were inadequate, despite what anyone said to the contrary. Maybe this feeling was partly due to our ages. I am told lots of teenagers feel useless.

During this time I, and other students, also attended a mainstream sixth-form college. At college, for some reason there was much peer group pressure to perceive ourselves through the eyes of the able-bodied, so that my feelings of uselessness were constantly reinforced, and indeed started, by my disabled friends. It's a sad fact that the disabled seem to internalise the labels which they think the able-bodied attach to them, and thus perceive themselves as stupid or useless or inadequate in some way, even when the exact opposite is clearly the case.

At sixth-form college I saw my first example of the lack of planning which dogs the 'integrated' disabled. The Student Union decided to change the seating in the canteen. At the time we were already restricted to one section of free-standing tables. In the interests of saving space in a room which was bulging at the seams these tables were exchanged for fixed seating. Anyone restricted to a wheelchair will agree how useless this is; if anyone had consulted us we would have pointed out that it's necessary to move a chair away in order to reach the table, but no one did. After all 10 of us had protested by eating in the corridor—justifiably, we thought, since we couldn't use the canteen—we were given two free-standing tables in the corner. We were offered a classroom but we refused—what price integration then?

Although there was no overt segregation at college, force of circumstance seemed to ensure that we were often segregated from the other students to some degree, particularly socially. For instance the squash in the canteen meant there was no longer any room for able-bodied friends to eat with us unless they sat on the table, and we needed the space! This may seem very trivial, but integration isn't about being in the same room as the able-bodied, it's about being part of the same group, having things in common. The gap between the disabled and non-disabled students was caused not by what we couldn't do together at college, but by what we hadn't done together away from it. Life in institutions can leave huge gaps in a disabled person's experience, especially those with no normal home life to redress the balance. For instance in my entire 19 years I have been to the bank three times.

People make friends naturally when they have opinions and experiences in common. Most non-disabled people have the same general experiences of life which enable them to find common ground. Taking this into account it is easy to see why we were angry at the layout of the tables in the canteen. The institutionalised disabled have little enough opportunity to make new friends outside institutions without having those we do have sabotaged. We were far more segregated by this loss of social contact than we were integrated by being taught together.

If the opportunities to meet people are there, I do not think the disabled make friends any differently from other young people. In fact I think people are ofter friendlier towards the disabled than they would be towards other people because they feel they ought to be. Sometimes it's a case of trying to squash well-meaning people I have no desire to be friends with—usually the sort who introduce themselves very seriously with gems like, 'I've never talked to a wheelchair before!'

There is another reason why contact with people outside institutions is so vital. Leaving Chailey was akin to leaving school and home in one go. I don't think those who have never had this experience can understand the magnitude of the break. Memories of my life before Chailey are distinctly hazy. I hated having to leave; and in my case the break was nowhere near complete. Both my homes are connected to Chailey, and not only did I have three of my best friends with me, I had a member of the teaching staff too. It was still awful. We missed the atmosphere of genuine caring of Chailey. I also found the formality and regimentation difficult.

I think the lack of choice in the lives of the disabled, particularly those who need physical care, is one factor which contributes to their low self-esteem. It's very easy to feel like a parcel and I don't think strict regimes help. Lack of facilities often means that the disabled are restricted as to where they can live and what they can do. This doesn't lead to a feeling of being in control of one's life. It has often seemed to me useless to decide that I will or will not go here or there or do this or that, because circumstances beyond my control will inevitably decide otherwise. It's very depressing to be reminded in the midst of rebellion that actually you have no choice!

To be disabled is to be resigned to an endless round of minor irritants. Like only seeing the bottom of National Trust houses, and being referred to as a wheelchair. They are small things, but are both indicative of the general attitude towards disability. No one would say to someone in a car 'I've never talked to a car before.' I am not a wheelchair, I am me! And why should I not want to see the top half of a National Trust property if I have seen the bottom? I think the disabled are so encouraged by circumstances and society to be grateful for the few rights and choices we are given, that we fail to notice how few they are. I think it's as necessary to change the attitudes of the disabled towards disability as it is those of the able-bodied. We are so used to being seen as second-class citizens, or even wheelchairs, that it seems ordinary. I don't think I protested at being called a wheelchair. I should have.

Vestiges of the old attitudes linger on. The lack of choice and arbitrarily dropped kerbs testify to that. I caused a 9-year-old distress when I called myself spastic; she said it was obvious that I wasn't stupid. I could not convince her that the two were not synonyms. And I did try.

Physical and mental handicap seem inextricably linked in the public mind. I hope this chapter has provided some insight into the differences between the two.

1. The baby and young child

*G.T. McCarthy   M. Cork   S. Crane   M. Jones
P. Russell   C.S. Young*

The birth of a baby with obvious physical abnormality evokes very strong feelings in parents and the staff caring for them. The staff may be unprepared and inexperienced; their reactions are remembered very clearly by the parents years after the event. A recent study on imparting the diagnosis of chronic and life-threatening illness in children (Woolley et al 1989) highlights the clarity of parents' memory of the interview.

It is important to develop a clear policy of management in the delivery room and to prepare junior medical and nursing staff who may be involved for the first time.

If the baby needs resuscitation after birth, this must be done speedily and effectively. If it is necessary to remove the baby for further treatment it is important for the mother to see her baby and if possible hold him, or at least touch him.

Paediatric help will be needed to assess the baby's condition, and an experienced paediatrician should speak to the parents. Most parents want to be told as soon as possible that something is wrong, even though doctors may be uncertain of the exact nature of the impairment (Quine & Pahl 1987). Most studies lead to the conclusion that delay and uncertainty are likely to cause additional distress for the parents and have a lasting effect upon the relationship between doctors and parents.

Obvious severe abnormalities like cleft lip and palate or absence of limbs will have an immediate impact on parents, while a baby with spina bifida for example may not appear to be physically very abnormal. The mental and physical state of the parents, particularly the mother, will inevitably affect the way in which they respond to the news that their baby has a problem. An understanding of the psychological responses to bad news of this sort is very important for the nursing and medical staff who are in direct contact with the parents (see Ch. 2).

It has been shown by follow-up studies that in the period of initial shock only a small fraction of the early information given to parents is retained. More than one session will be required for them to understand what they have been told and to respond with the questions they want to ask.

Basic guidelines for talking to parents include:

- The person to break the news should be the paediatrician
- Both parents should be told together
- A written report should be given to the parents after the initial interview which summarises what the paediatrician has said and gives details of future sources of help, including the name and telephone number of the parents' key-worker.

The help of an experienced member of the nursing staff, who is able to continue discussion and relay worries to the medical staff, is invaluable. Table 1.1 is a nurses' checklist of points to remember.

There is often the added trauma of separation of mother and baby if the baby requires transfer to a paediatric surgical unit before the mother is well enough to accompany him. In addition, there may be a period of indecision before surgery in babies with spina bifida; this is discussed more fully in Chapter 12. Spina bifida presents a particularly complicated picture and requires a multidisciplinary approach with the paediatrician coordinating care, particularly during the early years of life. Charney (1990), in a study of parental attitudes toward management of newborns with myelomeningocoele, showed that there was greater satisfaction expressed by parents to information given in the tertiary centre. Those giving the information were physicians, nurses and social workers with considerable experience in caring for infants with myelomeningocoele and their parents. Furthermore satisfaction was greater in those parents who recalled being actively involved in making choices about management.

If the physical abnormality is rare, such as limb deficiency or arthrogryposis, there is also the problem that the general paediatrician may have little or no experience of the condition. Early referral to a tertiary centre experienced in management is indicated so that the family can receive advice and perhaps also meet older affected children. Introduction to support groups or showing films or videos of children with the same condition at different ages can be helpful.

However, it is very important to be sensitive to the individual response of parents and not to rush them too quickly into learning everything about a particular disability. Not everyone can bear the full implications of their

Table 1.1 The early days: Nurses' Memo. (Reproduced with thanks to Karen Smith)

Talk to parents	Don't avoid them (or their eyes)
Be with them	During and after the paediatrician sees them
Accept	Parents, siblings and baby as a unit
Allow to grieve	Contact—Privacy—Caring—Retaining
Be helpful	Refer to specialist groups/people, answer 'foolish questions'
Be hopeful	It's happened before! Help is available! No prophecies!
Be aware	Of personal factors that make the problem seem even more devastating.

child's problems at first and it is better to give each family as much choice as possible and leave them to make it. However, it may be necessary to help parents move on through the stages of grief, as they may become fixed at one stage and unable to help the child. For this to happen the parents often need one person with whom to relate, and this key-worker, who may be therapist, teacher, health visitor, portage worker or doctor, should keep in contact with other members of the multidisciplinary team.

CHILD DEVELOPMENT CENTRES

In the United Kingdom, Child Development Centres have been set up over the past 20 years in an effort to provide a focus for the assessment and management of young children with disabilities. They vary in the composition of staff and in the way in which they relate to the local services. They may be community or hospital based, and directed by a community or developmental paediatrician. Many Health Districts have a Handicap Team which aims to coordinate care, and is based at the CDC.

In addition to medical services, the centre often provides group activities to stimulate young children and to encourage parents to be the main educators of their children. Therapy may be given in groups or on an individual basis, and home visits of teacher and therapist establish trust and an excellent working relationship.

For young children with special needs, between the ages of 2 and 5 years, the education authority has a statutory duty to provide early education. These are vital years for preparing the young child, particularly if there are plans for attendance at mainstream school. The combination of specialist groups and integration in a local playgroup is an ideal way of preparing the young child for school.

In a local area there may be several professional and self-help groups such as opportunity groups. Social services departments are setting up teams to work with disadvantaged families in their own homes as well as in day centres. This is a particularly imaginative way to help deprived parents who have to learn parenting skills. They often have no idea how to play with their children.

It is important that there is enmeshing of services so that full use is made of available resources. In the future the services for the under-5s should be better integrated as long as there is proper communication between the professional groups.

Regional Assessment Centres

These provide specialist help with difficult cases. They should also provide a district service for local children in order to see a cross-section of childhood disability. In addition, they should be a focus for research and development. It is all too easy to continue the same practice without questioning its validity. We need to constantly review, and share and discuss ideas in order to move forward.

DIAGNOSIS AND DEVELOPMENTAL ASSESSMENT

Dr Mary Sheridan (1973) defined a handicapped child as one who suffers from any continuing disability of the body, intellect or personality whi·h is likely to interfere with his normal growth and development or capacity to learn.

The skill of carrying out a full paediatric, neurological and developmental examination can only be acquired with practice, and the initial examination may not include a full developmental profile, although this is often possible in babies and young children. It is usually better to concentrate on the physical examination and arrange a separate session for developmental assessment.

Analysis of the examination is important as neurological problems may impair developmental levels, giving a false picture of cognitive potential.

The examination starts as soon as the mother brings the baby into the room. *Observation* of the way in which she responds to the baby, her confidence in handling, and their reponse to each other gives an enormous amount of information. Allow the baby to get used to you whilst you are talking to mother, then ask her to handle him for as much of the examination as possible. Watching spontaneous movement gives a great deal of information particularly in babies with postural disabilities. A skilled nurse who encourages the baby with appropriate toys is a great asset, as she will be able to divert attention at the right moment. Develop a system of examination, and spend time recording it as soon as possible afterwards. Baird & Gordon (1983) give a wonderful, practical, detailed description of neurological evaluation which amplifies this approach.

Children with multiple disabilities are particularly difficult to assess and it is important to gain a clear idea of their vision and hearing as well as assessing their motor function, manipulation, language and social development. This is discussed in more detail later in this chapter and in Chapters 3, 4 and 5.

DEFINING AIMS

Why has the baby been referred?

1. To determine whether a problem exists
2. To define the extent of the problem and diagnose the cause if possible
3. To determine the present implications for general health and development and make an informed guess about future implications
4. To provide genetic counselling
5. To develop a programme of management that includes family support,

continuing assessment by appropriate professionals and a willingness to let the family choose the way in which they wish to be helped.

Medical investigations

Medical investigations should be carried out early, with the aim of diagnosing the cause of the problem if possible (Table 1.2). It is also important to review the diagnosis from time to time in older children as new information may emerge.

Genetic counselling

This is best arranged after full investigation so that the Geneticist has as many facts as possible for the consultation. Genetic departments are usually based in teaching hospitals but many consultants carry out peripheral clinics, often held jointly with paediatricians. This allows information to be shared, teaches junior staff and gives much better communication. It is important to understand the dynamics of counselling, parents may have many different reasons for requesting counselling which need to be established at the time.

THE ROLE OF THE HEALTH VISITOR

As a health professional working in the community, the health visitor has an established role in visiting families in their own homes. She may thus be seen as more socially acceptable by the family with a handicapped child because they do not feel they are being singled out for her visits. Health visitors are now generally working as members of a primary health care team, and take their case load from the general practitioner's list. They have a knowledge of services within their local community and should therefore be able to provide valuable information about local support available for the family, such as parent self-help groups, playgroups, toy libraries, and the general health, social and educational services in the area.

Ideally the health visitor's initial involvement with the family should be in the antenatal period. This will allow a relationship to be established with the parents and for some insight to be gained into the family atmosphere before it has been affected by the trauma of the birth of a handicapped child.

If the handicap is diagnosed at birth, then a common reaction is one of grief at the loss of a 'normal' child (Gath 1982, Darling 1979). The parents may go through many of the stages associated with bereavement. These are outlined by Parkes (1975) and include shock and numbness, denial, anxiety and restlessness, searching, anger, and guilt.

When visiting the family following the birth of a handicapped child, the health visitor must be prepared for the parents' grief reactions and accept

Table 1.2 Causes of physical handicap, associated problems, genetic implications and useful investigations

Cause	Abnormalities: complications	Leading to	Investigations
Neural tube defects i.e. failure of fusion of neural tube	Spina bifida: meningocoele encephalocoele meningomyelocoele	Hydrocephalus Paralysis Loss of sensation Incontinence of urine/faeces	Skull and spine radiographs Brain ultrasound, CT scan Renal/bladder ultrasound Urodynamic studies, DMSA scan, GFR
	Spina bifida occulta	Weakness of legs Anaesthesia Bladder problems	Spinal radiographs Myelogram IVP; cystogram Urodynamic studies
Infection in utero 1. Virus infections, e.g. rubella, cytomegalovirus	Hepatosplenomegaly; purpura; pneumonia	Bleeding tendency	Virus antibody titres—baby and mother (Baby IgM antibody=intrauterine infection) Virus grown from urine or throat swab
	Microcephaly	Mental handicap Cerebral palsy	CT brain scan—malformation, atrophy, periventricular lucency, calcification
	8th cranial nerve damage	Sensorineural deafness (50%)	Radiograph bones—neonatal to 6 months to demonstrate demineralisation of lower femur
	Cataract; retinopathy	Visual handicap (30%)	
	Congenital heart disease (CHD)	Persistent ductus arteriosus (PDA) 50%; pulmonary stenosis; ventricular septal defect (VSD); atrial septal defect (ASD)	Chest radiograph; ECG; echocardiogram; cardiac catheter
2. Protozoal organisms, e.g. toxoplasmosis	Microcephaly Hydrocephalus Chorioretinitis	Mental handicap Cerebral palsy; epilepsy Visual handicap	Complement fixation test Sabin-Feldman test—requires living protozoa X-ray skull—calcification CT scan—periventricular calcification
3. Other viruses	Anterior horn cell damage	Arthrogryposis	Antibody titres—mother/baby

Table 1.2 (contd)

Cause	Abnormalities: complications	Leading to	Investigations
Drugs	*Thalidomide*: limb deficiency; deafness; congenital heart disease (CHD)		
	Phenytoin: limb anomalies		
Perinatal insults Hypoxia Hypoglycaemia Intrauterine growth retardation Haemorrhage: ante or intrapartum	Microcephaly Diffuse cerebral damage	Cerebral palsy Visual handicap Deafness Epilepsy Mental handicap	Skull radiograph CT brain scan Full examination of optic fundi
Jaundice (hyperbilirubinaemia)	Athetoid cerebral palsy High tone deafness		Audiological investigations Electrocochleography in some cases
Prematurity **Traumatic delivery**, e.g. Breech delivery High forceps Multiple birth Cephalopelvic disproportion	Intraventricular haemorrhage Periventricular leukomalacia Hydrocephalus Cystic changes	Cerebral palsy (especially spastic diplegia) Epilepsy Mental handicap Severe visual handicap —retinopathy of prematurity —cortical blindness Deafness	Ultrasound brain scan CT scan Electroencephalogram (EEG) Visual evoked responses (VER) Brainstem evoked responses (BSER) Electroretinogram (ERG) Audiological assessment Electrocochleography in some cases
Genetic syndromes	Typical collection of anomalies Upper limb abnormalities Congenital heart disease (CHD) Radial club hand; thrombocytopaenia Lobster claw	e.g. Down's syndrome Turner's syndrome X-linked mental retardation Holt–Oram syndrome Fanconi's syndrome Hand anomaly	Chromosome analysis: Trisomy 21 XO Fragile site on X chromosome Chest radiograph; ECG Full blood cell count; radiograph of arms Family history—three generations

Table 1.2 (contd)

Cause	Abnormalities: complications	Leading to	Investigations
Metabolic disorders	e.g. Lesch–Nyhan syndrome	Hypotonia: severe athetoid cerebral palsy Self-mutilation	Urine—uric acid: creatinine raised Hypoxanthine guanine phosphoribosyl transaminase (HGPRT) enzyme absent in red blood cells; X-linked Female carriers detected using hair follicles
	Other metabolic disorders	Hypotonia: severe developmental delay Epilepsy	Amino-acids in plasma and urine Organic acids in plasma and urine Mucopolysaccharides in plasma and urine Metachromatic granules in urine Enzyme abnormalities in WBCs Regional centres for investigation of rare recessive forms
Anterior horn cell disorders	1. Anterior horn cell degeneration (Werdnig–Hoffmann disease) (autosomal recessive)	Progressive muscle weakness before 6 months Areflexia; fibrillation; fasciculation of tongue. Death before 2 years. Some cases arrest with severe weakness and progress very slowly to death in late teens or early 20s	Electromyography (EMG) Creatine phosphokinase (CPK) (usually normal) Muscle biopsy
	2. Intermediate form (autosomal recessive)	Presents after 6 months Usually sit but need orthoses for standing and walking Progressive weakness secondarily to growth	Creatine phosphokinase (CPK) usually normal, may be slightly raised Electromyography (EMG) Muscle biopsy
	3. Late onset (Kugelberg–Welander disease) (autosomal recessive)	Usually ambulant, but weak; scoliosis may develop	Creatine phosphokinase (CPK) usually normal, may be slightly raised Electromyography (EMG) Muscle biopsy

Table 1.2 *(contd)*

Cause	Abnormalities: complications	Leading to	Investigations
Muscular dystrophy	Congenital	Early weakness—may be severe	Electromyography (EMG) Muscle biopsy Creatinine phosphokinase (CPK) raised
	Duchenne	X-linked: boys, present at 2½+ years	Creatine phosphokinase (CPK) very high EMG, muscle biopsy Carrier detection possible using DNA probes, CPK is raised in 70%
Skeletal disorders	Fragilitas osseum	Fractures Typical features	Radiographs—skeletal survey Carrier detection using fibroblast culture and studying connective tissue
	Osteodystrophies		Registers set up in many regional genetic centres to collect and pool information

that some of their anger and hostility may be directed towards the health professionals. In the past parents have been critical of health visitors for not responding appropriately to these normal grief reactions and withdrawing from the situation or keeping discussions at a superficial level, thereby not allowing parents to work through their grief (Ballard 1976, Hannam 1975). There is now an increasing emphasis on the health visitor's counselling role in relation to families with a handicapped child, and hopefully they will be able to meet the needs of parents more effectively.

If the handicap is not diagnosed at birth then the health visitor may be one of the first people the parents turn to if they are worried about their child's progress. Sheridan (1973) has stressed the need for health professionals to pay attention to any anxieties the parents may have—they are the ones in constant contact with the child, and if they are concerned about his development then he should be assessed. Increasingly, health visitors are being involved in programmes of developmental surveillance. They are therefore better equipped to respond promptly to any concern expressed by the parents. Even if the parents are not aware of any problems, the health visitor may detect developmental delay when carrying out routine developmental surveillance of the child. In either situation the health visitor has a responsibility to ensure that the child then has a full developmental assessment. The family will need continuing support from the health visitor while the child is undergoing tests, and when the diagnosis is made their reactions may be very similar to those of the parents whose child's handicap is apparent at birth.

In addition to the need to express their feelings, the family will want advice and guidance on the care and management of the child. The state of shock which follows the initial diagnosis may well result in the parents taking in very little of what is said to them about the extent of the handicap, prognosis and future care needs. The need to go over the implications of the handicap and reinforce information given is well recognised. It is when parents return home with the child and assume full responsibility for his care that many questions are raised relating to day-to-day management. The parents face the same problems of adjustment to new roles and responsibilities as all parents but, for them, problems may be exacerbated by feelings of inadequacy, fear of handling their handicapped child and hopelessness about their child's future.

The health visitor should be able to provide support and guidance for them during this critical period of adjustment. As a visitor in the home, she is able to be flexible both about the amount of time she spends with the family and the frequency of her visits. In the familiarity of their own home the parents may be more relaxed and feel more confident about discussing the realities of the problems they face. The health visitor may be able to offer practical advice on coping with everyday problems, such as feeding difficulties, the crying baby, and disrupted sleep patterns. Her knowledge of the handicapping condition may need to be augmented and advice sought.

If the health visitor's contribution to the care of the family with a handicapped child is to be fully effective, it is essential she has good liaison with the other professionals working with the family. It is often helpful if she can accompany the family on some of their visits to the hospital or assessment centre. This will allow her to hear the advice and guidance given and she can then reinforce this in her home visits. She can also help the family prepare themselves for these visits by drawing up with them a list of issues they wish to discuss; often, when faced with the stress of a hospital visit, parents forget many of the things they intended to ask.

Recently some health authorities have started to train health visitors as home advisors for the Portage Home Intervention programme. This programme is designed to teach parents how to help their child to develop specific skills. It involves an assessment of the child's present level of ability and then, in consultation with the parents, specific teaching targets are decided upon. These targets are broken down into small steps and a learning goal is set for each week. The Portage home advisor demonstrates how to teach the child the activity and then observes while the parent practises teaching the child. An activity chart is left with the family, outlining the particular skill that is being developed, the manner in which it should be carried out and the number of times the activity should be done per day. The chart also has space on which to record the child's progress over the week. The home advisor visits a week later to assess how the child has progressed with the activity and, if it has been mastered successfully, will introduce a new learning goal. Where health visitors have been involved with the programme, they have found it increases the effectiveness of their work (Mansell 1980).

The parents' need for a life of their own should be acknowledged and, if possible, the health visitor should try to find ways of providing short-term relief for the family. Liaison with social services is important here. In some areas it is possible to arrange a short-term admission to a hospital or residential unit. Alternatively it may be possible to arrange for foster parents to care for the child for the occasional weekend or while the parents and other children have a short holiday. Even arranging for a baby-sitter so that parents can have an evening out on their own can be invaluable in maintaining their morale and ability to cope.

The extent to which the health visitors provide support for families with handicapped children is variable. In many instances their involvement with the family ceases once the child starts school, particularly if he goes to a residential school. Warnock (1978) emphasises the importance of the health visitor in providing a link between the home and the school, and with the introduction of the 1981 Education Act health visitors may have an increasing involvement with the older child and his family.

The role of the health visitor can be very wide ranging. It encompasses information for the family about the handicapping condition, the services available, advice on the care and management of the child, and support for the family through periods of stress. She is also concerned with the physical, social and emotional health needs of all family members.

The specialist health visitor

The need for a health visitor with special expertise in relation to children with disabilities has been recognised. The emphasis is on the specialist being a resource person for the family health visitor and later the school nurse, particularly when the child is in mainstream school (Twinn 1981). She may be involved in joint visits to the family, or work intensely with them during a crisis period. However, it is the family health visitor who gives continuing long-term support.

In some health authorities there are specialist health visitors based in the children's hospital or in residential units or schools for the disabled. These health visitors provide an invaluable link between the hospital or school and the child's home. They are increasingly involved in training care assistants and teachers in mainstream schools and work closely with continence advisors. Parents value the support from someone with practical experience in the wide range of care that they have to learn to provide.

THE ROLE OF THE PHYSIOTHERAPIST

The paediatric physiotherapist often becomes involved with the handi-capped child and his family in the early weeks or months. A diagnosis may not have been established, but where there is delay in motor ability the physiotherapist can advise parents how to encourage the child to develop basic motor skills. There is also an important psychological role in giving parents confidence in handling their child.

Following the normal pattern of development parents can be shown how to help their child to achieve head and trunk stability, to become aware of their hands and feet, and to experience the feeling of normal movement. The role of the physiotherapist may overlap with that of the occupational therapist. Both will assess the child's level of ability and advise on suitable positioning, activities and equipment to enable the maximal development of functional skills.

To fully exploit each child's potential the physiotherapist should be skilled in handling children with neurological disorders. This ensures that the parents can be taught to handle their child correctly and with con-fidence. An experienced therapist will be able to suggest practical ways of overcoming problems related to the child's motor skills. It is important to take time to get to know the child and his family so that mutual rapport and a communicative relationship is firmly established. In this way the child can be clearly seen within the context of his family dynamics, and his problems assessed in the light of this. The preparation of an appropriate management programme can then be accurately tailored to the scope or limitation of the carers. It is vital that parents see management as a continuous process and carry it through to the home environment to encourage the child's maximum level of achievement. The physiotherapist must be both realistic about the child's abilities and potential whilst also being positive about solving problems. Often the therapist can help parents to adjust to the difficult realisation that their child may not achieve many motor skills and therefore management must be geared towards providing suitable equipment for daily living and to minimise deformity.

Assessment for the provision of orthotic equipment to enhance function and/or reduce the likelihood of deformity occurring may be an important part of the management programme, which is often coordinated by the physiotherapist.

Children who are developing and adding to their range of motor skills need to be reviewed regularly and progression of their management programme must be undertaken. It is helpful to see the child in his other environments, e.g. home, nursery, school, so that suggestions for his motor development can be incorporated into other activities.

Working with parents and children in groups—in addition to individual sessions—is often a valuable way to encourage motor development. The use of repetition and singing whilst breaking down complex movements into simple stages can be an enjoyable way to learn for children and parents. The additional benefit is the mutual support and encouragement the parents give each other. Similarly treating older children in a well matched group fosters peer support, encouragement and team work.

The physiotherapist is likely to be involved with a handicapped child and his family on a long-term basis during the early years of his growth and development.

The aim of the paediatric physiotherapist is to encourage each child to develop his potential so that maximum function is achieved, deformity is prevented or reduced and the effect of handicap is minimised. Encompassed within this is the need for the child to be securely established within the family and for the family to take its place within the community. Therefore it is important that the physiotherapist works as part of an integrated and coordinated professional team that provides a comprehensive and appropriate system of care. (See also Dunn et al 1990.)

THE ROLE OF THE OCCUPATIONAL THERAPIST

The occupational therapist (OT) also works as part of the multidisciplinary team and will focus attention on the child's functional abilities. The OT should be introduced to the family as early as is practical after diagnosis, although the baby's parents are likely to come in contact with a large number of professional workers while they are coming to terms with the diagnosis, and care must be taken to introduce each new face gradually.

A home visit should be carried out where the OT can meet the parents and siblings and discuss the baby's management while seeing the family home. Any practical problems that are troubling the parents can be discussed during the visit. The OT can discuss the methods of assessment used and the techniques indicated, so that the parents feel involved with the programme. Isolated sessions of therapy are of little use unless followed through by all who come in contact with the baby. The parents need to be shown how to handle the baby, and the activities and techniques recommended can be included in the Portage Programme if one is organised locally.

The initial assessment may be carried out as part of a multidisciplinary assessment organised in the local CDC or District Handicap Team. Once the initial assessment has been completed the OT will demonstrate positions, handling techniques and play activities related to the child's stage of development, which will help him to extend his skills. The programme of activities can be updated or amended by continuous reassessment to ensure that it remains relevant to the child's level of functioning.

Much of the OT's work is aimed at providing practical solutions to problems of day-to-day management. Advice is required on desirable positions for play, feeding, dressing, bathing and changing. These may be discussed with other team members. The OT frequently has access to a stock of equipment for short-term loan. Items such as wedges, supportive seating, potty chairs or special toys can be invaluable. The issuing of first items of equipment must be sensitively handled; it is important not to fill the family home with furniture and gadgets before exploring the child's ability to cope in a normal way.

When a new baby arrives, whether or not he has a disability, families often consider moving to a larger home. The OT can enable the child's parents to view the future realistically and choose a house which allows for mobility and access in the future.

Positioning

The baby with motor disability needs to be maintained in a variety of positions throughout the day. These should aim to encourage motor control and prevent incorrect patterns of movement. A correct sitting position is vital and it is important to ensure that the seat fits and is correctly padded to provide support whilst allowing active postural adjustment (see Ch. 25). The child needs to be able to see his hands and will require a tray at optimum height to encourage hand–eye coordination and give trunk support. A border to prevent toys falling off and a non-slip surface are helpful. Feet must be supported, and a grab bar will allow stabilisation with one hand while the other is used in play.

Occasionally two kinds of seat are indicated, one that provides little support and encourages the child to work at postural control, and another giving postural stability while the child works at fine play activities.

Similar padding, footrests and harness may need to be applied to car seats and baby buggies to ensure a safe, functional and symmetrical position.

Play

Play is essential for child development: it is part of the child's work, and through play the child learns about his world. For the baby and young child with physical disability, play is often distorted, frustrating and difficult to achieve. When the child is suitably positioned in prone or over a wedge or in a seat, play can be enhanced by selection of attractive, appropriately adapted and developmentally correct toys. Advice to parents about play should include selection of suitable toys and limitation of their number in order to encourage concentration.

Activities of daily living

Management of feeding is discussed later in this chapter. A range of shallow polycarbonate spoons, non-slip mats, scooper bowls and two handled beakers are useful during day assessment and for loan to the family.

The OT may advise on the selection of suitable clothes, not too tight-fitting and with generous openings. Dressing is the time when the child can be taught the names of different parts of the body and articles of clothing. The ideal position for dressing each particular child should be demonstrated to all his carers.

Bathing is usually the time when the baby or young child is most relaxed, with water partially supporting his limbs. If a bath aid is recommended, it should not be too restrictive but provide enough support for safety, leaving the parents' hands free for washing and playing. A contoured sponge pad is often sufficient. When transferred to the big bath, a non-slip mat and some head support might be necessary.

Toileting

Support, comfort and a feeling of total safety are important when considering potty training and a range of potties providing additional postural support is available (see p. 555).

THE ROLE OF THE SPEECH THERAPIST

A speech therapist may become involved in early management in two ways:

- If there are feeding problems
- If communication, language or speech are delayed or disordered.

Feeding difficulties often precede speech disorders, and communication and language development are often compromised before speech delay becomes apparent. Early intervention and support can have a major effect on the development of communication.

NORMAL DEVELOPMENT OF COMMUNICATIVE COMPETENCE

The infant is learning basic pre-verbal skills which will be the foundation upon which he will build later speech and linguistic abilities.

I Non-verbal methods of communication

- Facial expression: smiling, frowning
- Gesture and body posture: cuddling, arms out to be picked up
- Vocalisation: screaming, cooing, mimicking sounds, singing.

II Knowledge of the world

The baby learns about himself as a separate person from his carers. He learns about his environment using his senses, mobility, and by manipulating people. This knowledge allows the infant to understand objects, situations and events, and gives him ideas to express.

1. Objects. He learns about the object world—his environment—and his effect on that world:

a. Object permanence and search skills
b. Exploratory play
c. Relating two objects together
d. Cause and effect—means end—goal directed play
e. Construction—classification—symbolic imaginative play.

2. People and social play. He learns how to interact, to manipulate people, and to become a social being:

a. Responding to human contact/attachment
b. Seeking adult attention
c. Initiating contact for social gain
d. Turn taking
e. Imitating
f. Interacting and cooperating with adults and children.

3. Object–people play. He learns to combine objects and people in the same interaction:

a. Joint attention with an adult on the same object
b. Initiating object play for social contact
c. Use of a person to manipulate objects.

4. Sound and language knowledge. He learns to understand his language environment and formulate expressive ideas:

a. Listening and turning to sound
b. Discriminating, identifying and responding to meaningful sounds
c. Discriminating, identifying and anticipating routines and people
d. Tuning-in to speech
e. Learning to interpret gesture, facial clues, eye contact, gaze
f. Learning about speech in context with maximal clues
g. Responding to speech with minimal clues
h. True word understanding
i. Language understanding and internal formation of expression, e.g. *vocabulary, syntax* (grammar), *semantics* (meaning)
j. Memory and sequencing skills.

III The purpose of communication

- To start, maintain or end an interaction
- To ask questions, give or obtain information, fulfil a need, comment, etc.

IV The role of the carers

The care giver in turn is also learning about the infant's emerging skills' and is responding intuitively to reinforce and facilitate further development. Effective communication will only take place when both adult and child have some common understanding of the method being used to send the messages, some shared awareness of the subject, and perception that there is a purpose behind the interaction.

The normal infant develops skills not by specific structured teaching sessions but by everyday life experiences. One such recurring routine is feeding time. It is a very significant time for the earliest communication between mother and baby, a time for tuning in to speech, making eye contact, and receiving close attention. In addition it is the time for developing important physical and cognitive skills related specifically to eating and drinking.

NORMAL DEVELOPMENT OF FEEDING COMPETENCE

Mealtimes give the most natural and repetitive opportunity for the child to develop the skills necessary for eating and drinking and to integrate them into a functional system under voluntary control. By the age of 2 years most children will have developed the basic oral skills of the adult in eating and drinking. They may be messy and prone to slipping back to immature patterns, but can usually manage a wide variety of adult food presented in a range of sizes and consistencies, and from different utensils.

Oral developmental stages

1. Suckle/swallow stage. At birth the infant has a reflex suckle/swallow response to draw milk from a nipple or teat. Voluntary control develops but any other coordinated pattern of movement to deal with food is impossible. Sensory tolerance and range of movement are limited.

2. Weaning stage. The baby is presented with smooth semi-solid food from a spoon. New patterns of oral movement must be acquired to deal with the new utensil and the new food. Greater sensory tolerance to deal with the widening range of tastes, textures and temperatures is necessary. Yet more movement patterns are required when small lumps are introduced—they need more exploration than a simple squash and swallow will provide.

3. Chewing stage. The baby needs to learn how to crush food down and mix it with saliva into a consistency comfortable for swallowing. A far broader range of food requiring an even greater sensory tolerance is given. Progressively more complex oral activity is required to deal with each mouthful. The food is presented from different utensils—spoon, fork, on a stick—and each method requires different combinations of movement to be successful.

4. Drinking. Initially the infant uses reflex suckling on the nipple or teat. The mouth and lips seal around the nipple at the front and milk is drawn out, transferred along a grooved, rippling tongue and swallowed in one rhythmical, efficient, coordinated pattern involving lips, jaw, tongue, cheeks, palate and pharynx. As it is one continuous process from latch-on to swallow, the whole system breaks down or becomes less efficient if there is interruption or difficulty at any stage.

As the baby's drinking skills develop he is introduced to a cup. New skills are required for the lips to form a seal on the cup or feeder lid; the tongue to hold, mix and gather drinks into a lump (bolus) ready for swallowing; and to coordinate swallowing with breathing. New skills are also required for catching, transferring and swallowing dribble in association with removal of the cup.

The baby's ultimate achievements are to sip and swallow from any utensil offered; to gather and swallow saliva effectively without the assistance of dummy, cup or fingers, and independent of posture; and to suck maturely through a straw.

The functions of the voluntary stage of drinking are gradually mastered individually and become less dependent upon total oral patterns and reclining posture. Only the involuntary swallow stage stimulated when the bolus reaches the pharyngeal area remains purely reactive in adult life.

The five main areas of maturation of oral skills

1. Increasing *range* of oral movements

2. Increasing *fine motor* movements
3. Increasing *voluntary control* of those movements
4. Increasing *sensory tolerance*
5. Increasing *integration of motor and sensory skills* into a *functional system*.

The normal infant has an inbuilt adaptability and flexibility in his reactions which allows him to adjust to most varieties of food, utensils and techniques presented to him.

ASSOCIATED DEVELOPMENT AT MEALTIMES

I Health and growth

The infant needs reasonably efficient feeding skills in order to receive adequate and varied nutrition necessary for health and growth. An adequate fluid intake is also required.

II Social and language development

1. Bonding. Feeding time is most important for the early bonding between mother (and father) and baby. It is a time of intimate contact between two people where there is eye contact, vocalisation and natural communication. The baby begins to develop and shows basic feelings of satisfaction, delight, boredom and fear. The mother begins to identify her baby as an individual whom she can understand, care for and influence, and with whom she can communicate.

2. Social rules and integration. The older infant will gradually be included in family mealtimes and learn social rules and develop skills in turn-taking, coping with discipline, and sharing his mother with other people. As he becomes increasingly proficient his acceptability and integration into the family mealtime becomes greater.

3. Language. Mealtimes offer considerable scope for children to learn language. Particular concepts are regularly rehearsed e.g. more/no more, full/empty, hungry/thirsty, hot/cold, etc. The regular routine of mealtimes reinforces ideas of time—going to eat, eating, have eaten, finished; ideas of possession—mummy's cup, your spoon; and ideas of choice.

4. Social roles and functions. Mealtimes and activities surrounding food and drink offer an ideal time to learn about social rituals. Food and drink are often used in celebration and hospitality; to give rhythm and regulation to the day; and to help family/group maintenance. They are also used for comfort or respite and have a major function in establishing and maintaining relationships.

III Control and independence

The baby learns to exert control from an early age, for example he learns to stop suckling when full, to close his mouth firmly when he does not want the food, or to demand more if still hungry or wishing to maintain the social situation. Once able to be totally independent in feeding, the child can enter into new social situations without his care-giver, and can develop self-reliance.

IV Physical development

The feeding environment offers numerous occasions in which a baby can develop physical skills. He must master an increasingly upright and less supported posture when eating, greater hand and eye coordination for finger feeding and use of utensils, and ability to integrate several functions simultaneously, e.g. sitting, eating, listening, talking.

V Cognitive development

There are opportunities to learn the relationships of objects, e.g. spoon/fork, plate/cup; properties of objects, e.g. sticky, wet, crumbly, hot, cold, etc.; and how actions affect the world, e.g. tipping a plate, banging a spoon on a plate. Increasing ability to control actions, improve attention skills and develop conforming behaviour.

VI Discovering speech and non-speech sounds

The baby readily experiments with oral movement, oral control, and sound making when eating. For example he is most likely to learn about lip sounds when he is making noises with the spoon or his fingers in his mouth, e.g. raspberry blowing, 'p', 'b' and 'f' sounds. There is a strong link between the emergence of particular sounds and the development of specific oral movements in feeding. It is rarer for a child to master an oral movement first in sound making and this usually occur when there has been atypical eating experience.

REQUIREMENTS FOR DEVELOPMENT OF FEEDING AND COMMUNICATIVE COMPETENCE

The normal infant is able to respond efficiently and flexibly to learning opportunities open to him using the following systems:

- *Sensory system* by which he is aware of messages from his own body and the environment around him
- *Cognitive system* by which he can interpret the information supplied by his sensory system and formulate his response
- *Movement system* by which he can act on his environment
- *Language and social system* by which he can specifically interpret and respond socially.

In addition the infant's development can be enhanced or hindered by the *opportunities* to learn and respond which are provided by his environment and those around him.

EFFECT OF DISABILITY ON LEARNING SYSTEMS

Physical disability will always affect the movement system to a greater or lesser degree but there is often difficulty in one or more of the associated learning systems, which may be so severe that the physical problem ceases to be the most disabling factor. For example, a profound cognitive disability may mean the child will have difficulty learning to manage his physical problems; a severe sensory disability (blindness or deafness) will significantly increase the problems the physically disabled child has interacting with his environment.

EFFECT OF PHYSICAL DISABILITY ON COMMUNICATIVE COMPETENCE

Non-verbal methods of communication

Non-verbal methods of communication that are severely affected include:

- Problems responding and organising movements in the way desired
- Problems with unintentional responses
- Speech severely affected by poor control of breathing, voice and oral movements for speech.

Knowledge of the world

Object knowledge

Factors that severely affect the development of knowledge of objects include:

- Knowledge and control of own body is impaired
- Physical interaction with objects can be disrupted.

Learning is primarily passive by watching and being manipulated. Object knowledge remains limited, patchy and immature.

People and social knowledge

Social development is often delayed because:

- The child's responses are hindered by poor range, control and timing
- Adults may misinterpret, ignore or reject the child's attempts.

Highly successful once established but unsophisticated; succeeds only with known carers. The child may remain at immature level of demanding, manipulative or rigid social behaviour.

People and object play

Learning through people and object play may be affected by the following:

- Object play is often too limited to allow knowledge of what objects could do
- Problem-solving skills may not have developed.

People and object play is successful only when the child has been taught the possibility of using people as tools.

Sound and language knowledge

- Initial knowledge of what sounds signify and where they come from, may be limited by poor physical search and look skills
- Vocabulary/concepts limited by poor object, event and people knowledge.

Initial learning is hampered. Comprehension and internal language develop successfully towards the general cognitive level. Expression is severely hampered by poor means by which they can express themselves.

Environmental impact

- *Emotional*—grief for loss of normal child, distress, fear, anger, guilt, depression, tiredness, denial, drive to improve, conflict, etc.
- *Response to the child*—emotional distancing, over-protectiveness, under-challenging, over-pressurising, inconsistent response
- *Management*—family needs, time, finance, organisational skills, hospital appointments, intrusive equipment, little free time to relax as a family
- *Attitudes*—over-questioning about normality of the child's development, strong focus on the handicap, under-expectation because of the handicap.

EFFECTS OF ASSOCIATED DISABILITIES ON COMMUNICATIVE COMPETENCE

- *Sensory*—impaired monitoring of self, objects, events, people and language
- *Cognitive*—learning is slower, less flexible and restricted in capacity; disrupted ability to interpret experiences
- *Language*—specific difficulties have a major impact on child's ability to understand symbolic representation, rules, language and speech, and to formulate ideas. Remedial multi-channel teaching is severely restricted.

Purposes of communication

Limited opportunities and unreliable interpretation result in the following:

- The infant learns to be passive
- The range of reasons for communication become limited
- Overdemanding, inflexible communication may be adopted with minimal monitoring of the carer's response.

EFFECT OF DISABILITY ON FEEDING COMPETENCE

The child's development of feeding competence and the skills associated with mealtimes will be influenced by disturbances in the learning systems available to him.

Physical factors

1. Posture. The position in which a child is fed will influence posture generally, including that of the mouth and neck, and the degree of tension in the muscles used for eating, drinking and breathing. The greater the muscle tension the more the effort required for feeding, leading to fatigue and loss of coordination.

2. Physical disability. If the whole body is affected by abnormal muscle tone (either stiffness or floppiness) it can be very difficult to position the child correctly for eating. If the child is fed in a position which will exacerbate the abnormal tone, then the muscles used for feeding and swallowing will also be greatly affected. In many children with cerebral palsy the oral muscles themselves are affected leading to a poor range of movement, poor coordination and poor function.

3. Structural disorders. All structural anomalies affecting oral and associated structures are likely to affect feeding, e.g. cleft palate/lip, small lower jaw, large tongue, small tongue, total (but not partial) tongue tie.

4. Medical problems. Problems affecting the mouth, neck, breathing and digestion can interfere with eating and drinking, e.g. upper respiratory tract infections, gastro-oesophageal reflux, tooth decay. These problems may occur as a result of the feeding difficulties and compound them further, causing poor appetite, fungal infection (thrush), aspiration pneumonia, or contributing to constipation, and anorexia.

5. Problems of sensation. Some children with physical disabilities are under-responsive to food or utensils in their mouths, but it is more common to see excessive reactions. There are three types of sensitivity problems, all of which can coexist:

a. *Abnormal reflex action.* Hyper-reflexivity is seen when the normal primary reflexes, e.g. rooting, sucking, biting, gagging, are very strong and slow to disappear and normal inhibition of the reflexes is impossible. Hyporeflexivity leads to difficulties in establishing primitive feeding movements and later interference with the more mature reflex of chewing and the ongoing reflexes of swallow, gag and cough.

b. *Over-sensitivity* to touch, taste, temperature, texture or consistency of food occurs in some children, causing facial grimacing, eye flickering, tongue thrusting, gagging or vomiting, and eventual defensiveness, all of which they will be unable to suppress. Their fussiness is thus caused by actual physical reactions over which they may have little or no control.

c. *Over-defensiveness* may occur in children who are dependent on being fed with no control over the speed or presentation of the food. They often have had a bad experience whilst being fed, e.g. choking, feeder-induced vomiting, etc., and mealtimes are times of anxiety rather than pleasure.

Language and social factors

1. Behavioural problems. Many children exhibit behaviour problems at mealtimes, e.g. food refusal, faddiness, screaming, gagging and vomiting, playing about. It is important to try to define the cause of the behaviour, which may be rooted in fear, in the need to communicate, the need to have more control; or which may reflect the *developmental level* of his communicative competence.

2. Cognitive system. The cognitive level of the child, the ease with which he can learn new skills, and his degree of motivation can greatly influence how easily he can learn new feeding patterns and integrate newly acquired skills into the complexities of mealtimes.

Environmental factors

Many factors may affect the child's eating skills:

1. The utensils, food and techniques used by the feeder can influence feeding tolerance, feeding patterns, feeding expectations and mealtime independence.

2. General mealtime management such as distractions, time limits, availability of utensils/food in relation to the child, can have surprisingly adverse effects upon eating ability and should not be overlooked.

3. The emotions, attitudes and reactions of the carers can contribute to eating and drinking problems. Fear, control issues, preferences and expectations can hinder progress and over- or under-pressurise the child during feeding.

4. The nature of the child's feeding problem and physical disability may hamper his social integration at mealtimes, his opportunities to communicate and learn, and the choices available to him.

INTERVENTION

When there is suspected physical disability, early referral to a speech therapist allows the provision of support, advice and therapy to promote the child's development. The speech therapist can help limit inappropriate development and bad habits, which are so often seen by the time a late referral (e.g. 2 years old) is made for poor speech development.

Early intervention

Why?

- To limit the effect of the child's disability on his development
- To facilitate/promote normal or appropriate alternative development in communicative and feeding competence
- To support the family and thus influence, where possible, the environment of the child.

How?

1. Team approach—through feeding therapy

— A high proportion of physically disabled infants have feeding problems
— Early feeding intervention is usually acceptable
— Early referral for communication/language or speech is often met with anxiety, denial or hostility
— Feeding referrals are usually earlier than those for communication problems
— Mealtimes offer ideal opportunities for advice on communication and interaction, in addition to eating/drinking and oral skills
— A holistic approach is best achieved through the support of a team of professionals as outlined in this chapter. The team must be self-supporting as well as supporting the children and families.

2. Key workers

— Can assist in coordination of services
— Can act as an advocate for the child and family
— Professional overload on the family can be limited.

3. Home-based advice and therapy can be focused through the family's everyday routines, events, environments and interactions.

4. Parent/carer centred approach helps to limit the loss of control and identity suffered by parents and carers in the hospital environment.

5. Problem-solving approach encourages parents to take control of and plan appropriate means of dealing with problems, and limits professional prescriptive strategies that may not suit parental style or environment. Such an approach also uses professional time effectively.

Table 1.3 Stages in infant learning and relation to professional intervention

Learning stages	Example	Level of communicative competence	Developmental facilitation
		Pre-intentional communication	*Parent/carer centred*
Reflexive	Particular patterns of behaviour are set off by outside stimulus. The child is at the mercy of the stimulus	Sounds produced in reaction to natural functions, e.g. feeding, sleeping, pain, filling nappy	The child does not mean to send a message	Therapist discusses generally, or in association with regular activity (e.g. mealtimes): identification of behaviours which could become communicative: interpretation of 'abnormal' infant responses which the baby is gaining control over and is likely to develop as communicative
Voluntary control	The child takes control of behaviour which remains largely unmodified. Can start and stop behaviour. Child tries it out to develop knowledge of his own body	Learns to stop and start the vegetative sounds voluntarily. Sounds undergo some slight changes. Sound production not associated socially or dependent upon people.	The adult interprets and responds as if child did mean to communicate	Facilitating the baby's physical/cognitive development to broaden range of behaviours available to the child
Modified control	The child has more control; he adds other actions to the behaviour and integrates it with other skills. He is still carrying out the behaviour for his own knowledge	Wider range of sounds controlled and produced for own entertainment. Now incorporated with other activities, e.g. sound play when eating, playing, moving. Sound play occurs with other people intentionally, but not for social interaction.	Cause-and-effect awareness is thus developed in the child	Advice on activities and environments to facilitate range and development of skills

Advice on adult responses to enhance cause-and-effect communicative development |

Table 1.3 (contd)

Learning stages	Example	Level of communicative competence	Developmental facilitation
		Intentional communication	*Parent/carer centred*
Trial and error	The child tries the behaviour out socially and sees what happens	Child tries out sounds socially with people but unsure of results. Initially any sound will do for any situation	Therapist discusses activities to encourage: *imitation* (child/adult), *repetition, opportunities, choice, specific skills.* Some
Planned	The child plans a behaviour knowing what the effect will be	Pre-verbal communication The child *means* to send messages. Often the communication is idiosyncratic but he is also adopting some conventional signals of the surrounding adults	direct child/therapist activities to help with conventional symbol expressions (signs, speech) to establish prerequisites for augmentative communication
	Child plans particular sounds for particular situations as communicative social act, e.g. raspberry for dislike of food, whining in protest, 'eh' for yes, 'mumumumum' for comfort from mother		
		Verbal communication	*Therapist/parent centred*
Linguistic planning	The child plans words, sentences and a form of expression—usually speech—appropriate for the situation	Child plans particular words/ sound sequences for specific situations. 'Mum' for Mum, 'Dad' for Dad	Language and oral skills/speech augmentative communication work.

6. Support services

— Self-help groups and therapy groups, which limit isolation
— Equipment and information services, e.g. toy library
— Care and respite services, e.g. link families.

FACILITATING THE DEVELOPMENT OF COMMUNICATIVE COMPETENCE

The speech therapist's role in facilitating development depends very much on the stage of learning achieved by the infant. In the early months the therapist is likely to work entirely through the carers, exploring with them what the baby is doing and what to look for, interpreting the baby's behaviour, and discussing ways of broadening, developing and generalising development. At a later stage, when the baby is ready to use skills in an intentional way, the therapist may focus on and demonstrate specific skills or environmental needs to allow the infant to progress.

Only when the child has achieved some reliable intentional parent/child communication will it be appropriate for work between the therapist and child, alongside the parent, to take place.

Table 1.3 shows the stages in the baby's learning and how they relate to the professional intervention offered.

FACILITATING THE DEVELOPMENT OF FEEDING COMPETENCE

Early intervention aims:

1. To facilitate the development of feeding patterns and sensorimotor oral skills to ensure effective and adequate intake and maturation as a factor in future sound production and dribble control.

2. To limit or prevent the development of inappropriate oral patterns and secondary problems.

3. To facilitate the emotional and interactional social aspects of development during the feeding process or in alternative environments when necessary.

4. To enhance the potential of the mealtime for communication, language and cognitive development.

5. To enhance the potential of the mealtime for development of independence.

The administration of effective early intervention requires:

- A feeding team with medical, physiotherapy, occupational therapy, dietetic, health visitor, social work, clinical psychology and specialist speech therapy members
- A key worker system to minimise professional overload

- Fast acute service response time
- Flexible hours to accommodate infant eating times
- Back-up medical investigation service, e.g. radiography
- Access to a range of feeding equipment
- Budget arrangements to allow for rapid purchase and replacement of feeding equipment
- Home-based service for outpatients
- Staff awareness and cooperation for in-patients.

HOW IS EARLY INTERVENTION IN FEEDING UNDERTAKEN?

Comprehensive team assessment

1. Giving detailed knowledge of what happens during feeding
2. Considering aspects of feeding which concern the carers, those they wish to change and those they do not, noting particularly any differences of opinion, attitude, beliefs and approaches between the adults involved
3. Drawing up a profile of factors which may be causing or contributing to the feeding problem—likely to be in the form of hypotheses which can be evaluated during therapy
4. Considering the reasons for intervention, e.g. oral skills, nutrition, development of communication skills, independence, etc.

Planning therapy with the primary carers

1. Appropriate explanation and discussion about the assessment, with the parents, carers and professionals involved
2. Deciding upon aspects and priorities of the feeding problem to be tackled. The setting of only a few goals and small steps allows attainable objectives and easier evaluation
3. Setting strategies and techniques as appropriate for the infant and the carers, clearly outlining the roles of the different professionals
4. Setting up easily accessible support mechanisms for the carers, with discussion opportunities for differences to be resolved
5. Establishing methods of evaluation.

Therapy strategies and approaches

Behaviour and emotional management

The implementation of feeding therapy is frequently hampered by the young child's strong emotional and behavioural responses of fear, refusal and self-assertion. In addition the child's difficulties may provoke or reinforce anxieties, behaviours, beliefs and approaches in the main carers and professionals, which further hinder intervention. The psychological difficulties need to be tackled first, for which a clinical psychologist is likely to play a principal role. Various techniques are available including:

- Counselling for the carers and professionals to explore the effects of their emotional and belief systems
- Relaxation and stress management
- Situational desensitisation techniques for phobic reactions
- Specific teaching approaches, e.g. small steps, backward chaining, etc. (Backward chaining is the term used to describe the process whereby a child learns a task by firstly accomplishing the final step of that task, then the penultimate step, and so on until the whole sequence is achieved.)
- Behaviour modification techniques
- Time and environmental management to facilitate a more relaxed situation
- Advice on interaction to facilitate social, play and choice aspects of the feeding session.

Professionals must be careful not to take over the feeding of the young infant in such a way that they are seen to succeed in nurturing the baby when parents are failing. Under such circumstances it is natural for parents to feel inadequate, distressed, anxious and resentful, which hampers their feeding attempts further. Where possible, feeding therapy should be conducted through the parents, helping them to achieve even if progress is more difficult. However, it is important to establish a mechanism to give parents relief from the relentless exhausting process of continuous problem mealtimes.

Dietary management

If there is concern about the infant's low weight or food intake then the carers main concern will be to get food into the child by whatever means possible. The introduction of therapy is likely to provoke additional anxiety about nutrition and may lead to poor cooperation in new approaches. A dietitian will work with the feeding team to assess the nutritional status and requirements of the infant and advise accordingly, for example:

- Monitoring and advising on nutrition during new feeding therapy
- Advising on additional variety to balance the diet
- Advising on food and methods of preparation to concentrate nutrients into the smallest bulk possible
- Use of special supplements to enhance protein, calorie, vitamin and mineral levels
- Use of thickening agents to establish the consistency of food the child can manage
- Dietary management of constipation

- Management of nutritional aspects of alternative routes of feeding, e.g. nasogastric feeding, button gastrostomy.

Food management

Appropriate planning of the taste, texture, temperature and thickness of food is helpful in the following ways:

- It reduces adverse sensorimotor reactions in the infant
- It makes the food more manageable for the infant's poor eating mechanisms and aids independent eating skills
- It facilitates the development of sensory and motor competence.

Particular techniques used with infants include:

1. Thickening of milk and drinks to allow more controlled swallowing and to minimise reflux, posseting and vomiting.

2. Very gradual introduction of extra textures into totally smooth baby food (commercially available baby foods provide too great a sensory and motor transition from stage 1 to stage 2 for most infants with oral problems).

3. Introduction of dry, easily chewed pieces of food, snacks and fun-foods even whilst multi-textured semi-solid foods are still causing difficulties.

4. Strict thickness, consistency and texture control to enhance development.

5. Planned meal and snack times to facilitate development in different skills at different times.

Postural management

The occupational therapist and physiotherapist must work together with the speech therapist to establish a good sitting posture for the infant. Correct positioning has a fundamental influence on oral competence and patterns of movement. The most advantageous posture is one of partial flexion, especially at the neck with the chin tucked in. The shoulders should be forward and the arms forward and stable, the hips flexed at 90°, the knees bent and apart, and the feet supported. The position must be controlled, stable and comfortable for the child and carer, and relatively easy to reestablish. It must also be possible to release the child quickly in case of choking or vomiting. Where it is desirable to maintain the closeness, comfort and security of the mother's lap, various positions for the young infant include:

1. A semi-reclined or upright position on the feeder's lap. Strong hip flexion is maintained by sinking the infant between the feeder's legs whilst the cradling arm maintains shoulder flexion, arms forward, a gentle chin tuck and some jaw control.

2. Positioning in an adapted soft or moulded small baby seat held in the feeder's lap.

3. Side-lying on the feeder's lap in a partially flexed position has the additional advantage that food does not fall to the back of the throat and the airway remains clear. This position is frequently used in the early stages of intervention with a feeding phobic infant to break up the position-associated fear reaction.

Adapted and special seating is recommended as early as possible to reduce the variations and inconsistencies of the previous posture.

Medical management

Members of the medical team will advise on aspects of the feeding problem requiring medical management, for example:

- Radiological investigation for hiatus hernia, gastro-oesophageal reflux, aspiration
- Drug therapy, e.g. for reduction of excessive muscle spasm, constipation, treatment of acid reflux, etc. (see Ch. 10)
- Advice on drug side-effects, e.g. on appetite, arousal, salivation, etc. also checking for alternative forms, e.g. liquids or crushed tablets instead of syrup
- Surgical management, e.g. gastrostomy, palatal surgery, tracheostomy, dental surgery, hiatus hernia repair
- Alternative/augmentative feeding systems, e.g. gastrostomy, nasogastric tube feeding, parenteral feeding, supervised withdrawal from alternative feeding
- Orthodontic appliances, e.g. palatal training devices
- Allergies and food intolerance, eczema, asthma
- Advice on the medical stability of the sick infant, e.g. the premature infant, infants with heart defects or chronic chest infections.

Feeding techniques

Advice on feeding techniques focuses on three main approaches:

1. Reducing the speed of presentation of the food and producing a predictable rhythm for the infant
2. Modifying the amount of food presented to facilitate optimum oral control
3. Modifying the angle of presentation to reduce the effects of gravity and maximise oral development.

Utensil management

Utensil management serves three purposes:

1. It reduces inappropriate techniques used by carers. The size, shape and capacity of utensils can greatly influence the angle of presentation and amount of food.

2. It facilitates patterns of eating and drinking. The size, shape and texture of spoons, teats and cups can either help or hinder the acquisition of competent feeding patterns.

3. It facilitates independence: the occupational therapist can advise on padded handles, special plates, plate guards, non-slip mats, the use of forks, etc. (see Ch. 33).

Sensitivity management

Formal systematic desensitisation techniques involving firm stroking around the face, lips and inside of mouth is often poorly tolerated by young children. However, much desensitisation can be facilitated through messy play with sand, water, face paints and food, and through face play whilst singing adapted nursery rhymes. Similarly, appropriate positioning and handling can minimise total body reactions. Behaviour management can help to build up tolerance, and food management can diminish unwanted sensorimotor reactions.

Oral control techniques

The speech therapist will be able to advise on various special techniques of holding, utensil use, food use, and physical stimulation both to inhibit unwanted oral movements and to facilitate appropriate patterns. Advice can be given on gradual reduction of the adult role in order to develop the child's voluntary control. However, many of the techniques are highly intrusive. Care must be taken not to work excessively on oral control at the cost of behavioural, emotional and sensitivity reactions in the infant or carer. Considerable groundwork must be undertaken to develop tolerance if such indispensable techniques are to be used to the full.

Summary

Early intervention in the development of feeding and communicative competence in the disabled infant is a complex process involving the infant, parents, the wider family, and many professionals. Care needs to be taken to support and empower parents as they undertake the day and night task of nurturing their child. The professionals need to be sensitive and flexible, imaginative and inventive. They frequently need to compromise between what they think is ideal and what is practical in the circumstances. They also need to learn to cope with the strong emotions surrounding early feeding problems and newly diagnosed disability. It is vital that the professionals involved act as a true team where they can offer positive and practical support to each other, if they in turn are to help and support the infant, parents and family.

THE SOCIAL WORKER'S ROLE: WORKING WITH FAMILIES OF YOUNG DISABLED CHILDREN

What does it mean to this person to have this handicap;
At this time in his or her life;
With these care givers;
In this environment;
In this locality; With this peer group;
And with these professionals?

Professor Joan Bicknell 1981

The birth of any child can be a frightening as well as a happy event for the family concerned. Parenthood brings new responsibilities and concerns, as well as pleasures. When the new baby has a disability or any special need, the initial diagnosis may devastate the parents. Research by Cunningham and others clearly demonstrates the need to recognise the impact of disability on parental expectations and self image, but confirms that active support and appropriate services can minimise trauma and dramatically improve parental acceptance and enjoyment of their child. As Hewitt noted in 1970, 'the general tendency to characterise parents of handicapped children as guilt ridden, anxiety laden . . . over-protective and rejecting beings' is a reflection not of real feelings and attitudes but of the absence of coherent local practical support, which gives dignity, respect and appropriate services to the whole family when a child has a learning disability or other special needs.

Since 1970, major shifts in opinion have led to parents being perceived as 'partners' and as having not only a voice but also direct skills to utilise in meeting their child's special needs. Recent studies (Davis & Cunningham 1985, Brimblecombe & Russell 1987) emphasise the importance of supporting professionals as well as parents, and of perceiving a child with disabilities as a child first, and disabled second. Government reports (Court 1976, Warnock 1978) emphasise the duality of parents and professionals and the importance of developing a dialogue which offers parity of esteem between service providers and family consumers. A genuinely multidisciplinary service will focus upon the whole family. Many traditional services for children with disabilities have failed to facilitate the normal experience of parenting because of the absence of a focus on good quality child-care. The same services have often ignored the psychological and social aspects of disability within a family. *Childhood* offers an opportunity to initiate on-going assessment; to involve families rather than exclude them; and to initiate a continuum of care based within an agreed framework for mutual support and interactions between parents and professionals. Collaborative planning and goal setting is a problem in adult services. Many *children's* services already liaise effectively, and legislation such as the 1981 Education Act and the 1989 Children Act offer challenges (and opportunities) to 'get it right' from the start.

PARENTS AS PARTNERS: RELATIONSHIPS WITH PROFESSIONALS

The majority of service providers for families with children who have disabilities now acknowledge the need to encourage active partnership with parents for the benefit of the family and of the child. Partnership, however, cannot be assumed to be present simply because professionals are working with parents, or because parents wish to be more fully involved in the care of their child. Professionals are generally currently endeavouring to 'demystify' their work and to be more openly accountable. Integration, as a social as well as an educational policy, recognises that severely disabled people will live in the community.

Since the majority of children with disabilities will continue to live in their own homes, the family must be seen as having a more pro-active relationship with professionals. In a time of scarce resources it has also been suggested that the 'economics' of intervention in the family will be cost effective, since teaching the parents to pass on new skills will be less time-consuming than working with the child in a separate environment. Additionally parental involvement in the care and education of *all* children has become more widely supported and it is recognised that 'home' plays a critical role in the development and education of young children (Wolfendale 1987, Mittler & McConachie 1983). The voluntary sector has additionally emphasised the *right* of parents to be involved and (with the new open access to information provided by the Education Act 1981) it seems probable that many more parents will not only be involved in assessment but will actually know the basis for future professional judgements.

The growth of professional willingness to work in partnership with parents must be put in the context of individual family dynamics, and the support which is given to parents who may be playing multiple roles. All young children are demanding. Wolkind (1981) has shown the high incidence of depression amongst young mothers living in inner city areas where traditional family support may be lacking and where poor housing, lack of services and unemployment may exacerbate the usual problems of rearing young children. In these circumstances the birth of a disabled child will put the family in double jeopardy.

Oakley (1974) noted that 'motherhood has a single long-term goal, which can be described as the mother's own eventual unemployment. A successful mother brings up her children to do without her'.

Unfortunately the pathways to independence may not be so clear when a child has a disability. Disability and lack of practical help may delay the achievement of developmental milestones and provide fewer tangible rewards for hard work and effort. Studies by Glendinning (1987) found that 50.1% of 361 severely disabled children over 5 years old could not be left alone for even 10 minutes during the day. In these circumstances practical support and help—and involvement in educational programmes— must be matched with wider support and recognition of existing family structures. Wilkins (1979) emphasised the particular burden placed upon mothers with little support from neighbours or relatives.

A factor for consideration in service development must also be the special needs of one-parent families. Cooke & Bradshaw (1986) noted that disabled children are more likely than other children to experience at least one spell in a one-parent family. These spells are longer for disabled than non-disabled children, and families with a severely disabled child are less likely to be reconstituted. In effect the single parent carer must have special support in order to act as an effective partner and as a relaxed and positive parent of a disabled child.

The Honeylands survey (Brimblecombe & Russell 1987) shows the importance of not only involving the *whole* family in treatment, counselling and support, but also of the necessity to avoid assuming that stable local communities and extended families will automatically support parents with a handicapped child. Pahl & Quine (1984) have emphasised the need to recognise *whole* family dynamics when recommending treatment. A report on the Carraigfole Paediatric Support Unit in Northern Ireland (Barnardo's Irish Division 1984) mirrors these conclusions and notes that:

The importance of family networks was apparent in the course of our work. The extended family often shared in the care of the child and provided emotional support. But sometimes this also brought emotional complications. While giving some emotional support, all parties were under strain as they (the extended family) lacked the necessary information to be able to help adequately.

The Honeylands evaluation, and that of Pahl and Quine (1984) of services in Kent, similarly found that a 'holistic' approach was impossible without a recognition of the emotional and practical needs of grandparents and siblings. Likewise the Carraigfole team concluded after their first two years, 'We learned as the months went by that the unit should be a 'family support' unit in the widest possible sense'. Such family support will require effective coordination involving communication and mutual respect between and within professionals and services in the community.

Research at the University of Manchester (McConachie 1982, Cunningham 1988) has also shown that families may prefer different styles of involvement in the care of a child with a disability, some liking a highly structured approach, others favouring a more 'natural' parental style or finding systematic efforts difficult to sustain. Davis's work at the London Hospital Medical School (1985) has confirmed the importance of matching early intervention to individual family needs and lifestyles, and the necessity of providing counselling and emotional support as essential components in any treatment programme.

THE PARENT AS EDUCATOR

The increasing popularity of the Portage Home Teaching scheme for parents of preschool handicapped children has demonstrated the importance of a known trained and supported home visitor making regular visits to a family in order to monitor the child's progress, and to identify goals and structure simple teaching programmes in order to reach them. Portage has been a major source of skills training for *professionals* as well as for parents. Health visitors, community nurses, home liaison teachers, psychologists and (in some instances) volunteers have learned through using Portage how to work as a team; how to work directly with parents and share skills and expertise and, most importantly, to be able to offer parents positive action at a time when they may feel depressed and pessimistic about happy outcomes (Wolfendale 1987, Cameron 1985). Cameron (1985) has indicated that a positive *educational* role for parents of young children will enhance later partnership and raise expectations about the child's development and progress.

Portage has been successfully modified for use in local authority and NHS residential and day-care settings with adolescents and young adults, involving the young people in goal setting and programme plans (Brimblecombe & Russell 1986). However, the role of the parent as 'educator' is not that of a cheap treatment resource for hard-pressed statutory services. Cunningham & Davis (1985) note the need to reinforce parental competence; to ensure resource availability and accessibility; to provide accurate comprehensible information; and to ensure continuity and effectiveness rather than one-off interventions

Since the implementation of the 1981 Act, a number of evaluations of parental satisfaction with special educational provision have been initiated. All reiterate the importance of providing clear, coherent and relevant information to parents, and of acknowledging the pain and trauma surrounding identification and assessment of a special need. As the House of Commons Select Committee emphasised (1987), parents frequently under-utilise opportunities for participation in their children's education and development because of perceived inequality as decision makers. However, early evaluation of a number of parent advocacy projects show that it is possible to reinforce parental confidence and develop strategies for learning from—as well as giving support to—children with special needs and disabilities.

THE ROLE OF VOLUNTARY ORGANISATIONS

The role of voluntary organisations (whether local groups, national organisations like MENCAP, or self-help groups for 'mixed' handicaps such as those run by Contact a Family) is still under-exploited by health, education and social services when helping families with children who have learning disabilities. There is high potential in the voluntary sector for a variety of roles, ranging from befriending and counselling to shared social and leisure activities, practical help and involvement in professional decision-making. Many parent groups can not only act as self-advocates in participating in the development of new patterns of care, but can also monitor and evaluate what is already being provided. A number of voluntary organisations are also acting as advocates for young people. Shared accountability will mean better services. But it will also entail more mutual respect, honesty and willingness to change. The responsibility for a healthy and positive voluntary sector rests partly on professionals. Referrals to voluntary bodies will increase membership (as well as provide individual support). However, the OPCS Reports (Meltzer et al 1989) showed that only 38% of parents knew of relevant voluntary organisations. The duties laid on DHAs to inform parents of relevant voluntary organisations under Section 10 of the 1981 Act seems to have been neglected. *All* services working with families should ensure they know of relevant voluntary organisations—including those working with 'ordinary' families in local communities—and recognise their unique contribution to family support.

Acknowledgement

We would like to acknowledge the contribution of Kathie Gerard's work on the development of Communicative competence.

REFERENCES

Baird H W, Gordon E C 1983 Neurological evaluation of infants and children. Clinics in Developmental Medicine 84/85. Spastics International Medical Publications, Heinemann, London

Ballard R 1976 Sharing the pain. Help for parents with a handicapped child. Health Visitor 49: 395–396

Barnardo's 1984 Carraigfole Paediatric Support Unit: the first two years. Barnardo's Irish Division

Bicknell J 1981 Right from the start. Royal Society for Mentally Handicapped Adults and Children

Brimblecombe F, Russell P 1987 Honeylands: developing a support service for families with handicapped children. National Children's Bureau

Cameron R J 1982 Working together: Portage in the UK. NFER Nelson

Cameron R J 1985 Parents as educators: learning from Portage. In Pugh G (ed) Partnership papers III. Working together with special educational needs: implications for pre-school services. National Children's Bureau

Charney E B 1990 Parental attitudes towards management of newborns with meningomyelocoele. Developmental Medicine and Child Neurology 32: 14–19

Cooke K, Bradshaw J 1986 Family dissolution and reconstitution. Developmental Medicine and Child Neurology 28: 610–616

Court S D M 1976 Fit for the future: report of the Committee on Child Health Services. HMSO, London

Darling R B 1979 Families against society. Sage, London

Davis H, Cunningham C 1985 Working with parents: frameworks for collaboration. Open University Press, Milton Keynes

Department of Education and Science 1978 Special educational needs: report of the Committee of Enquiry into the education of handicapped children and young people. The Warnock Report. HMSO, London

Dunn C L, Williams V S, Young C S, 1990 Paediatric physiotherapy: guidelines for good practice. Association of Paediatric Chartered Physiotherapists

Gath 1982 The effect of a handicapped child on the family. Midwife, Health Visitor and Community Nurse

Glendinning C 1987 Unshared care: parents and their disabled children. Routledge and Kegan Paul, London

Hannam C 1975 Parents and mentally handicapped children. Penguin, Harmondsworth

Hewitt S 1970 The family and the handicapped child. George Allen and Unwin, London

House of Commons Select Committee (Education, Science and Acts Committee) 1987 Report of the Select Committee on the implementation of the 1981 Education Act. HMSO, London

Mansell C 1980 Portage: not just another course. Health Visitor 53: 426–427

Meltzer H, Smyth M, Robus N 1989 Disabled children: services, transport and education. HMSO, London

Mittler P, McConachie H 1983 Parents, professionals and mentally handicapped people. Croom Helm, London

Oakley A 1974 The sociology of housework. Martin Robertson, Oxford

Pahl J, Quine L 1984 Families with mentally handicapped children: a study of stress and service response. Canterbury Health Services Research Unit, University of Kent

Parkes C M 1975 Bereavement. Pelican, Harmondsworth

Quine L, Pahl J 1987 First diagnosis of severe handicap: a study of parental reactions. Developmental Medicine and Child Neurology 29: 232–242

Sheridan M D 1973 Children's developmental progress from birth to five years: the Stycar sequences. NFER, Windsor

Twinn S 1981 The specialist health visitor for handicapped children: luxury or necessity? Health Visitor 54: 478–479

Warnock M 1978 Special education needs. Report of the Committee on the Education of Handicapped Children and Young People. HMSO, London

Wilkins D 1979 Families of mentally handicapped children. Croom Helm, London

Wolfendale S 1987 The parental contribution to assessment. National Council of Special Education

Wolkind S 1981 Depression in mothers of young children. Archives of Disease in Childhood 56: 1

Woolley H, Stein A, Forrest G C, Baum J D 1989 Imparting the diagnosis of life threatening illness in children. British Medical Journal 298: 1623–1626

SPEECH THERAPY—FURTHER READING

Crane S 1987 Feeding the handicapped child: a review of intervention strategies. Nutrition and Health 5(3/4): 109–188

Ellis R E, Selley W G 1989 Method for monitoring the co-ordination of neonatal feeding. What is cleft lip and palate? A multidisciplinary update. (Ed) Kriens O. George Thieme Verlag, Stuttgart, 89–91

Evans Morris S, Klein M D 1983 Pre-feeding skills. Available from Winslow Press, Oxford

Logemann J A 1983 Evaluation and treatment of swallowing disorders, College Hill Press, Santiago, California

Morris S E 1982 Pre-speech assessment scales: a rating scale for the measurement of pre-speech behaviour from birth through two years. J A Preston Corporation.

Morris S E 1977 Programme guidelines for children with feeding problems. Childcraft Education Corporation, Wisconsin

Mueller H A 1972 Facilitating feeding and pre-speech. In: Pearson P H, Warner J (eds) Physical therapy services in the developmental disabilities: Helping the handicapped child with early feeding. Winslow Press

Selley W G, Flack F C, Ellis R E, Brooks W A 1990 Co-ordination of sucking, swallowing and breathing in the newborn; its relation to infant feeding and normal development. British Journal of Disorders of Communication (in press)

Wilson J 1977 Oral function and dysfunction in children. University of North Carolina

2. Mechanisms of coping with handicap

D.C. Taylor

The handicapped child is, at the same time, its parent's child and also not the child they would have wished for. No parent would have wished for a child burdened by imperfections. So the child that exists is not the child they will have imagined they would have, unless it is the realisation of their worst fears. Yet the child that exists is the child they have made; the child whose life they are responsible for; whose advocate they should be; and whose outcome, at whatever odds, they will feel is a measure of their capacity as parents. Every public engagement with their child is a potential retelling of their painful story; every contact with the caring services is a public engagement.

The difference between acute and chronic disorders is the extent to which the chronic disorders become intimately interwoven in the fabric of life itself. Assessment and treatment become bound in as measures of the emergent child and the functioning of his family, and consequently these are issues of great sensitivity. Professionals might be regarded as being concerned 'less with how we are, than what we are'. For these among other reasons, professionals dealing with the chronically handicapped will experience different relationships with patients, parents and families than with those whom they know from their more acute work. Not everyone can work to the sorts of rewards that care of the handicapped provides.

HAVING CHILDREN

There are powerful drives towards having children which safe contraception now allows to be distinguished from sexual gratification. One measure of this is the distress of the involuntarily childless, and the excess of enthusiasm for adoption over availability of children to adopt. Having children is now an exercise of choice and this heightens the tragedy if things go wrong. There are a wide range of motives given for having babies but they all reflect some form of self-actualisation by the parents expressed at various degrees of sophistication. Having a baby represents a considerable investment in effort and money, as well as in the physical resources of the mother and the psychological resources of both parents. Usually a return upon those investments is looked for, but in addition there are other needs to be fulfilled. There is a social, or transgenerational expectation to maintain the lineage; the parents' need to test and display their capacity to love and nurture, to provide continuity of their own biological substance, and to represent their synthesis with each other. At the very least, children are an adornment, an achievement, or even just a useful chattel. Only when these various purposes are understood can the effect of frustrating them be understood. The handicapped child might disappoint most of these purposes. He will represent the parents' failure to meet a social expectation, a potential problem rather than a contributor to the breeding group. He will sometimes put such capacity for love and care as the parents have to the most extreme tests, even beyond the limit of their endurance. He will not represent their happy synthesis nor offer continuity of their biological substance: not an adornment, no achievement, but a stigma; not even a useful chattel, but a burden.

LOSS AND GRIEF

What is lost is the child who would have existed and who could have realised those expectations for the parents. However, unlike a death, what is gained is a child who might yet achieve some of them, but at various degrees of extra cost of effort and resource. The child cannot be mourned, its presence precludes a proper grief. It is the potential for lovely ordinariness that is mourned. It is hard to experience a proper grief without a sense of diminishing their handicapped child by their sorrow. Sorrow implies an unfair criticism of their child. It is even harder for parents to discover that such an abstraction is the source of pain. The pain of loss follows the course of ordinary grief with these exceptions. The continuity of the handicapped child gives a sense of guilt to grief, and it will repeatedly provide powerful reminiscence of that original pain of the first discovery of differentness.

Parents will be encountered in various stages of their grief, a grief which is easily acutely rekindled by the professional activity itself. The grief will be countered by various defence mechanisms so that the combination of the stage of grief reached and the modes of defence used will produce a variety of presentations of distress within parents. Professionals must come to recognise these. Some parents are very hard to help. That must be realised just as much as the fact that some handicaps are hard to help.

Professionals are easily placed in a difficult position. They must at the same time recognise and respect the handicapped child as a completely valid member of the social group, and yet at the same time maintain their active empathy for what has been 'lost'—for what the child might otherwise have been. Angry or sad parents can so readily knock professionals off the tightrope they walk that the professionals must have an active awareness of their own predicament and know something of their own motivation. They must actively work to seek to understand their own hurts rather than behave quite as directly as they might in other professional or social situations. The cohesive body of professional staff actively working together and sharing their experience of their problems is some help towards keeping appropriate responses towards patients and their families.

Shock

The first stage of response to bad news is shock, similar to the effects of a severe fright. It numbs the senses, impairs recognition of the scale of the news, and produces apparently inappropriate social responses. Parents are in shock as they receive their bad news and it is for this reason that they need to be supported by each other as they receive it so that information can be further discussed equally between them, and what they believe they heard can be confirmed or corrected by each other. Shock also occurs in later consultations; all information should be made plain more than once, and where possible confirmed in a written form.

Denial

Denial emerges from the numbness of shock but is a longer continuing of an inability to believe the news, a failure of acceptance that it is so. It is sometimes episodic—a sudden sense that it has all been a bad dream, that it will mend, recover, that the doctors are mistaken, that the outcome will be better than predicted. Denial also shelters hope, so it must be carefully managed if hope is to survive. Denial is the repudiation of reality. Professionals will not believe it possible for parents to maintain beliefs which so directly controvert what is objectively incontrovertible. But it is so. Denial is a 'defence' as well as a stage in grief; it must never be stormed by angry professionals anxious to be understood. It is so robust it will last for years. If it is to be moved it must be replaced by better defences.

Anger

There will be a variety of targets for rage. Many can rail against unkind tricks of nature or of God, but others will need nearer and more realistic targets. The doctors and the hospitals where the bad news originated offer themselves for this, but so do current services. Some rage is directed against the handicap itself; the very thing may produce disgust: the withered limb, the emaciation, the rash, the odour. One of the benefits of precise medical diagnosis of the basis of a handicap is that the anger can be more precisely directed, whether in pursuit of legal redress or by recognition of the intrinsic fallibility of the reproductive process. Being angry provides an activity which diverts people from thinking too much about themselves. It shields a little against helplessness, guilt, depression. It can be transmuted into effective action.

Depression

As anger recedes there arises the opportunity to consider the self, one's potential share in the blame, the sense of helplessness and hopelessness about the future. Self-blame can reach delusional proportions. Depression involves a realisation, even a heightening, of the loss of esteem created by being responsible for a handicapped child. The depression too can last for many years and be exacerbated by reliefs that should lift it, such as respites of care and improvements of service, since these can also reveal once again a glimpse of how things might otherwise have been.

Guilt

Guilt arises from the facts, and the mental states of grief. Unacceptable reactions to the fact of the handicapped child—murderous feelings, wishing at least the child was dead or would soon die, feeling like injuring the child—are not all defended against, and parents feel guilty in consequence. Some feel generally guilty that their seed is somehow tainted and they have passed on a bad part of themselves. Then there are reminiscences of reasons to deserve punishment: former pregnancies that have been terminated, former children who were healthy but given away for adoption, children sired with other women or pregnancies that might have come in other relationships. One parent may have pressed much more for the pregnancy than the other who felt the family already happily complete. Hence, for professionals to gauge the likely nature of parents' reactions or to understand their difficulties, it is necessary for them to be informed in some way, derived from obtaining a very detailed account of family development, its life and its structure. These demand high levels of skill and sensitivity. Incompetent prying for information may leave a parent or a family deeply wounded. Working psychologically with a family requires special skills but it can enable them to ease out their story and state their various pains at their own pace. Professionals working with chronically handicapped children might wish to acquire some of these skills. But patient and assiduous listening, and the giving and receiving of information, also create a relationship between the hearer and the heard, and that will need skilful management. The psychiatrically or psychologically trained member of the team is the person to help other professionals with these issues.

COMING TO TERMS

It is commonly said that the grief of the loss of children is never assuaged. However, any enquiry about the lost child reveals him in the mind with attendant pain, but with time he may ordinarily occupy the mind less and hence produce pain less often. Grief is modified in sorrowing about the handicapped child, first because there can arise considerable ordinary joys.

Then the expectation of perfection can be negotiated to coincide more with the reality; that is, 'the child-valued-for-what-he-is' is perceived within the handicapped child's frame. Love, as they say, is blind; or at least it is blind to defects. And the continuity of dependency in the child calls out a continuity of service from parents which can provide them with some satisfaction.

On the other hand the continuity of the child precludes winding up grief and leads on to chronic sorrow. Some handicaps include the repeated stress of potential sudden loss of life. Others provide the 'Damocles' effect: the inevitable fact of eventual loss which can include the excruciating thought of wishing it would all end now. All handicapped children markedly increase the labour of parents; the sheer grind of lifting, pushing, carrying, dressing, bathing, feeding, which goes on and on, in some cases without hope of ending, are additional to what would have been. This labour often goes quite unrewarded, within the partnership, within the family, by professionals, and also intrinsically because the child appears to make no material progress as a result. Then there is the continuity of stigma, the second glances, the quizzical looks, the attempts to give sympathetic smiles, the gaze avoidance and the looks of frank distaste to be coped with daily.

Defences

The defences as considered here are taken to mean those used by all people in ordinary life to maintain their psychological integrity. Just as people have powerful physical structures—such as the skin and the immune system, which defend the body against alien intrusion by viruses, bacteria, or foreign material—so too the self needs not to be at the mercy of its environment. Parents' and handicapped children's defences are the main issue here. But the professionals will have their defences too and they must be conscious of what they are using.

Loss can be recognised and shared by others as a notable absence of something from the outer world; but loss requires a readjustment towards that which existed only within, the personal image of that lost object. A death will create different degrees of loss in different people, determined by what the lost person meant to them. Given the loss of an abstraction like 'the child we hoped he would have been', it is very probable that there will be greatly varying degrees of loss experienced even in a closely-knit, caring family. As professional helpers reach out to understand that loss empathically, so their own psychological system must come into play. For they can only realise empathically what they themselves understand such a loss to mean.

Repression

The simple basic defence is simply not to think about things that are difficult and painful to deal with. This is a defence of both parents and their handicapped children, a basis of procrastination of decisions, a mode of maintaining an apparent calm and control. It can be applied to the fact of the handicap itself and to those feelings that arise in consequence of it. Parents and children who very actively 'forget' their appointments, programmes, diets, but do not argue with the doctor about them, could be said to be repressing, actively. What is repressed cannot be worked upon by the people concerned. When bad news is given and apparently understood, and feelings appear to be untouched, repression is actively keeping it out of mind. The truths will need to be brought into mind again and again with kindly patience by the professionals if there is work that must be done.

Denial

Repression comes close to denial. How many professionals have been told 'I'm so grateful to you for this consultation, you are the first person who has ever 'told' us anything'? These parents will still be waiting to be told after that consultation too, and for as long as their denial lasts. Denial is the repudiation of fact. 'You don't mean [i.e. I won't believe] there's something wrong with his brain, do you?' can be offered by apparently astonished parents many years into the management of a problem related to cerebral disease. Denial will also preclude, or materially interfere with, any treatment. Denial may relate only to some aspects of the diagnosis, such as its severity, its lethality, its persistence, its unresponsiveness to treatment. Thus denial can allow frantic searches and irrational attachments to therapies because the lack of change or benefit is also denied.

Denial operates widely and to some extent is very necessary in coping with chronic handicap. 'Human beings', T. S. Eliot remarked, 'cannot bear too much reality'. Care is needed in confronting established denial; an alternative solution has to be available.

Projection

Projection is a means of ascribing to others those characteristics, actions, or wishes in one's self that one does not dare to own. Fearing, for example, for the well-being of the child left in what ordinarily would be regarded as appropriate care, might arise from those unexpressed personal wishes that harm should come to the child. Such persons may be very quick to detect the weaknesses of professionals or the inadequacies of their organisation. It occurs likewise between parents and within families. 'We don't like to leave him with the little one, for fear, you know . . . .'

Another aspect of projection is projective identification. In work with the handicapped this is usually seen when rather positive characteristics are attributed to a handicapped person who does not possess them. It is common in ordinary life. A person might even say of their cat that 'he understands every word I say'. In some ways it maintains hope, but it stands in the way of realistic appraisal and coming to terms appropriately. Parents of very severely handicapped children with multiple impairments are prone to projective identification.

Reaction formation

'I'd like you to know, doctor, that I won't allow him to go into a home' could be a clear statement of considered opinion but could represent the defence of espousing the opposite viewpoint to one which is owned but regarded as unacceptable. It matters because it renders the basis on which negotiation can take place rather more difficult. It is not a matter of persuading in reality, but of coming to terms with the disowned feelings. Similarly 'Doctor, we are interested in exploring every possible avenue of treatment' actually includes the important fact of not following any given one of them and implies the opposite of what it seems to suggest. 'I love and hate', wrote Catullus, 'and I don't know why, and it's excruciating'. Very strong negative and destructive feelings may need to be balanced by even stronger, total and overweening preoccupation and concern with the person in question. Sometimes this strength of feeling can be married to another defence (see 'Sublimation' below) and release considerable beneficial creative energy. At other times a collusion of totally exclusive preoccupation with a handicapped person will be seen by professionals to realise neither participant's full potential and indeed they may see that such overweening is destructive. These situations are hard to change and, when they do, the change in the dynamic can reveal the latent hostility.

Displacement

An English proverb has it that 'He who cannot beat the horse, beats the saddle'. The real objects of the powerful feelings of the parents and their handicapped children may be quite unacceptable places to locate them: parents dare not rage at their son, and he dare not blame them for his hereditary disease. Their energies must be located elsewhere. The parents of a severely handicapped child with seizures travelled a long distance to seek yet another 'top opinion'. There were many negative aspects to their management, which became apparent but were not commented upon in the consultation. Their response to detailed diagnosis and a proper management plan was to vituperate at the consultant and declare that they had utterly wasted their time in seeking his worthless analysis. Having given vent to their destructive anger rather more profitably than when directed towards their handicapped child and her handicap, they proceeded to follow the consultant's 'worthless proposals' to their considerable benefit.

Displacement can result in tireless pursuit of legal action, and endless complaints and letters about the quality of what is being provided. In the real world there is no problem in finding a reality basis for these. But they are displacements none the less.

Rationalisation

Rationalisation is what provides the justification for behaviour which is not, on the face of it, very sensible. 'Good reasons' arise for extreme forms of actions, diets, regimens, treatments. Vehement defences are required to justify behaviour that is irrational and for which there is no valid empirical evidence. Strong affects and fixed positions will be recruited in lieu of such evidence. For these reasons money and time and more money and more time can be spent in attempting to alter the individual behaviour and indicate the false premise. Professionals who stand in the way of these powerful beliefs (however false and however transient they may prove) will be swept aside and other opinions sought until a congruent view can be found, or until the defence is worked through by therapy. Rationalisation can be another basis for 'shopping' for opinions.

Sublimation

The energy of the original hurt and pain, and also that arising from the continuing sense of grievance and loss can be funnelled into useful work. The work can directly concern the handicap or might be usefully directed elsewhere. There are numerous examples of this form of tireless, selfless giving that come into the public domain. These selfless defences are socially desirable but not necessarily the very best for the individual concerned. They are hard to broach—it is possibly even offensive to enquire whether so deep a commitment to a cause may not betray an unresolved problem. But coming to terms through sublimation, through a vigorous and protracted effort does allow the self the satisfaction of having laboured against the source of such pain. Such a mechanism explains how dedicated work can continue even when the beliefs are illusory and the effort wasted.

Problematic coping styles

Professionals will recognise that the greatest amount of effort is expended upon those families who cope less well, whose defences are unbalanced or frail, who are dealing with additional hazards that tax their defences, or who have themselves experienced problematic development even before the stress of the handicapped child's birth. Stress is a nonspecific term and it identifies its weaker victims at lower levels. From the foregoing, however, can be discerned the sorts of ways in which all people will respond eventually, provided the stress grows strong enough. It is unprofitable to consider problem families as constituting a group with disorders in a dimension other than those of stress and defence, though inevitably every person will react in ways fashioned by their personality, and where these were formerly problematic they can be exacerbated. Referral to experts with psychiatric or psychological training is appropriate if it is obvious that the reactions in the parents or the handicapped person go well beyond what is useful to them or manageable by others.

Professionals who rarely refer to psychiatrists will be disappointed regularly if they set their sights too high. That is akin to saying there are distresses which are beyond the reach of all help. A regular link forged with a psychiatrist will allow the team to discover where and when the psychiatrist can help most.

DISEASE, ILLNESS AND PREDICAMENT

It is worth having a framework of logic upon which the various components of sickness can be organised so that the different thinking modes required for dealing with them can be deployed. These three components occupy different philosophical categories: things, behaviours, and states of affairs. To confuse them will confound one's efforts.

Disease

Handicapping conditions usually arise from disorders of structure which can be visualised, described, named, and understood in structural terms. But it needs to be known that much of the sickness of diseased persons is not directly entailed by their disease. Thus, much of the effect of having tuberose sclerosis is not determined by the presence of the gene or the brain or peripheral lesions, but by whatever process it is that determines whether early epilepsy supervenes. The microbiology of Down syndrome does not yet adequately account for the variability in the real-life problems of persons so described.

'Disease' should be a term confined to describing abnormal structures which are, in principle, accessible to the sense organs. This helps avoid making presumptions about how people are, simply on the basis that they suffer a nameable disease, and the presumption that relief is only possible on the basis of curing the disease. It allows recognition of the fact that growing up with a disease could place constraints on development that are not recovered from simply by relieving the disease.

Illness

Illness is a useful term for the social behaviour of the sick. For example, the subjective experience of nausea with a mounting propensity to vomit is accompanied by recognisable signals such that others may accurately guess the subjective state of the ill person and act accordingly. But as this behavioural syndrome can also be simulated, we can recognise a dissociation between 'illness' and 'disease'. There are very strong, 'pathognomonic', as well as very weak illness manifestations that will guide physicians in the effort to discover disease processes. Where handicaps are manifest there is likely to be impairment, which may or may not produce a disability or an 'illness'.

The illness repertoire of a disease can also vary in severity over time and between persons. Something more is therefore required of diagnosis than a label about impaired structure, albeit a detailed label. Illnesses are possible which cannot accurately be given a disease label: for example, dystonia musculorum deformans describes a dreadful condition of completely unknown aetiology; coryza politely (and pointlessly) renames the common cold.

Predicament

People's predicament is defined by the precise moment-to-moment inter-connection of their social networks, their esteem within them, the meanings ascribed to their behaviour, and the sense in which people are understood. It is more precise and local than their 'environment'. Everyone is in a predicament all of the time but mostly it is comfortable enough to cope with. It can become extremely uncomfortable very abruptly, given, say, the sudden threat to the life of one's child, or even a catastrophic revelation that threatens one's self-esteem such as giving birth to or becoming a severely stigmatised person. These predicaments do not entail personal illness or disease but they are likely to be registered in somatic changes and often facilitate a physical distress. Predicaments also work chronically, especially for the chronically ill. For example: 'Knowing that she can only be moved out of her wheelchair by an assistant whom she dislikes and feels dislikes her, creates further physical and mental distresses for Julia'. A further example: 'The fact that his parents are angrily divorced means that his father can no longer be enjoyed in the house that was specially adapted for John'.

Unachievable aspirations are neither illnesses nor diseases but they may be among the most excrutiating limitations in a handicapped life. Realistic self-appraisal and assessment of a life situation should not necessarily be demeaned by being regarded as 'depressive' if the predicament is very severe. Predicaments are generally unstable and can be altered by altering the perspective which is taken of them. This underlies the application of psychological treatments to people involved with chronic physical illness. Simply put, things can be seen in a better light; entrenched positions can be altered if everyone agrees to do something about their discomfort.

Whereas diseases require biotechnological evaluation, and illness may be pathognomonic or may at least be palliated by medicines and deserve medical attention, the diagnosis of predicaments is a matter of discernment that is available to any appropriately aware professional. Empathic skills, the capacity to promote the telling of the history, to listen intently and to promote real change in the structure of the predicament can ease the plight of a handicapped person substantially.

ADOLESCENCE

As handicapped children grow and mature, the focus of concern turns more and more from those problems experienced by or interpreted by parents and caregivers to those expressed or enacted by the young handicapped people themselves. Adolescence is the fulcrum of this change as it is in non-handicapped people. The adolescent period over which the pubertal and maturational changes occur in a population occupies a decade or more, but the adolescence of an individual is, importantly, a briefer period within that decade. From a social and biological perspective adolescents are new recruits to the breeding group and there are very old, established cultural attitudes towards them. These are not necessarily diminished by the presence of handicap. All the professionals intimately concerned with the handicap recognise both the reality and the fantasies that surround emergent sexual capacity. The management of menses and the potential embarrassment of ejaculation, each so often referred to in the literature, are also the cardinal signals of the potential 'danger' of sexuality. In reality, sexuality is much more likely to be diminished and physically difficult to enact. It is much more likely that the adolescent metamorphoses give rise to a new form of anxiety among caregivers relating to the actuality of the constraints upon the young people's emergent identities and opportunities. There is, within nearly all species, an epoch of special deference to the young. The end of this protective period, for the handicapped, can be very painful. Adolescence is, in any event, marked by a sharp increase in depressive disorders, suicide and suicidal behaviours, which can be taken to imply very negative self-evaluations of the emergent identity, 'I don't like who I am'. Indeed many handicapped adolescents will experience developmental difficulties and limitations on their experiences, which will constrain their identity development. The task of maximising experience and opportunity for growth is one of education, in its wider sense, with the best enabling of the handicapped young person from earliest childhood. But handicap will generally place restrictions upon the sorts of explorations that are necessary for the fullest form of self-actualisation. The basic tasks are 'work', 'independence' and 'love'. The constraints upon them will vary with the handicaps but also with the whole manner in which the handicapped person has been managed and treated, and enabled. The quality of life will be a direct function of the sort of personality that has been formed. Within even the most unpromising frame, the light of a person can shine brightly to ensure its own continuity.

FURTHER READING

Blum R W 1984 Chronic illness and disabilities in childhood and adolescence. Grune and Stratton, London

Dobbing J, Clarke A D B, Corbett J A et al 1984 Scientific studies in mental retardation. The Royal Society of Medicine. Macmillan, London

Dowrick S, Grundberg S 1980 Why children? Women's Press, London

Hannam C 1975 Parents and mentally handicapped children. Penguin, London

Kimball C P 1981 The biopsychosocial approach to the patient. Williams and Wilkins, London

Locker D 1981 Symptoms and illness: the cognitive organization of disorder. Tavistock, London

McCarthy G T 1984 The physically handicapped child: an interdisciplinary approach to management. Faber and Faber, London

Milne P 1982 John David: the child that changed their lives. Virago, London

Prugh D G 1983 The psychosocial aspects of pediatrics. Lea and Febiger, Philadelphia

Taylor D C 1981 Psychosexual development. In: Davis J A, Dobbing J (eds) Scientific foundations of paediatrics, 2nd edn. Heinemann London

Taylor D C 1982 Counselling the parents of handicapped children. British Medical Journal 284: 1027–1028

Taylor D C 1982 The components of sickness: diseases, illnesses and predicaments. In: Apley J, Ounsted C (eds) One Child. Spastics International Medical Publications, Heinemann London

3. Assessment of the child with multiple disability

C. Zergaeng   J. Cattermole   R. Cartwright   M. Jones
G.T. McCarthy   V. Moffat

A multiple disability by definition involves more than one area of function. As almost all physical disabilities involve some central neurological impairment, it is rare to find a child with a physical disability who does not also have some other form of disability. Most commonly learning, vision, hearing and visual perception are affected to some degree.

In addition physical disability restricts the child's interaction with the environment, his ability to explore and play with objects, and his interaction with parents. If a child is non-verbal he may be less likely to be spoken to and he is unable to learn about language and his world through asking questions as normal children do. Therefore a physically disabled child is often deprived of normal learning experiences which can lead to the child's development being retarded generally or in certain areas. When assessing the needs of the physically disabled child it is therefore important to consider the nature of other modalities and areas of development which are affected.

AIMS OF ASSESSMENT

The objective of assessment is to produce as full a profile as possible of the child and his family at a particular time, linking the findings with the past and using them to plan for the future. Assessment is carried out to establish a developmental and functional level by drawing up a profile of the child's strengths and weaknesses in order to:

- Plan therapy, treatment and equipment
- Plan educational programmes and future placement
- Provide support for the family both practical and emotional.

LENGTH OF ASSESSMENT

This will vary according to the aim of the assessment:

1. *Day assessment.* This may be a preliminary assessment used to answer specific questions, e.g. Should a child attend a particular school? It may well be preliminary to a long-term assessment.

2. *Outpatient assessments.* These are usually for a specific reason, e.g. new equipment or help with communication systems. They may not be multidisciplinary but, like a day assessment, they may lead on to a more in-depth assessment. Outpatient assessments are invaluable for disabled children in mainstream or local special schools.

3. *Short-term assessment.* A few centres offer a short-term residential assessment for up to a week, e.g. The Wolfson Centre or Chailey Heritage. These assessments require provision of appropriate accommodation for child and family, preferably in an adapted flat or bungalow. The bonus attached to this is the unlimited access staff have to the child and their parents during their stay. Reports and advice must then accompany the child back to the referral source with copies to the relevant disciplines involved. Short-term assessment may be repeated as needs change to give a clearer idea of the child's rate of development.

4. *Long-term assessment.* It is often impossible to obtain a clear view of the child's cognitive and physical potential in a day or even a week. Subsequent or continuing assessment may be needed to determine the child's rate of learning, which is as important as the child's level of development. Long-term assessment/placement may be necessary if the child needs training or equipment before assessment can be carried out, e.g. in eye pointing or use of switches.

WHO ASSESSES?—THE MULTIDISCIPLINARY TEAM

Assessment is often necessary before a Statement of Educational Needs can be drawn up, and for young, severely disabled children this can be very difficult. The first statement may simply indicate the child's need for fuller assessment. This will include advice from a multidisciplinary team either directly or indirectly. The team outlined in Figure 3.1 is an example of the possible permutations.

It is in the interest of the child and family for this assesment to be carried out at a single centre if possible. Not all team members outlined in Figure 3.1 will be involved, and many of their functions may overlap. It is also useful for two or three team members to see the family together, not least because it cuts down the number of questions the family are asked, but also because if one team member is playing with, or testing, a child the other can be recording or observing. Thus teacher, speech therapist and psychologist might all be working together on the assessment of the child's understanding of language.

THE SOCIAL WORKER'S ROLE

A severely disabled child must be seen firstly as a *child*, with the same needs for physical and emotional care as other children. He or she is a member of a family and a wider community who seek to meet those needs. It is important for the social worker to approach assessment by considering the common needs of all children and parents, but also to understand the implications of the disability for the child and family, and to have an extensive knowledge of available community resources.

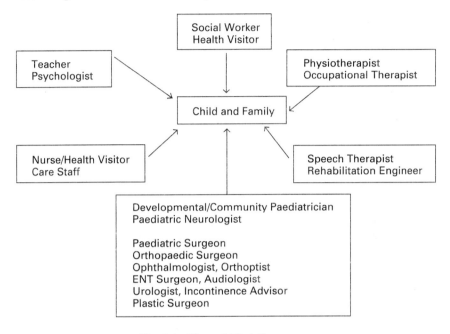

Fig. 3.1   The multidisciplinary team.

Initial assessment

This seeks to give a clear picture of the whole family. It is helpful to include information from professionals already known to the family. A clear account of family relationships is important to assess strengths and weaknesses and to identify the needs of all members. Practical details of housing, finance, and employment should be noted. It is also important to assess the understanding the family have of the disability, and the attitudes and responses of all family members. How well are the family meeting the needs of the disabled child, of their other children and of both parents? What are their short and long term plans and aspirations?

If the assessment is for a particular establishment, how clear and realistic are the family about their child's particular needs? Are they clear about provision offered by other establishments, and do they consider the particular placement is right to meet the needs of their child and family?

Long-term assessment

Assessment will always need to be ongoing. It is rarely possible or appropriate to obtain all relevant information initially. The initial information forms a baseline upon which the social worker in long-term contact with a child and its family will need to build. At varying stages in a child's life there can be a re-awakening of the initial shock, guilt, grief and loss or rejection experienced earlier. There will also be changes in the child in response to its own disability and to the family, requiring varying levels of support and information from the social worker.

The ultimate aim of long-term social work is to enable the child and family to live their lives as fully as possible, meeting the changing needs of all members. In some cases this may include providing a substitute family for the child when the needs of all concerned cannot be met in any other way.

Areas to be assessed initially and reviewed throughout long-term contact

Family structure

1. *The nuclear family*—details of all members
2. *The wider family*—Are they accessible? How often are they in contact? Are they able to offer practical and emotional support and do they understand and accept the child's disability? Are there other disabilities within the family/Do the family have friends who are able to offer support?
3. *Legal status*—including past marriages and partnerships.
4. *Other household members*—status, connection and function within the family, e.g. lodger, au pair, mother's help.

Family functioning

1. *Finance*—employment, commitments, rights and allowances available.
2. *Housing*—ownership, suitability for the whole family including the disabled member. Grants and loans from local authorities and charities. Extensions and adaptations. Accessability to placement under consideration.
3. *Transport*—ownership of a car and its suitability. Mobility allowance, Motability, Orange Badge. British Rail provision and local transport schemes for the disabled. Wheelchairs, buggies, adapted cars.
4. *Home aids*—telephone availability, washing machines and household equipment. Special equipment and adaptations.
5. *Respite care*—family aides for home support from local authorities or charities. Baby-sitting services. Night care provision in the home. Short-term respite care outside the home in establishments or via family link schemes. Carers' organisations. Holidays for the child or the whole family. Holiday play schemes and outings. Boarding school in some cases.
6. *Community involvement*—local church, uniformed organisations, play-

groups, mother and toddler groups, PHAB (Physically Handicapped and Able-Bodied) clubs, opportunity playgroups.

7. *Disability groups*—parent support groups, voluntary organisations such as the Spastics Society, the Association for Spina Bifida and Hydrocephalus, the Muscular Dystrophy Group, etc.

8. *Parent directed treatment*—Are the family involved in groups based on conductive education, the Portage project or patterning programmes?

9. *Professional help*—health visitor, general practitioner, local social services department, voluntary organisations, hospital based services for children with special needs.

Family plans

Changing or leaving school—Is the current placement meeting the child's needs, and if not what else is available? Have the family seen other units? What help have they received to investigate other possibilities? Courses at local colleges. Independence courses. Day care and sheltered work provision. Sheltered accommodation. Independent living schemes. Residential establishments offering nursing care.

Where is the child/young person to be based? Is the family able to meet his/her needs and wishes? Should a substitute family be sought? Is the school-leaver to be based at home or in an establishment or independent accommodation? Is this a long-term aim if the short-term base is to be at home?

MEDICAL ASSESSMENT

By the time the child is seen for assessment it is likely that a number of doctors will have been involved in his care. It is helpful to have as much past medical information as possible. In practise, however, there is often very little written information, particularly if the educational statement is the main source. It is therefore helpful to take a full history from the parents. This also enables one to observe the family interaction and to gain some insight into their understanding of their child's disability. The following headings may be used to obtain a full history:

- Parents' understanding of the reason for assessment
- History of the disorder
- Perinatal history
- Developmental history
- History of vision or hearing problems, epilepsy
- Chronological list of surgical operations (amplified from previous hospital notes)
- Intercurrent illnesses, immunisations
- Medications: past and present

- Present abilities
- Present worries
- Examination—physical and functional (see appropriate chapters). It is helpful for the examination to be carried out with the physiotherapist and occupational therapist
- Referral for specialist opinion, e.g. orthopaedic, opthalmological, ENT, etc.

The use of problem-orientated case records for children with continuing physical problems can be very helpful. A chronological chart of surgical operations and radiological investigations should also be made—many children are exposed to a high number of radiographs. Height, weight and head circumference charts should be started. Finally the medical and functional aims should be made clear.

PLANNING THE INDIVIDUAL ASSESSMENT

THE SEVERITY OF THE CHILD'S DISABILITY

The type of assessment will depend on how the child is able to respond.

The child who has speech and hand function

It is possible to use techniques of assessment available for able-bodied children, e.g. observation of play. Also a wide range of norm-referenced tests are available which compare the child's performance with a sample of the general population. The Wechsler Intelligence Scale for Children, British Ability Scales and McCarthy Scales are all batteries of tests designed to investigate such skills as verbal reasoning, vocabulary, short-term memory and visual perceptual skills. The Reynell Developmental Language Scales measure expressive language and verbal comprehension. These tests are standardised on the able-bodied population and therefore great care must be taken when interpreting the results obtained from a disabled child. (See Table 3.1.)

This type of assessment can be used as a measure of the child's present skills, but may not reflect the child's potential. However it can be used to provide a profile of the child's present strengths and weaknesses, which can be used to devise an educational and therapeutic programme. Repeating the tests over a period of time will also give an indication of a child's rate of learning.

The child with no speech and/or hand function

This group of children are very difficult to assess, particularly as many may have a sensory impairment and nearly all means of expression may be impaired.

Table 3.1 Standardised tests for use with children who have speech and/or hand function (* indicates all or part of test can be used with a child who is non-verbal) (see also Table 3.2)

Modality	Age range (years)	Main users
General ability		
*British Ability Scales Authors: C D Elliot, D J Murray, L S Pearson. Pub: NFER	2½–17½	Educational and clinical psychologists
*Leiter International Performance Scale Battery for children (non-verbal test) Author: R Leiter. Pub: NFER	2–18	Educational and clinical psychologists
*Wechsler Intelligence Scale for Children (revised) Author: D Wechsler. Pub: NFER	6–17	Educational and clinical psychologists
*McCarthy Scales of Children's Abilities Author: D. McCarthy. Pub: The Psychological Corporation	2–8½	Educational and clinical psychologists
Play		
*The Symbolic Play Test Authors: M Lowe, A Costello. Pub: NFER	1–3	Speech therapists educational and clinical psychologists
Language		
*Reynell Developmental Language Scales Author: J Reynell. Pub: NFER	1–7	Speech therapists
*The Token Test for Children Author: F DiSimoni. Pub: NFER	3–12	Speech therapists Teachers
*Illinois Test of Psycholinguistic Abilities (revised) Authors: S Kirk, J McCarthy, W Kirk. Pub: NFER	2–10	Speech therapists Clinical psychologists
Developmental assessment checklist		
*The Schedule of Growing Skills Authors: M Bellman, Cash Pub: NFER	0–5	Health visitors Doctors
Stycar Chart of Developmental Sequences Author: M Sheridan. Pub: NFER	0–5	Health visitors Doctors
Griffiths Mental Development Scales Author: R Griffiths. Pub: The Test Agency	0–8	Doctors Psychologists
Portage Early Education Programme Pub: NFER		
Vineland Adaptive Behaviour Scales Authors: S Sparow, D Balla, C Cicchetti. Pub: NFER	0–8	Teachers Psychologists Occupational therapists

Table 3.1 (contd)

Modality	Age range (years)	Main users
Pre-verbal Communicative Schedule Author: C Kiernan, B Reid. Pub: NFER	Children and adults	Teachers Speech therapists
Developmental Hand Dysfunction Author: M P Erhaut. Pub: Winslow Press.	1–15 months	Teachers Occupational therapists
Bayley Scales of Infant Development Author: N Bayley Pub: Psychological Corporation	2–2½ years	Doctors Psychologists

Although the child may have control over the eyes or facial expression, training may be necessary to establish a reliable means of answering questions. Cognitive potential may be masked by a severe physical disability, and extended assessment is recommended for this group of children. The remainder of this chapter focuses primarily on the practicalities of assessing the child with a severe physical disability, but many of the principles involved will be found useful for the less disabled.

ORGANISATION OF ASSESSMENT

Preparation and organisation of the assessment is important and a coordinator is helpful.

1. Initial information. Obtain all relevant information from appropriate professionals. This gives the team some idea of the type of approach which can be used on the day and cuts down on preliminary questions. It may also highlight any sensory/perceptual difficulties that need to be clarified prior to the assesmment day.

There is sometimes the need to visit the child in a familiar setting, e.g. playgroup or home, to give time for discussion with present staff and to meet the parents. It is vital that the child be relaxed and comfortable during the day so that familiar equipment needed must be brought along, e.g. chair, wheelchair with tray, communication chart, spoon, cup, and should be requested in the invitation letter to the parents informing them about the day.

2. Type of day. Although the day needs to be carefully planned, there is a need for flexibility. Some children will not be cooperative, especially with strangers. The best approach is to use a mixture of informal and formal time, working with one or two team members. It is also important not to talk over the child's head, and to involve him as far as possible.

3. Environment. Just as the day needs to be a mixture of formal and informal activities the environment also needs to be varied. The child in a busy classroom or dayroom can be observed watching what is going on, but for more formal tasks a quiet room is necessary. A two-way mirror is very useful as several team members can observe without distracting the child or family.

Care must be given to the lighting, not too harsh but bright enough, making sure it does not reflect on the table surface or the pictures being used. The furniture needs to include a chair and table with adjustable heights, different size wedges, and several pillows or towels which can be useful for maintaining a good functional position.

If the child needs a sleep during the day this must also be taken into account.

4. Positioning. Talk to parents about positions currently used and preferred. Observe the position the child is in on the parent's lap while a history is taken. Decide which will be the most appropriate for the particular assessment activity.

Look at the child in lying, sitting, standing. Consider the following:

- Comfort
- Relaxation
- Eyes to hands
- Use of hands
- Symmetry
- Stability, i.e. feet supported firmly, pelvis stable.

It has been shown that the position a child is in has an effect on their cognitive function (Green 1987). The best position is seated upright with feet firmly placed and head upright. If the child is responding by eye-pointing, the eyes must be clearly seen by the examiner.

When sitting is not possible, prone lying over a wedge (Chs 33, 25), supported by straps and with hands onto the floor to encourage propping and play, can be an alternative, ensuring that toys are placed within sight and reach. However, eye to eye contact and observation is not easy in the prone position.

Side-lying is another position that can permit the child to see his hands. It is often found that side-lying on one side is preferable to the other with regard to hand function. A prone stander, standing frame, box or table can sometimes give the child an opportunity to demonstrate a different quality of hand function in the upright position. Support may be given with orthoses or gaiters.

When assessing the child at home, the assessor will need to use ordinary furniture or portable positioning aids that are not bulky. Examples include:

— Small chair with range of foam pads
— Feet on floor/box
— Long-sitting on the floor, using cushions/pillows to make corner seat shape
— Bed, table or tray with folding legs for work surface.

For side-lying, rolled towel or pillows (often with support from the helper) can be wedged to maintain stability. Prone-lying can be supported by piling pillows in a wedged position—care must be taken to avoid encouraging spasm in the child with cerebral palsy. A helper's hands will generally be needed to maintain the position.

PARENTAL INVOLVEMENT (See 'The social worker's role' above)

Information about the child must be obtained from the parents if a full picture of the child is to be made. The following are some of the questions it might be useful to consider. Remember that if the child is present throughout an interview, he/she should be included in the conversations as much as possible.

Medical case history (See 'Medical assessment' above).

Personality. What sort of a child (outgoing, timid, etc.) is he? Level of determination, concentration, distractibility, motivation. The child's relationships with other members of the family.

Physical capabilities (See 'Positioning' above). Which parts of the body does he have best control over (if any) and how does he use his body? Can he perform any movements on command? How mobile is he? What positions are preferred?

In order to start the assessment, a knowledge of the preferred hand, eye and position of objects in play is necessary, although experimentation with new positions is likely to be part of the assessment.

What equipment is in use, how successful is it, and what equipment has been tried?

Independence skills. Eating, feeding, toileting, dressing. What techniques and equipment have already been tried? What has been successful? (See Ch. 33.)

Communication. How does the child communicate?—e.g. vocalisations, expression, eye pointing, gesture, speech. How does he make his needs known? Does he make choices? How? Does he have a yes/no response? What does he understand?—e.g. situations, words, sentences. How do parents know he has understood?

Play/interests. Favourite activities or pastimes. Favourite toys, games, books, music. Does he have any pets or belong to any clubs?

The parents should be actively involved in the assessment, not merely by a list of questions, but by encouragement to *participate*.

Observation

Observation plays an important part in assessment, especially with a child who cannot or will not cooperate in more formal tasks. Experienced staff can learn a lot by observing the child in various situations. For this to be useful, a sound knowledge of normal child development is required so that observations can be put into a developmental context, thus giving an understanding of the child's level of functioning in various areas (see Table 3.1 for development assessment checklist). This also gives a wider view of the child than his performance in a formal test situation.

The following pointers have been found useful, both in structuring the type of activities used and in making sense of what is observed:

Parent–child interaction

Watch parents handle the child. What is the level of language used with the child? (This can give an indication of what the parents may perceive the child as understanding.)

How much is done for the child? Do parents expect the child to answer/touch an object? Do they give plenty of time for the child to respond?

Watch parents working or playing with the child. How does the child react with parents? How do both child/parents cope with a short separation (not forced!)?

Interaction with other adults and children

- Ability to make and sustain eye contact
- How does the child communicate?—facial expressions, looking, gestures, noise, speech, yes/no response
- Talk to the child—expect an answer/response, but give plenty of time to respond
- Can the child obey a simple command?—e.g. look at the teddy, touch the switch, look at daddy. (Such commands must be within their physical capabilities and appropriate to their age and level of development)
- Ability to understand situations, e.g. preparation of drink
- Ability to make choices, e.g. What would you like to drink?—orange or milk. How is choice made?—eyes, fist, yes/no
- Ability to anticipate other people's actions, e.g. knows when about to be picked up.

In group sessions, observe the child's ability to anticipate his turn, take turns, track objects around the group, take interest in other group members.

Child's interest in environment/play situations

An assessment box containing a range of appropriate toys and items is required. This will include: everyday objects, e.g. spoon, cup, for the assessment of the understanding of the function of objects and symbolic play; visually stimulating materials, e.g. torches, luminous toys, tinsel; noisy toys such as balls with bells; a variety of cloths and textures; some doll's-house people and furniture; novelty toys, e.g. musical pop-up box and some simple switch-operated toys. The box will need a wide variety of toys and equipment suited to various ages, abilities and needs.

Using the above materials it will be possible to observe:

1. The child's ability to track objects vertically, horizontally and randomly
2. The range of the visual field and the preferred position for toys
3. The ability to anticipate in simple games, e.g. One, two, three, here comes the ball . . .
4. The ability to imitate (within the child's physical capabilities, e.g. tongue thrust)
5. Understanding of object permanence—Does he look where the ball has gone once it has fallen off the tray?
6. Understanding of cause and effect—Can he operate a simple switch?
7. Understanding of simple concepts, e.g. big, little, broken, in play situations
8. Enjoyment and participation in symbolic play, i.e. simple make-believe play or miniature doll play.

Formal assessment

Following observation of the child, it is possible to consider whether a more formal assessment is either possible or necessary, and this will depend not only on the child but also on the aims of the assessment. A formal assessment will involve either the use of standardised or criterion-referenced tests which will enable the examiner to formulate a more accurate idea of the child's level of development at that particular time.

A formal assessment will not always be necessary, especially if the assessment is a preliminary to a longer term assessment. For a formal assessment to be possible, the child must have some way of reliably responding to a question. If the child cannot speak and has little control over his hands, the questions must involve a multiple choice for the child to be able to select the correct response. There are three main ways of responding: eye-pointing, which involves the child looking at the object/picture; fist or hand pointing; or a yes/no response. Table 3.2 shows those tests and assessments that may utilise eye or fist pointing. The practicalities of using these methods of responding are discussed below.

Eye-pointing

A child who has little control over other parts of the body may well have good control over the eyes. During observation it will have been possible to see if the child can look at objects, pictures, or people on request. It is important to consider the child's vision. Do objects have to be placed in a particular place to be seen? If a child has a squint, is one eye used more than the other?

Table 3.2   Tests and assessments that can be used/adapted for eye/fist pointing or yes/no response

Modality	Age range (years. months)	Main users
Language		
English Picture Vocabulary Test (preschool version) Authors: M A Brimer, L M Dunn. Pub: Education Evaluation Enterprises	3–4.11	Speech therapists Educational and clinical psychologists Teachers
Peabody Picture Vocabulary Test Author: L M Dunn. Pub: American Guidance Service (NFER)	2.6–adult	as above
British Picture Vocabulary Scale Authors: L M Dunn, C Whetton, D Pintilie. Pub: NFER	3–5.6	as above
Sentence Comprehension Test Authors: K Wheldall, A Hobsban, P Mittler. Pub: NFER	3–5	as above
Test for Reception of Grammar Author: D Bishop. Dept of Psychology, Manchester Univ.	4–13	Speech therapists
Reynell Developmental Language Scales Author: J K Reynell. Pub: NFER	1.6–6	Speech therapists Educational and clinical psychologists
The Word Finding Vocabulary Test Author: Catherine Renfrew (useful for signers) The Renfrew Action Picture Test (Both from C E Renfrew, North Place, Old Headington, Oxford)	3–3.6	Speech therapists
Other tests		
Colombia Mental Maturity Scale Authors: B B Burgemeister, L H Blum, L Lorge. Pub: NFER (Scale claims to measure general reasoning ability using 'odd man out' type items)	3.6–10	Clinical and educational psychologists
British Ability Scale Visual Recognition. Basic Number Concepts. Pub: NFER	2–17	Educational psychologists
Boehm Test of Basic Concepts Author: A Boehm Pub: NFER (A test designed to test mastery of certain concepts, e.g. most, middle, every)	4–6 N/A	Teachers Psychologists Speech therapists

Table 3.2   (*contd*)

Modality	Age range (years. months)	Main users
Pre-Symbol Assessment—Bliss Symbolics		Speech therapists
Picture Aided Reading Test Author: N Hamp	5–10	Teachers

Note.   These norm-referenced texts were not standardised on a disabled population, and caution should be used in interpreting the results. The tests should be used as part of a wider overall functional assessment of the child's strengths and weaknesses.

Position of the child

The child needs to be in a good functional position (see 'Positioning' above) where the examiner can see his eyes, but facing away from the light source.

Position and size of objects/pictures

The size of objects or pictures needs to be considered if the child has poor vision. They must be placed where the child can see them, remembering that shiny pictures reflect light.

The number of objects or pictures used will depend on the child's ability and skill in eye-pointing and the examiner's skill in knowing where the child is looking: four or five objects are usually enough. The objects can be placed on the child's tray, a table, or on an 'E' tran frame. The latter device is shaped rather like an empty picture frame held in the vertical. The examiner sticks objects or pictures around the frame with Blu-tac and has a clear view of the child's eyes in the middle of the frame. Perspex board can also be used. The position of the correct object must be alternated as children often respond to a preferred position.

Testing procedure

Make sure the child has looked at all the items (if necessary by pointing to each in turn) before asking him to look at one. If possible ask the child to look at the examiner in between items so that it is known where he is starting from. Also make sure that the child understands the question asked, e.g. 'Look at the big car', or 'Where's the big car?'

Advantages of eye-pointing are that the responses can be very quick and it is not very tiring for the child.

Disadvantages include:

- It is a skill that may have to be learned
- It can be easy for the examiner to give non-verbal clues by looking at the correct item

- The examiner needs to be a skilled observer as some children look at objects only fleetingly.

Fist-pointing

Some children who have the physical capability may be very motivated to fist-point (or use some other part of the arm or hand). Again a choice of items is needed, placed near enough for the child to touch, alternating the position of the correct item.

Disadvantages

- It is often very tiring for the child
- It may take a long time for the child to respond
- The physical exertion and organisation involved may interfere with the child's memory of what you have asked him to do
- There may be incoordination between eyes and hands because of reflex activity. A child who is trying to touch something may look in the opposite direction and therefore forget where he was looking or touch the wrong item
- It may be so unreliable that it is difficult to know if errors are due to poor coordination or lack of understanding
- Objects get knocked over.

Yes/no response

If a child has a reliable yes/no response, the examiner can do the pointing and the child can respond to the correct item, e.g. by looking up or smiling. The examiner must point slowly to allow the child to respond, and be careful not to give non-verbal clues by looking at the correct item, varying their intonation (e.g. Is it *this* one?) or hesitating when pointing.

Advantages

This method is less tiring for the child, and can be very quick depending on the child's reaction time. It can also be used to check the child's response to eye-pointing or fist-pointing.

In all methods, it is necessary to establish a routine so that the child is clear about what the examiner is expecting of him, as too many instructions are confusing.

DEVELOPMENTAL ASSESSMENT

Developmental assessment compares the child's behaviour in the context of normal developmental processes, and many test batteries are available to do this, e.g. Griffiths Mental Development Scales, Schedule of Growing Skills, Bayley Scales (see Table 3.1).

The disadvantage of these scales for assessing the multiply disabled child is that most rely heavily on the child being able to use his hands and use expressive speech. It is often necessary, therefore, for the team to devise their own assessment materials based on normal child development, but geared to the specific population involved.

Criteria-referenced tests

These can be designed to measure the child's performance in a particular skill area, e.g. eye–hand coordination or symbolic play. This assessment involves describing in detail those aspects of a task that the child has mastered, and those which he needs to learn, usually in the form of a checklist.

There are many checklists available, e.g. Portage, Cathy Gerard Pre-Verbal Communication Schedule, but none of these caters entirely for the needs of the severely disabled child and therefore it is usually necessary to make a checklist which can be used by the team.

Thus the checklist is not only a detailed record of the child's achievements at a certain time, but also forms part of the curriculum and is used to set aims and objectives for the child's programme.

RECORDING THE ASSESSMENT

Staff need to devise their own record forms that will be able to record clearly the material collected from parental interviews, observations and informal assessment. It is therefore necessary before the assessment for the staff to have a clear idea what they are looking for, and this will be evident in the record form.

Norm-referenced tests have their own record forms available and checklists are easily filled out. Observers, e.g. behind a two-way mirror, may find it useful to have a checklist of behaviours which they can tick off as observed. Video recording may also be helpful.

ACTION TAKEN FOLLOWING ASSESSMENT

After an assessment has been carried out there should be full discussion with parents and team members to complete the profile and to define aims for therapy, educational, medical and social work involvement. Priorities need to be drawn up and the decision made about who will carry out the action. If necessary, referral should be made to other agencies, and full discussion with reports made available to the GP and other professionals involved. Requests will be sent for funding if a placement is sought, and for equipment as needed.

LONG-TERM ASSESSMENT

The above techniques will also form part of a long-term assessment.

A day or short-term assessment may not be sufficient to establish the child's educational needs, especially if the child has a severe multiple disability. In these cases it is often necessary for a long-term assessment to take place.

Advantages of long-term assessment include the following:

1. The child can be properly seated and given other necessary equipment (such as glasses or switches) that will enable him to function at an optimum level.

2. Staff have time to get to know the child, and he has a chance to settle and feel confident with the adults around him.

3. Training can be given in eye-pointing, or other effective methods of communication. This is vital for assessment to be carried out successfully.

4. By keeping careful records of the child's progress over time, the child's rate of learning can be measured. This often gives a clearer view of the child's cognitive and physical potential.

REFERENCE

Green E M 1987 The effect of seating position on cognitive function in children with cerebral palsy. 59th annual meeting of British Paediatric Association. Abstract G: 158, 108

4. Assessment of vision and management of visual problems

A. Harden   V. Raynar-Smith

An ophthalmic examination is an essential part of the assessment of the handicapped child. It is only when the whole picture has been established that constructive decisions can be taken on the child's management. *Visual problems are a hundred times more common in children with physical handicap, particularly those with a neurological basis.*

The skills of an ophthalmologist and an orthoptist are needed for visual assessment, often requiring two or three visits before definite conclusions can be drawn. The importance of gaining the confidence and cooperation of the parents cannot be overemphasised. A full history is essential, with particular attention to the perinatal period as well as any family history of any visual disorder. Useful information can be gathered from birth, although the younger the child the harder it will be to draw conclusions.

Visual development depends on the maturation of the visual pathways. The more sensory input the developing child receives the better. When visual function is known to be poor every effort must be made to maximise the visual stimulus from the earliest age, to achieve the best visual potential for the child.

Visual information is an essential part of the learning process: it is used in the development of the upright posture and balance (Butterworth 1983); in perception of shape and space; in recognition of familiar people; and, crucially, in social development and play. In the presence of other abnormalities it is all too easy to overlook severe visual problems that may be compounding the disability.

Assessment of vision

The normal visual milestones are as follows:

0–2 weeks — Large coloured objects are fixated
— Head will turn to a light or window
— Erratic following movements are made
— The baby shows reduced motor activity with fixation and brightening of the face to visual stimulation
— Optokinetic nystagmus (OKN) can be demonstrated
2–4 weeks — Re-fixation from one object to another develops

2–3 months — Visually directed reaching begins
               — Convergence develops
               — Eye contact is made

3–5 months — Blinking to threat response is present
               — Examination of own hands and feet begins

By 6 months — Any intermittent squint should disappear

By 5 years — Binocular vision is established.

At the first assessment of a child with possible visual problems note carefully what the parents say about the child's vision: they are frequently right. 'A smiling baby is a seeing baby' is a good rule of thumb. All babies should respond to their mother's visual stimulus from 2–3 weeks.

The examiner should be clear about the difference between visibility and resolution. Visibility implies an ability to see but does not give any clue about resolution (the ability to discriminate). For example, the child sees a white ball (visibility) but how clearly (resolution)?

TESTING OF VISION

0–12 months — Catford Nystagmus Drum (a test of visibility rather than resolution)
               — Coloured scarf (to demonstrate fixation and refixation)
               — Optokinetic nystagmus
               — Forced-choice preferential looking (FPL) using static sinusoidal gratings
               — Photo-refraction (Atkinson & Braddick 1983)
               — Ability to overcome base-out prisms

8–12 months — Worth balls
               — '100s &1000s' and Smarties

2–3 years — Ffookes symbols

2½ years — Picture tests

2½–3½ years — Sheridan-Gardiner single optotype test

3½–5 years — Linear visual acuity assessed with matching letter test.

Linear visual acuity should be obtained as early as possible because a single optotype may give a false impression of good acuity. In astigmatism and squint a linear presentation of letters may induce the 'crowding phenomenon', which may reduce the visual acuity by 2 lines in astigmatism, and 4 or 5 lines in squint.

Visual evoked potentials

The use of visual evoked potentials (VEPs) is helpful in visual assessment. The test gives a good indication of the presence or absence of an intact visual pathway, and also shows the latency (time taken between flash stimulus and occipital cortical activity). Repeated VEPs may show a change in latency, as for example in delayed visual maturation.

OCULAR EXAMINATION

The pupils should react to direct and indirect light. ('Indirect' here refers to the reaction whereby light shone into one pupil produces a reflex constriction in the other pupil.) The ocular media should be clear, manifesting a red reflex when viewed with an ophthalmoscope. If the ocular movements are not full an adequate explanation must be determined.

The fundus should be examined under mydriasis, using cyclopentolate 0.5% or 1%, to exclude any pathology of the optic disc, fovea or retina. At the same time retinoscopy can be performed to determine whether a refractive error is present (long sight, short sight or astigmatism).

In some circumstances it may be pertinent to try to assess a child's field of vision with the 'flashing light test' or Worth balls.

The orthoptist's role is to:

- Assess the visual acuity of each eye independently
- Diagnose the presence of ocular muscle imbalance or squint (strabismus)
- Determine the state of development of binocular vision
- Ascertain in children with squint whether binocular vision can be restored or whether cosmetic improvement only is achievable.

NEURO-OPHTHALMOLOGY

In cerebral palsy and related conditions with poor motor development and coordination, squints are common and often have a paralytic element. Optic atrophy of varying degree also occurs. (For a fuller discussion of visual disorders in cerebral palsy see Ch. 6.)

Optic atrophy is also seen in hydrocephalus, secondary to chronically raised intracranial pressure. It may also give rise to oculomotor palsies of which the 6th cranial nerve is the most vulnerable due to its long intracranial course. An ocular motor sign of raised intracranial pressure (ICP) is the 'setting sun sign' where the eyes are held or frequently move into depression, disappearing below the lower lid, usually associated with poor elevation caused by pressure on the brain stem.

The optic discs may be swollen (papilloedema) due to raised ICP. After closure of the fontanelles the degree of swelling may be much greater, although often the presence of optic atrophy makes it difficult to interpret.

Trauma and tumours may present or be associated with ocular manifestations, mainly as pupil abnormalities, palsies of the 3rd, 4th and 6th cranial nerves, and optic atrophy, but also with blurred discs, retinal haemorrhages, field defects and a fall in visual acuity.

Abnormalities of the eye may accompany many of the rare neurological syndromes because the eye is an extension of the nervous system.

Neurotropic organisms (those attracted to nerve tissue) like toxoplasmosis, cytomegalovirus and rubella, cause chorioretinitis often with profound visual consequences.

Cataracts may also occur, for example in rubella and Down syndrome.

As premature low-birth-weight babies survive, further ocular problems become manifest. Squints and refractive errors, especially myopia, are much more common than in the normal population. In about 5% of cases major visual defects occur, usually with nystagmus, due to complications of retinopathy of prematurity, resulting in blindness in a few.

In musculoskeletal and metabolic diseases the eye is commonly involved, which adds to the child's handicap.

MANAGEMENT OF VISUAL PROBLEMS

It is essential that every handicapped child has a full ophthalmic assessment at a time deemed appropriate by the paediatrician—usually at an early stage. Without this, visual problems may be missed and the opportunity to direct and advise how best to help the child may be lost, e.g. knowing which eye sees best, whether there is a field defect, or whether glasses should be worn.

Once under the care of an ophthalmologist the time for discharge will vary according to the diagnosis. By the age of 8 years the visual system has reached maturity and achieved maximal acuity.

Teachers or care assistants should be present at ophthalmic assessments of older children with visual problems because they are able to help and advise about the best way to deal with a child in order to obtain maximal performance.

Where there is major visual disability, help and advice from the Rehabilitation Officers for the Visually Handicapped (ROVH) should be sought. Case conferences should be arranged, where all disciplines can plan management and objectives over a period of time.

Counselling of parents may be necessary and genetic counselling offered. Frequently in the early stage blind registration is best postponed until the parents are ready psychologically. The ophthalmologist must beware of making instant judgements in view of the many parameters that need to be considered. Other disciplines as well as the parents should be prepared for several visual assessments before direction on management and treatment is given.

Management rests primarily with the diagnosis and control, where possible, of the neurological disorder. In hydrocephalus, problems with the shunt may occur resulting in a rise in ICP and a return of cranial nerve palsies (especially the 6th nerve), blurring of the disc margins and a fall in visual acuity. Regular visual assessment is essential.

The eye, optic nerve and brain may show remarkable degrees of recovery, often over a period of many months—particularly following head injuries, and periventricular leukomalacia.

PARALYTIC AND NON-PARALYTIC SQUINT

Delayed or impaired motor development is likely to be associated with the development of squint. The handicapped child may have so many other problems that a squint may be ignored. It should be appreciated that early treatment is necessary if long-term amblyopia is to be avoided. However, in children with gross handicap a positive decision may be taken by parents and ophthalmologist to leave the amblyopia untreated.

Management of squint

The aim of treatment is to develop good visual acuity in each eye and to realign the eyes so that binocular vision is able to develop. Good visual acuity may be restored by wearing glasses, but more often occlusion is required. Glasses and occlusion alone will straighten the squint in a few cases, but surgery is necessary in the majority of cases.

Glasses. When glasses are indicated a child will normally be encouraged to wear them from the age of 2½ years. However, in high degrees of refractive error associated with the development of a squint, they should be worn earlier. Glasses at this age are a therapy, not just a visual aid, and should be worn constantly throughout the development period (8 years).

Occlusion. The better eye is occluded to stimulate the vision of the amblyopic eye. A baby under a year will normally tolerate occlusion much longer than a child in the second year of life. Therefore it is essential to make as much progress as possible at this young age. It is important to explain to parents that the occluder is being worn to improve the vision of the squinting eye and not to correct the squint, that a squint does not occur in one eye but affects the balance of both eyes, and that if a squint is noticed in the other eye following the use of the occluder it is an indication of improvement. In children with gross amblyopia and in babies the occluder is usually stuck to the face. Initially it should be used for approximately 2 hours a day (less with small babies) and that period will be reduced as the acuity improves, or increased if there is no improvement.

Surgical correction. If there is potential for binocular vision the squint should be corrected surgically as soon as good visual acuity has been established in each eye (but not before the age of 6 months because of the complications of general anaesthesia in small babies).

The shorter the duration of the squint and the later the onset, the greater the possibility of restoring binocular vision. If only a cosmetic result is expected surgical correction can be postponed until the squint becomes a social problem. The parents should be warned that it may take two or more operations to straighten the eyes. Beware of operating on a child with a squint for cosmetic reasons when the child is not aware of the problem, unless it is undoubtedly affecting non-verbal communication. A sympathetic but frank discussion with the parents will usually remove both doctors' and parents' 'need to be seen to be doing something'.

REFERENCES

Atkinson J, Braddick O J 1983 Assessment of visual acuity in infancy and early childhood. Acta Opthalmologica, Suppl. 157: 18–26
Butterworth G 1983 Structure of the mind in human infancy. Advances in Infancy Research (11): 11

FURTHER READING

Atkinson J 1986 Methods of objective assessment of visual functions in subjects with limited communication skills. In: Ellis D (ed) Sensory impairments in mentally handicapped people. Croom Helm

5. Assessment of hearing and management of hearing problems

G. Baird

PREVALENCE OF HEARING LOSS IN CEREBRAL PALSY

The prevalence of deafness in cerebral palsy is falling. Studies of prevalence in older cerebral palsy populations give figures of 25% in the 40s and 50s (Fisch 1955) and 12.5% by 1970 (Robinson 1973).

Robson, reviewing children born after 1970, concluded that 5% had sensorineural deafness—those with athetosis were still the largest group, with 1.6%–3% in other types of cerebral palsy (ACHSHIP reports, DHSS 1981). In the total child population of West Sussex, five children with cerebral palsy (2%) have a hearing loss (Abra, personal communication).

Most at risk are premature babies who have had anoxic seizures with jaundice, and children exposed to the prenatal infections of rubella and cytomegalovirus (Preece et al 1984, Crewers 1989).

In addition, children who have gross malfunction of the oropharyngeal structures may be at greater risk of middle ear catarrh.

ASSESSMENT

The age of diagnosis of deafness in cerebral palsy tends to be older than in the non-handicapped population. Of recent referrals to Guy's tertiary service in 1989, only three children who have cerebral palsy and deafness and no other defect were diagnosed at over 3 years of age. Children with cerebral palsy who are deaf have a 65% chance of another defect—mental, visual, or epilepsy. All of these factors make accurate behavioural testing of hearing extremely difficult; in addition, parents and professionals may be concentrating on what is seen as the primary defect or disability.

Testing can be divided into methods appropriate for successive developmental ages as with non-handicapped children.

THE NEONATAL PERIOD

The total population of babies may be screened, or an at-risk group (decided on the basis of various perinatal risk factors) may be selected.

Methods

At the moment neonatal screening is still at the stage of evaluation but is likely to become increasingly widely used.

- The auditory response cradle (Report of a Kings Fund Seminar on Infant Hearing Screening 1984). This is a behavioural response method relying on various reflex measures like respiratory rate, head jerk, head turn and gross activity level to narrow-band noise of high intensity.
- Brainstem evoked responses (BSER).
- The click evoked acoustic emission—a cochlear 'echo'.

The last two methods seem the most reliable, and a recent paper (Stevens et al 1989) compares both methods. Acoustic emission is quicker and as reliable as BSER. Both are non-behavioural methods. Problems include:

1. The reliability of threshold measures in the newborn period—the nearer to term they are recorded the better.

2. There may be improvement in the threshold response during the first year: even if tested twice in the neonatal period, a significant number will 'fail' who do not later appear to be hearing impaired (Murray 1985).

3. Hearing loss may become worse in the first year of life (particularly if associated with rubella and CMV) (Peckham 1985).

4. Facilities for audiological centre testing and parental support are required, which are not at present adequate.

TESTING IN THE FIRST 18 MONTHS

Neonatal screening with careful clinical follow up may be the method of choice for the future but, at present, neonatal screening has not been carried out in most children, and the detection of hearing loss relies on parental suspicion, often supplemented by a behavioural questionnaire and *distraction test* at 7–8 months (McCormick 1983). When the first few months of life are taken up with the additional problems of difficult feeding, hypotonia, and possibly general delay in responsiveness and poor health the judgement about hearing may be very difficult to make by parents or professionals.

Methods

- Blinking to a loud sound (70 dB above threshold)—the APR may be observed and may be an indication of *some* hearing although it is a reflex response and does not give an accurate threshold
- Distraction test—a behavioural response.

In the distraction test, widely used to screen for hearing loss in the total child population, the child sits on the parent's lap and turns to sounds made at ear level out of the visual field, the child's attention having been briefly caught, but not held, by a distractor (see McCormick 'Paediatric Audiology 0–5' for a fuller description of the test technique). The sounds used can either be traditional sound sources—e.g. cup and spoon, high frequency rattle, voice or sibilant (hiss), which if presented at *minimal* levels are frequency limited (except for cup and spoon, which is employed by some as an 'interesting sound')—or frequency modulated 'warble' tones.

The integrated turning and visual location of a sound made at ear level (described by Touwen (1976) as present in over 90% of normal term babies by 8 months) and the location below and above the ear by 8–9 months, depends on multiple factors, all of which may be abnormal in the child with cerebral palsy:

1. The hearing may be defective.
2. The integration of auditory and visuomotor responses may be very much slower, i.e. cortical processing and motor execution time.
3. Developmental and cognitive defect—the response to sounds has a developmental progression. It is linked to a general cognitive level including: listening to sounds within an area which increases from a few inches to several feet from the baby; sufficiently mature auditory attention to be distracted by any new dominant audiological stimulus, rather than 'fixed' by a visual stimulus as would a 5-month-old baby; and an increasing interest in unfamiliar sounds rather than familiar (increases from 4 months–10/12 months). Mental retardation will delay the behavioural responses regardless of hearing level.
4. The motor disorder may prevent full head turning; this ability is dependent on good *trunk* control (check the head turning ability visually before starting testing). It is also clear that the alertness of response to sound can be affected by the degree of uprightness of posture (see Ch. 8). The age of sitting unsupported may be delayed in prematurity, as well as normal motor variants, and can contribute to difficulties of testing and interpretation of responses. If it is impossible to achieve enough head and trunk control in sitting, then hearing can be tested in supine, but care must be taken to avoid the visual fields. The sounds need to be 15–30 cm away at 3–4 months and 30–45 cm away from the ear at 6 months, at ear level (Sheridan 1960). Again a check should be made that the child has sufficient voluntary head control to turn and is *not* trapped in reflexes like the asymmetric tonic neck reflex .

If developmentally it is thought that an integrated audio-visuo-motor turn to locate is not possible (i.e. pre 4 month development level) other signs, e.g. eye widening, or alertness to sound can be used but reliability is very uncertain and one can delude oneself and others. The sounds used should be 'familiar' ones at this developmental level—the child's own toys may be used and the intensity used carefully measured, but they will not have a known frequency.

5. Visual defect—This may be a disorder of gaze (as part of the motor disorder when visuomotor integrated location of sound may be delayed), an acuity defect, a *field* defect, or all three.) *Severe* functional visual loss removes the reward obtained by turning and locating sounds; instead the child adopts an alert and listening posture. A field defect, even due to severe squint, may cause a delay in turning to that side which can sometimes lead to the suspicion of unilateral hearing loss.

In view of the complexities of testing it is suggested that children with cerebral palsy should have their hearing tested by a specialist team, particularly if there is any doubt expressed. The auditory channel/potential for language comprehension and thinking may be the only one spared in this condition, and therefore assumes massive importance.

'Objective' tests

If clinical testing yields equivocal results, or confirmation is required, brainstem evoked responses (BSER) may be used. Careful interpretation is needed as brainstem function may be abnormal. Occasionally, in the very severely physically handicapped who are also mentally subnormal and visually unresponsive, there may be no BSER responses and yet parents and care staff are sure that there is some responsiveness to sound. Electrocochleography will at best establish if the cochlea is responding to sound (a source of anxiety if amplification is being considered). Cortical abnormalities of hearing, unlike visual cortical blindness, are not well described or understood.

Visual reinforcement audiometry

This is a technique of assessment using sound location, well suited to handicapped children. The child and parent are in the test room, audiologist outside and the sounds are presented through loudspeakers. Correct source–location responses are rewarded by a visual reinforcing stimulus (see Bamford 1989 for a further description). Potential difficulties with this technique are as described under 'distraction'.

TESTING AFTER 2 YEARS

Speech tests can be used from a mental age of 18 months upwards, using large toys at first, then smaller ones, exactly as described with non-handicapped children. Lay out the toys on the table, ensure the child knows the names, and ask the child to indicate them; use a measured, quiet voice, and cover your mouth to prevent lip-reading. Again the important test tips are:

- Posture—sitting upright, able to see; table at the correct height

- If eye pointing is used, sufficient space for accurate observer detection but avoid giving eye-point or gestural clues
- Time for response
- Limited number of toys in a row, for scanning (not exhaustion) to take place—assist scanning by physical demonstration yourself, pointing across the toys.

Conditioning may be used from a mental age of 2½ years. The first thing to establish is whether the child can make any regular repetitive controlled movement: knocking bricks off a table with any part of the body is acceptable. Then the conditioning processing, using a free field hand-held audiometer, can be attempted in the same way as with other children. If successful, pure-tone audiometry closed circuit can be proceeded with very quickly.

MANAGEMENT OF HEARING IMPAIRMENT IN CEREBRAL PALSY

Accurate diagnosis must be the first requirement of management, and subsequent general principles are the same as those of the non cerebral palsy child. Using a 'team' approach with the parents as integral members, the first step is to give them the skills to promote the child's development. (Coping with parental and sibling feelings of grief, etc. is part of the professional support, as elsewhere in the book.)

AMPLIFICATION

Appropriate aids based on established formulae are chosen. Most children use post-aural aids now; advantages include ear-level sound reception, convenience and appearance. In high noise levels, for example in a classroom, a radio aid may be used with the personal aids to ensure a satisfactory signal-to-noise ratio.

Difficulties may be experienced with physically handicapped children if they are lying down more frequently or moving jerkily, as the aids will be rubbed or knocked off. Uncontrolled movements may mean greater reliance on double-sided sticky tape.

Difficulties of transport to centres contribute to problems in getting ear moulds made frequently enough. (See Evans 1988 for further description of aids and amplification.)

EDUCATION AND THE PROMOTION OF COMMUNICATION AND LANGUAGE

In children with cerebral palsy the greater emphasis will be on promoting *comprehension* of verbal language and *communication* by methods which may be verbal or non-verbal (signs and symbols). The teacher of the deaf will have to collaborate with the speech therapist and others to plan the most relevant individual programme for any particular child. Integration in ordinary school will present extra challenges to communication and special skills on the part of the ordinary teacher. See Wood (1986) for an excellent description of teaching communication. The dependence of the partially hearing, cerebral palsied child means that many more people will have to understand the principles of wearing and looking after hearing aids, as well as the influence of the suboptimal acoustic environment.

Particular problems and difficulties are usually due to the additional defects of severe mental handicap, where it becomes impossible to judge the response to amplification. Our approach is usually to try *cautious* use of amplification and judge the response to familiar sounds over time.

In summary, although the finding of an additional defect—deafness—in a child who is already disabled may be an overwhelming blow for parents, it represents a deficit for which there is a well tried and effective management and treatment strategy with good results. For the professionals the challenge is that of integrating one's skills with *other* professionals and finding the most appropriate educational setting in which to meet the child's needs.

REFERENCES

Bamford J 1988 Visual reinforcement audiology. In: McCormick B (ed) Paediatric audiology 0–5 years. Taylor and Francis, London
Crewers 1989 Causes of sensorineural hearing loss. Journal of the Royal Society of Medicine 82: 485
Evans P 1988 Hearing aid systems. In: McCormick B (ed) Paediatric audiology 0–5 years. Taylor and Francis, London
Fisch L 1955 The aetiology of congenital deafness and audiometric patterns. Journal of Laryngology 69: 7
King's Fund Seminar on Infant Hearing Screening 1984 Report: The Auditory Acoustic Cradle
McCormick B 1983 Hearing screening by health visitors. Health Visitor 56: 449–451
Murray A 1985 Prognostic validity of auditory brainstem responses in newborn infants. American Journal of Otolaryngology 6: 120–131
Preece P M, Peckham C S, Pearl K N 1984 Congenital cytomegalovirus infection. Archives of Disease in Childhood 59: (12) 1120–1126
Robinson R O 1973 The frequency of other handicaps in children with cerebral palsy. Developmental Medicine and Child Neurology 15: 305
Robson P 1981 ACHSHIP Reports, DHSS
Sheridan M 1960 The developmental progress of infants and young children, HMSO
Stevens J C et al 1989 Click evoked otoacoustic emissions compared with brain stem evoked responses. Archives of Disease in Childhood 64: (8) 1105–1111
Touwen B 1976 The neurological development of infants. Clinics in Development Medicine 58 (Published by SIMP)
Wood 1986 Teaching and talking to deaf children. John Wiley, Chichester

6. Cerebral palsy: definition, epidemiology, developmental and neurological aspects

G.T. McCarthy

Cerebral palsy is not a single condition. The term is used to describe a disorder of posture and movement, which is persistent and caused by a non-progressive brain lesion, arising before or around birth, during the time of rapid brain development. It implies that there has been an event or process causing a change in brain development, and hence subsequent function, at least as far as the control of movement and posture are concerned. The lesion is permanent and static and the condition is lifelong, but there are inevitable changes which occur as a result of maturation and growth.

It is rare for the brain to be damaged purely in the motor areas. Brain structure and function may be changed affecting cognition, vision and hearing, and sometimes causing epilepsy.

The ways in which the baby and young child are handled can have profound effects upon the severity of the condition in adult life. There have been a number of notable people who have increased our understanding of the condition and developed ways of helping children to overcome their disabilities. Most agree that they have learned from experience and have modified their management over the years. 'It is never the technique, but the response of the child to the technique which is the most important' (Bobath 1980).

CAUSES OF CEREBRAL PALSY

In spite of improved obstetric care the incidence of cerebral palsy is not falling. Population studies in Britain (Emond et al 1989), Australia (Blair & Stanley 1988) and the USA (Nelson 1988) have led to similar estimates of the proportion of cerebral palsy that might have been caused by intra-partum damage (3–13%).

Perinatal asphyxia is not the only, nor the commonest, cause of cerebral palsy, especially in full-term infants (Hall 1990, Aylward et al 1989, Emond et al 1989). Recent large studies by Nelson & Ellenberg (1988) in the USA, Blair & Stanley (1988) in Western Australia, and Hagberg et al (1984) in Sweden, showed that there were correlations between abnormalities of pregnancy and cerebral palsy, but there was little association with abnormalities of labour.

It is probable that infants with cerebral abnormalities antedating labour show signs of birth asphyxia which may be caused by their brain anomaly and wrongly regarded as the cause of the cerebral palsy. In the majority of cases the cause is still largely a matter of speculation.

Vascular occlusion or haemorrhage in the fetal or infant brain is a cause of cerebral palsy—occlusion of the middle cerebral artery or internal carotid artery may cause infarction and cyst formation and is associated with hemiplegia. Embolism may also cause infarction, particularly in the surviving member of a monovular twin pregnancy (Asindi 1988, Schinzel 1979, Yoshioka 1979).

Pre-term infants

In pre-term infants most adverse outcomes seem to have a multifactorial aetiology. The immature brain is vulnerable to insult from non-traumatic intracranial haemorrhage, which develops in 40% of all newborn infants of <1500 g birth weight (Wigglesworth 1984). Bleeding occurs from capillaries, being most frequent in infants with hypercapnia and metabolic acidosis, as may occur in respiratory distress syndrome. Intraventricular haemorrhage occurs when the initial bleed ruptures through the ependymal layer. The extent of haemorrhage and subsequent damage is very variable; there may be extensive spread into the cerebral substance or obstruction of CSF drainage resulting in hydrocephalus.

Ischaemic damage of the newborn brain may also occur, probably due to hypotension during apnoeic attacks. The periventricular region in the pre-term brain is a boundary zone between arterial territories and it is in this area that damage occurs. These lesions may destroy future white matter and prevent the development of the corticospinal pathways resulting in spastic hemi- or quadriplegia. Destruction of the visual pathways may interfere with visual function.

The final effects of these lesions depends on their severity and position. There may be capacity for remodelling during later development.

Other causes of cerebral palsy

Anomalies of cortical development and metabolic disorders, some of which are familial, must be considered as causes of cerebral palsy. Inheritance may be autosomal recessive, X-linked, or dominant. Chromosomal abnormalities may also be associated with maldevelopment of the brain. Lissencephaly (smooth brain) is an abnormality of brain development characterised by incomplete neuronal migration and a smooth cerebral surface. It is sometimes seen in association with chromosomal abnormalities (Dobyns et al 1984). Lesch–Nyhan Syndrome, a rare X-linked disorder of purine metabolism, is associated with severe dystonia and self-mutilation (see p. 180). Intrauterine infection with rubella virus, cytomegalovirus or *Toxoplasma* may also result in cerebral palsy.

INCIDENCE OF CEREBRAL PALSY

Incidence means the number of new cases of a disorder occurring during a certain time period in a defined population at risk. Since cerebral palsy is a heterogeneous condition that may arise at different stages of intrauterine or early infant life, it is difficult to produce meaningful stastistics. Many severely affected infants do not survive the neonatal period.

Prevalence is the number of cases of the disorder present during a certain time period. The infantile prevalence is expressed as the number of cases of cerebral palsy per 1000 neonatal survivors.

If children with cerebral palsy are defined as those with stable motor handicap who are alive at the age of school entry and who require services, a prevalence of 2/1000 live births in industrialised nations can be taken as a reasonable estimate (Paneth & Kiely 1984). In a comparison between two national cohorts in 1958 and 1970 the prevalence of cerebral palsy in the neonatal period remained static, but there was a pronounced increase in the prevalence at age 10, from 1.9/1000 in 1968 to 2.6/1000 in 1980 (Emond et al 1989).

Another major difficulty in definition in epidemiological studies arises from lack of standardisation in the description of types or severity of cerebral palsy. In an attempt to overcome this problem a group from Oxford have produced a record form—*Standard recording of central motor deficit*—intended to be used in prospective population studies. This record form is reproduced in full (with permission) at the end of this chapter. The form moves away from the confusing use of neurological terms, which have different meanings to different people, and encourages a more accurate description of the child's performance on the day. The distribution of involvement is recorded in detail giving a more accurate picture of the child's difficulties, and a description of unwanted movements and what the examiner actually feels when assessing muscle tone. The record form was produced by a multidisciplinary working group who met over a period of years in order to standardise the responses as much as possible. It is designed to be used by relatively inexperienced professionals to observe a population over time. It should produce more accurate figures of the degree of disability at different ages, and be a useful tool in planning for services.

MOTOR AND POSTURAL DEVELOPMENT

Normal development involves complex interaction between the child and the environment dominated by gravity. It depends upon the development of sensory responses—vision, hearing, touch, taste, smell—and crucially upon the interaction between the baby and the mother, who facilitates each stage. If the process is disrupted by abnormal responses a vicious circle of failure and depression may result.

In essence motor development entails development of the ability to mix flexion and extension components of movement and to maintain fixation and balance in an increasingly upright posture. The ability to carry out a skilled movement depends upon stabilisation of the trunk and the proximal segments of the limbs using vestibular and visual information. It also requires smooth relaxation of antagonist muscles as the agonist muscles contract (see later). The anticipatory postural responses are centrally driven complex reflex pathways, which are invoked when skilled activity takes place. They have been shown to arise from the periphery in response to movement of the limbs.

Marsden et al (1976, 1977, 1980) have demonstrated these responses in adults. It is likely that they develop in infancy and early childhood and are responsible for the increasingly sophisticated motor performance seen as children develop. Postural development starts from birth and can be seen developing in babies in the lying positions of prone and supine (Pountney et al 1990) before sitting, crawling and walking can be achieved.

Sensory systems involved in postural control include vision, vestibular, kinaesthesis and touch. Butterworth & Cicchetti (1978) showed that the effect of discrepant visual feedback was greatest in the first 3 months after acquiring the ability to sit or stand. Butterworth (1983) concluded that it is likely that there is an innate sensory–motor relationship, where prestructured visual feedback is used as a means of gaining control over posture. Older children between 5 and 15 years are able to correct conflicting input.

Other authors (Shambes 1976, Williams et al 1983) have studied the developing control of balance and movement in young children of different ages, showing the gradual reduction in muscle activity required to maintain upright posture as the nervous system matures.

Sutherland et al (1988) have studied the development of mature walking in normal children using sophisticated techniques of gait analysis. These studies show how the walking pattern changes as a result of greater muscle control and changes in angles of the long bones, which occur with growth.

Kinaesthesis has been defined as the sense of movement and position (Laszlo & Bairstow 1980). It includes the discrimination of the position of body parts, and movements and amplitude of movement of body parts, both actively and passively produced. It is based on information other than visual, auditory or verbal (Howard & Templeton 1966). There are four classes of stretch receptor contributing to the sense of kinaesthesia: joint receptors, tendon organs, muscle spindles and skin receptors. The position sense is mediated via the posterior columns of the spinal cord. In children with cerebral palsy impaired kinaesthesis may be a hidden cause of learning difficulty both motor and cognitive (Parfitt 1990). This is an area which needs further investigation (see also Elliott et al 1988).

THE EFFECTS OF DAMAGE ON THE DEVELOPING CENTRAL NERVOUS SYSTEM

Cerebral palsy is rarely associated only with motor and postural disability.

Since the brain is damaged early in its development it follows that there will be interference with the normal integration of function that flows naturally during development. At birth the neural mechanisms for vital functions such as breathing, rooting, sucking and swallowing, crying, spatial orientation, sleeping and waking are fully developed as very complex control systems and not as simple reflexes. Prechtl (1981) describes these processes in detail, pointing out the fallacy of regarding the infant brain as simply a brainstem without the functional capacity of the cortex and cerebellum.

If the cortical areas of the brain are damaged the normal motor and sensory pathways are unable to develop. The motor pathways pass from the cortex via the corticospinal tracts (the upper motor neuron), through the spinal cord, and exiting the cord via the anterior nerve roots and peripheral nerves (the lower motor neuron) to the individual muscles. It is likely that the supraspinal connections modulate the spinal cord neurons and maturation of the pathways.

Koh & Eyre (1988) have studied the maturation of the corticospinal tracts in normal infants and children using electromagnetic stimulation over the motor cortex, and measuring evoked muscle action potentials at the periphery. They showed a progressive increase in the index of conduction velocity within the descending motor pathways up to the age of 11 years, when adult values were reached. This correlates well with the continuing acquisition of motor coordination during childhood. Since myelination is complete by age 3 years, these data suggest that there is an as yet uncharacterised process of maturation that leads to an increase in conduction velocity within the corticospinal tracts beyond completion of myelination. This may in part be due to maturation of interneuronal synaptic connections both in the cortex and at spinal cord level.

It has been recognised for some time that the spastic stretch reflex in children with cerebral palsy differs from that seen in adults with acquired spasticity following stroke or brain injury. Children with cerebral palsy lack reciprocal inhibition necessary for smooth coordinated movement. In a study of the stretch reflex in children with cerebral palsy using the H reflex, Leonard et al (1990) showed that they were unable to inhibit soleus and gastrocnemius before activation of the anterior tibial muscle, as occurred in normal children and adults with spasticity following stroke. (The H reflex is elicited by applying a mild electric current to a peripheral nerve, which causes an electromyographic potential, H response, within the muscle being stimulated. It may be regarded as the electrical equivalent of the stretch reflex.) These findings suggest lack of control from supraspinal centres, though they conclude that it is not possible to exclude impairment of spinal mechanisms.

The demonstration of a supraspinal element to reciprocal inhibition is of particular clinical relevance since it shows the potential influence of cognitive and emotional factors in treatment. In normal children Leonard (1990) showed it was possible to demonstrate activation of anterior tibial muscle contraction before gastrocnemius and soleus activation when children were rising on their toes from standing, i.e. it was an anticipatory postural response (APR). This did not occur in children under 4 years, in mentally retarded children, or children with cerebral palsy.

This information suggests that automatic APR, similar to voluntary movement, also uses reciprocal inhibition to prevent excessive antagonist co-contraction. The children with cerebral palsy did not have the normal pattern of H reflex changes before plantar flexion, nor did they activate the pretibial muscles before plantar flexion. These results show how supraspinal damage results in inability to perform coordinated movement, and there could also be spinal cord damage.

Skilled motor activity is consciously learned and becomes automatic after a period of practice: there is transfer of control from conscious to unconscious mechanisms. Figure 6.1 shows diagrammatically some of the nervous pathways which may be impaired in the developing nervous system of children with cerebral palsy.

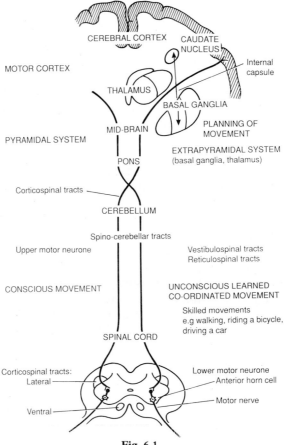

Fig. 6.1

CENTRAL VISUAL DISTURBANCES IN CEREBRAL PALSY

Impairment of visual perception has been recognised as a complication of cerebral palsy for many years; Foley (1987) reviewed the subject in detail. It is particularly common in children with diplegia and those who have suffered severe hypoxia, who have periventricular leukomalacia. This can be explained by the damage caused by ischaemia in 'watershed zones' where arterial territories meet. Two triple watersheds are in the parieto-occipital areas and over the body of the caudate nucleus. Other factors involved are the concentration of lesions in the posterior parts of the hemispheres and delayed myelination which accompanies early lesions (Dubowitz & Bydder 1985).

Damage to the optic radiations is likely to occur as they sweep around the ventricles interrupting the *primary visual system*, which links to the area striata of the occipital cortex. The *second visual system* is the colliculo-pulvinar parietal projection, thought to be responsible for the detection of events and the direction of gaze, so that the primary system can identify the object brought into sight (Denny-Brown & Fischer 1976, Zihl & von Cramon 1979). This system operates subconsciously and explains the ability of some blind children to be aware of movements.

An inability to detect (visual inattention) or to aim, despite normal acuity, is not uncommon in children with brain damage. This forms part of Balint's syndrome, which is caused by bilateral parieto-occipital lesions in the watershed areas. This can be used as a model to explain the difficulties often seen in people with cerebral palsy: difficulty in sorting objects from background, piecemeal vision, difficulty in tracing and tracking, and inaccurate reaching or placing.

Visual perception is an active process in which the eye must actively scan the image. The occipitofrontal fasciculus runs forward just above the roof of the lateral ventricle to the frontal eye fields and is vulnerable to periventricular leukomalacia. This accounts for the frequency of defects of voluntary eye movements in children with diplegia and quadriplegia (Abercrombie 1964). Difficulty in initiating saccades is common in such children. They are not able to make voluntary eye movements to follow or look at an object, but they are able to move their eyes automatically as in optokinetic nystagmus.

The disorders described are of higher visual function and explain why children with the 'spastic' cerebral palsies often have learning difficulties associated with visual perception. Menken et al (1987) compared a group of children with cerebral palsy with normal controls using a motor-free perception test; they showed the cerebral palsy children had a significantly lower mean perceptual quotient than the controls.

In a study of 50 children with cortical visual impairment Jan et al (1987) highlighted the variable and inconsistent visual performance including visual acuity. The children were able to see better in familiar environments (i.e. those requiring less interpretation), and to identify colour better than form. Many turned their heads to the side when reaching, as if using their peripheral visual fields (and perhaps also their asymmetric tonic neck reflex). They appeared to have great diffi- culty with the cognitive evaluation of visual perception in spatial terms. All of these findings suggest impairment of visual processing and interpretation.

The difficulty of assessment of these children is self evident and it is important to stimulate vision and encourage parents to observe visual performance in different situations. Visual maturation undoubtedly occurs and can be another reason for underestimating potential in the young child (see. p. 83).

CLASSIFICATION OF CEREBRAL PALSY

The varieties of cerebral palsy are traditionally defined according to the type and topography of the positive signs, and pay no attention to the important negative signs (see later). There are three main types of cerebral palsy. The spastic group amounts to about 70% of the total. The athetoid or dystonic group (dyskinesias), showing involuntary movements as the main feature, comprises 20-25%. The less common cases of ataxia show imbalance and diminished muscle tone. A mixture of types is often found in one child.

Topographical classifications are an attempt to describe what is seen clinically according to the part of the body involved. 'Pure' cases of athetosis or ataxia usually involve the whole body and therefore description by topography is used only for the spastic or mixed cases. Commonly described are:

- *Hemiplegia*—one side of the body is primarily involved
- *Diplegia*—the lower half of the body is primarily involved
- *Quadriplegia*—the entire body is involved.

Many clinicians use the term bilateral (or double) hemiplegia to describe asymmetrical quadriplegia. Unfortunately these classifications contribute to the tendency to concentrate on the limb involvement, and pay little attention to the involvement of the trunk, head and neck, which is fre- quently of more significance.

The specific diagnosis or classification of a child gives little indication of his actual level of ability. A child with cerebral palsy may be one who is totally dependent and posturally disorganised, or one who is able to talk, walk and even run with little hindrance. There are, however, characteristics—including those of associated disorders—that typically relate to specific types of cerebral palsy, and it is very important to be aware of their occurrence.

CLINICAL SIGNS OF CEREBRAL PALSY IN THE BABY

- Feeding difficulties—inability to suck or swallow, lack of interest, very slow feeding.
- Abnormalities of gaze—failure to fix when feeding, delayed smiling
- Abnormalities of tone—reduced or increased
- Abnormalities of behaviour—irritability, anxiety, lack of interest in sounds or visual cues, sleep disturbance
- Delayed postural development—lying ability (persistent asymmetry), head and trunk control, balance reactions
- Development of asymmetry of movement or tone
- Delayed motor development.

THE NATURAL HISTORY OF CEREBRAL PALSY

It is important to realise that there is a natural history to the condition. It is of course partly dependent upon the severity of the cerebral lesion, but also upon the effects of growth and maturation which occur in all children.

Beals (1966) showed that the motor performance of children with spastic diplegia changed up to the age of 7 years, and the improvements seen are not necessarily related to treatment. The biomechanics and dynamics of walking need to be better understood. It is becoming increasingly possible to investigate the walking pattern by gait analysis (Gage et al 1984) (see later). This facilitates the effectiveness of surgical intervention, and allows for a concerted effort postoperatively.

The early stages of the child's life are concerned with diagnosis and active therapy to encourage motor development alongside other areas of deficit. If the child has the potential to walk, every effort is directed towards that end. The child's own motivation is a major force in the eventual outcome. There comes a time when it is important to move on to alternative strategies of mobility and to acknowledge the need to accept a change in emphasis. Often it is the parents who need to change and this can be part of the acceptance of the child as he is.

DEFINITIONS OF NEUROLOGICAL TERMS

Spasticity

Spasticity is a disorder of tone characterised by an initial increased resistance to stretch which may then lessen abruptly. The degree of spasticity varies with the child's general condition, emotional state, temperature and health; it also depends on correct positioning and the degree of support of the child.

If the spasticity is severe, the child is more or less fixed in a few typical patterns due to the severe degree of co-contraction of the involved parts, especially around the proximal joints (shoulders and hips). Some muscles appear weak due to tonic reciprocal inhibition by their spastic antagonists; for example, the gluteal and abdominal muscles by spastic hip flexors, the quadriceps by spastic hamstrings, and the dorsiflexors of the ankles by the spastic triceps surae. True weakness may develop in some muscle groups from longstanding disuse or immobilisation in plaster casts or apparatus.

Dystonic choreoathetosis

Involuntary movements (choreoathetosis) are so frequently combined with dystonic posturing that they are conveniently classified together. Here the brunt of the damage has fallen on the basal ganglia. Although much overlapping pathology exists, choreoathetosis is most frequently found with damage to the caudate nucleus and putamen, and dystonia with damage to the globus pallidus. Since kernicterus as a cause for this has receded, the mechanism is obscure in the remainder, but probably involves subacute regional hypoxia rather than acute total asphyxia (which gives rise to brainstem and thalamic damage), or periodic hypoperfusion (which gives rise to damage in the 'watershed' areas).

Athetosis is defined as irrepressible, slow writhing movements, the result of which is imperfectly coordinated activity of agonists and antagonists, exacerbated by attempting voluntary movements. Choreic movements are rapid involuntary jerks present at rest, and also increased by voluntary movements.

Dystonia is defined as a disorder of muscle tone, expressed as postural abnormality, intermittent contractile spasms, and complex action dystonias where purposeful movements are deformed.

Voluntary movements are partially or totally disrupted anywhere in the body including the lips and tongue. The tone varies with age: the baby is usually markedly hypotonic, and exhibits athetosis in the second or third year; the adult may develop increasing muscle tension, which helps to control posture.

Ataxia

This is a relatively uncommon form of cerebral palsy which is usually characterised by generalised cerebellar signs. These are: disturbance of balance, incoordination, dysarthria, intention tremor, hypotonia and sometimes nystagmus. Ataxia may occur as part of a dysmorphic syndrome, or be associated with intrauterine infection. Mixed ataxia and spasticity may occur in a diplegic pattern and be caused by prolonged hypoglycaemia in the neonatal period.

REFERENCES

Abercrombie M L J (ed) 1964 Perceptual and visuomotor disorders in cerebral palsy. Clinics in Developmental Medicine 11: 135, SIMP/Heinemann

Asindi A A, Stephenson J B P, Young D G 1988 Spastic hemiparesis and presumed prenatal embolisation. Archives of Diseases in Childhood 63: 68–69

Aylward G P, Verhurst S J, Bell S 1989 Correlation of asphyxia and other risk factors with outcome: a contemporary view. Developmental Medicine and Child Neurology 31: 329–340

Beals R K 1966 Spastic paraplegia and diplegia: an evaluation of non-surgical factors influencing the prognosis for ambulation. Journal of Bone and Joint Surgery of America 48: 827–846

Blair E, Stanley F J 1988 Intrapartum asphyxia: a rare cause of cerebral palsy. Journal of Pediatrics 112: 515–519

Bobath K 1980 The neurophysiological basis for the treatment of cerebral palsy. Clinics in Developmental Medicine 75, SIMP/Heinemann

Butterworth C, Cicchetti 1978 Visual calibration of posture in normal and motor retarded Down's syndrome infants. Perception 7: 513–525

Butterworth G 1983 Structure of the mind in human infancy. Advances in Infancy Research 2: 11

Denny-Brown D, Fischer E G 1976 Physiological aspects of visual perception II: The subcortical direction of visual behaviour. Archives of Neurology 33: 228–242

Dobyns W B, Stratton R F, Greenberg F 1984 Syndromes with Lissencephaly I: Miller Dieker and Norman Roberts Syndromes and Isolated Lissencephaly. American Journal of Medical Genetics 18: 509–526

Dubowitz L M, Bydder G M 1985 Nuclear magnetic resonance imaging in the diagnosis and follow up of neonatal cerebral injury. Clinics in Perinatology 12: 243–260

Elliott J M, Connolly K J, Doyle A J R 1988 Development of kinaesthetic sensitivity and motor performance in children. Developmental Medicine and Child Neurology 30: 80–92

Emond A, Golding J, Peckham C 1989 Cerebral palsy in two national cohort studies. Archives of Disease in Chilhood 64: 848–852

Foley J 1987 Central visual disturbances. Developmental Medicine and Child Neurology 29: 110–120

Gage J, Fabian D, Hicks R, Tashman S 1984 Pre- and post-operative gait analysis in patients with spastic diplegia: a preliminary report. Journal of Pediatric Orthopaedics 4: 715–725

Hagberg B, Hagberg G, Olow I 1984 The changing panorama of cerebral palsy in Sweden. Acta Paediatrica Scandinavica 73: 433–440

Hall D M B 1990 Birth asphyxia and cerebral palsy. British Medical Journal 299: 279–282

Howard I P, Templeton W B 1966 Human spatial orientation. John Wiley, Toronto

Jan J E, Groenvald M, Sykanda A M, Hoyt C S 1987 Behavioural characteristics of children with permanent visual impairment. Developmental Medicine and Child Neurology 29: 571–576

Koh T H H G, Eyre J A 1988 Maturation of corticospinal tracts assessed by electromagnetic stimulation of the motor cortex. Archives of Disease in Childhood 63: 1347–1352

Laszlo J I, Bairstow P J 1980 The measurement of kinaesthetic sensitivity in children and adults. Developmental Medicine and Child Neurology 22: 454–464

Leonard C T, Moritani T, Hirschfeld H, Forssberg H 1990 Deficits in reciprocal inhibition of children with cerebral palsy as revealed by H reflex testing. Developmental Medicine and Child Neurology 32: 974–984

Marsden C D, Merton P A, Morton H B 1976 Stretch reflex and servoaction in a variety of human muscles. Journal of Physiology 259: 531–560

Marsden C D, Merton P A, Morton H B 1977 Anticipatory postural reflexes in the human subject. Proceedings of the Physiological Society, pp 47–48

Marsden C D, Traub M M, Rothwell J C 1980 Anticipatory postural reflexes in Parkinson's Disease and other akinetic-rigid syndromes and in cerebellar ataxia. Brain 103: 393–412

Menken C, Cermack S A, Fisher A 1987 Evaluating the visual perceptual skills of children with cerebral palsy. American Journal of Occupational Therapy 41: 646–651

Nelson K B 1988 What proportion of cerebral palsy is related to birth asphyxia? Journal of Pediatrics 112: 572–573

Nelson K B, Ellenberg J H 1988 Cluster of perinatal events identifying infants at high risk for death or disability. Journal of Pediatrics 113(3): 546–552

Paneth N, Kiely J 1984 The frequency of cerebral palsy: a review of population studies in industrialised nations since 1950. In: Stanley F, Alberman E (eds) The epidemiology of the cerebral palsies. Blackwell Scientific, Oxford

Parfitt Y 1990 Personal communication

Pountney T E, Mulcahy C M, Green E M 1990 Early development of postural control. Physiotherapy 76(12): 799–802

Prechtl H F R 1981 The study of neural development as a perspective of clinical problems. In: Maturation and Development: biological and psychological perspectives. Clinics in Developmental Medicine, ch 10, pp 77–78

Prechtl H F R (ed)1984 Continuity of neural functions from pre-natal to post-natal life. Clinics in Developmental Medicine 94, Blackwell Scientific, Oxford

Schinzel A A G L 1979 Monozygotic twinning and structural defects. Journal of Pediatrics 95: 921–930

Shambes G M 1976 Static postural control in children. American Journal of Physical Medicine 55(5): 221–251

Stanley F J 1987 The changing face of cerebral palsy. Developmental Medicine and Child Neurology 29: 263–265

Sutherland D H, Olshen R A, Biden E N, Wyatt M P 1988 The development of mature walking. Clinics in Developmental Medicine 104/105. Mac Keith, Blackwell Scientific, Oxford

Wigglesworth J 1984 Brain development and its modification by adverse influences. In: Stanley F, Alberman E (eds) The epidemiology of the cerebral palsies. Blackwell Scientific, Oxford

Williams H G, Fisher J H, Tritschler K A 1983 Descriptive analysis of static postural control in 4, 6 and 8 year old normal and motorically awkward children. American Journal of Physical Medicine 62(1): 12–26

Yoshioka H 1979 Multicystic encephalomalacia in a liveborn twin with a stillborn macerated co-twin. Journal of Pediatrics 95: 798–800

Zihl J, von Cramon D 1979 The contribution of the second visual system to directed visual attention in man. Brain 103: 835–856

STANDARD RECORDING OF CENTRAL MOTOR DEFICIT
and associated sensory and intellectual deficit

Name of child _____ Sex M/F _____

Date of birth _____

Date of examination _____

The purpose of the form:

This form is intended primarily as an epidemiological tool, for collecting accurate date on impairment and disability in children with a motor deficit of central origin.

Its development was necessary because the terms in common use, e.g. spastic, athetoid, dystonia, diplegia, were not used in a consistent way. As a result, comparison of outcomes from different centres was difficult.

The form is **not** intended to be a complete clinical description of the child. Rather it provides the data necessary to identify groups of children with similar motor deficits.

This will:

a) enable case counting and monitoring of trends in the frequency of central motor deficit in differing geographical areas;

b) allow pooling of similar cases as a basis for aetiological studies;

c) identify children with similar disabilities who have special health needs.

FOR COMPLETION GUIDELINES SEE NEXT PAGE

GUIDELINES FOR COMPLETION

This form is intended to provide a "snapshot" of the child at the time of examination and should not take aetiological or prognostic considerations into account.

It can be used for children of all ages but it is most applicable to children of 3 years and over.

Most of the form is self-explanatory. The following comments apply to the items marked *.

Section 1.

Inco-ordination – this should be recorded only where this is the predominant motor deficit and not when it is secondary to increased, decreased or variable tone.

Section 3.

This section will allow the examiner to record differences in the level of increased or decreased tone in the limbs. Children whose distribution of involvement cannot be fully categorised in this way can be described in the comments section.

Sections on functional severity (5–7)

These sections are particularly important in epidemiological studies. The categories in each section are hierarchical and are graded so that the division between the 2nd and 3rd categories defines the threshold below which 100% of cases will almost certainly come to the attention of the clinician or services. Difficulties in comparison arise in the less severe cases, where the level of ascertainment will vary.

This approach has resulted in very broad divisions of severity of disability, which are appropriate for epidemiological purposes, though they may not fulfill all clinical needs.

Section 7

Some children with obvious unilateral impairment, which is unlikely to be missed, may manage to achieve the 2nd category i.e. below the expected level of full ascertainment. Their impairment will, however, be described in other sections (e.g. 2 & 3).

Comment on and suggestions on improving the form are welcomed.
Please send these to:-

O.R.C.D.P. Office, Level 3 Maternity Department, John Radcliffe Hospital, Headington, Oxford OX3 9DU. Tel. Oxford (0865) 817289.

PLEASE COMPLETE EACH SECTION - TICK ✓ BOXES AS APPROPRIATE
(Items marked * see 'Guidelines' on previous page)

NATURE OF MOTOR INVOLVEMENT

WITH THE CHILD IN ANY COMFORTABLE POSITION

1. **OBSERVED** (Abnormal unwanted movements)
Tick ✓ as appropriate

	At rest	With excitement or goal-directed movement
None	☐	☐
Short and jerky	☐	☐
Slow and writhing	☐	☐
Tremor	☐	☐
Flexor/extensor spasms	☐	☐
Inco-ordination* (tick only if this is **NOT** secondary to increased tone or weakness)		☐
Abnormal postures or grimacing resulting from voluntary movement elsewhere in the body		☐
Other (please describe) _____		

COMMENTS: _____

_____

2. **FELT (Tone)**
Tick ✓ one box for each limb

	Right upper limb	Left upper limb	Right lower limb	Left lower limb
Within normal range	☐	☐	☐	☐
Increased	☐	☐	☐	☐
Decreased	☐	☐	☐	☐
Varying between increased and decreased (with time/position)	☐	☐	☐	☐

Contractures present?   Yes ☐   No ☐

If yes, describe: _____

_____

COMMENTS - e.g. adductor spasm, thumb in palm, clonus, operative procedure such as tendon release.

_____

_____

_____

_____

_____

3. DISTRIBUTION OF INVOLVEMENT*   Tick ✓ one box for each question

	Yes	No	Uncertain
Is there obvious R/L asymmetry of tone or function present?	☐	☐	☐
If yes, which side is worse? _____			
Are the upper limbs more affected than the lower limbs?	☐	☐	☐
Are the lower limbs more affected than the upper limbs?	☐	☐	☐

COMMENTS: _____

_____

_____

4. MOUTH   Tick ✓ one box for each question

	Yes	No	Uncertain
Is there a problem with articulation of speech? (Developmental age appropriate)	☐	☐	☐
Is there a swallowing problem with either food or drink?	☐	☐	☐
Is there excessive drooling or dribbling during waking hours?	☐	☐	☐

COMMENTS: _____

_____

_____

5. FUNCTIONAL SEVERITY*

AXIS - HEAD AND NECK (with shoulders held)   Tick ✓ one box

Normal head control	☐
Abnormal head control but adequate to hold head up for extended periods of time	☐
Poor head control but can hold head up for very short periods of time	☐
No obvious head control	☐

- TRUNK

No apparent problem when sitting on stool with feet on floor	☐
Can sit unsupported but less secure and stable than a normal child of same age	☐
Cannot be left in sitting position unless supported	☐
Very severe impairment: difficult to place or maintain in sitting position (includes inability to sit because of deformity)	☐

COMMENTS: _____

_____

_____

6.   LOWER LIMB FUNCTION - GAIT (Applicable 3 years of age and over)

	Yes	No	Not applicable
Aids usually used to facilitate walking? Tick ✓ one box	☐	☐	☐

Tick ✓ one box

No significant problem with gait; walks fluently   ☐

Gait functional but non-fluent   ☐

Gait obviously abnormal, reducing mobility and/or restricting life style   ☐

No independent walking   ☐

COMMENTS: _____

_____

_____

_____

_____

7. UPPER LIMB FUNCTION (Applicable 3 years of age and over)

Tick ✓ one box

No apparent problem with bimanual tasks   ☐

*Some difficulty using both hands together, but dresses self
(age appropriate)   ☐

Physically incapable of putting on vest or T-shirt without help,
but **able** to feed self with one or other hand   ☐

Physically incapable of putting on vest or T-shirt
and **unable** to feed self with either hand   ☐

COMMENTS: _____

_____

_____

_____

_____

8.   DIAGNOSIS, as recorded in medical notes, including underlying disease entities

_____

_____

_____

9.   CURRENT MEDICATION: _____

_____

_____

_____

Children with cerebral palsy often have defects in other systems which are important clinically and epidemiologically. Sections 10-14 are included in order to describe these associated defects in broad terms. These sections have not been subjected to repeated inter-observer trials during development as have sections 1-7.

——————◆——————

OTHER ASPECTS

	Yes	No	Uncertain
10. Is **intellectual impairment** present? Tick ✓ one box	☐	☐	☐

Date of last assessment ————————

Method and results of assessment ————————————————————————————————

COMMENTS: ——

	Yes	No	Uncertain
11. Is a **visual or eye defect** of any type present? Tick ✓ one box	☐	☐	☐
If **YES**: Does the child use spectacles or other aids to vision?	☐	☐	☐

"Usual vision" (with spectacles/aids if worn)	Tick ✓ one box
Normal or near normal	☐
Moderately impaired	☐
Severely impaired	☐
No useful vision	☐

	Yes	No	Uncertain
Is there a squint present?	☐	☐	☐
Has the child had an operation for squint?	☐	☐	☐
Are there abnormal eye movements?	☐	☐	☐
Does the child have a problem with fixation?	☐	☐	☐
Does the child have a problem with tracking?	☐	☐	☐

COMMENTS: (include test results if available)————————————————————————

	Yes	No	Uncertain
12. Is **hearing impairment** present? Tick ✓ one box	☐	☐	☐
If **YES**: Does the child use hearing aids?	☐	☐	☐

"Usual hearing" (with aids if worn)	Tick ✓ one box
Normal or near normal	☐
Moderately impaired	☐
Severely impaired	☐
No useful hearing	☐

COMMENTS: (include test results if available)————————————————————————

	Yes	No	Uncertain

13. Are communication difficulties present? Tick ☑ one box
(Exclude isolated articulation defect - see section 4)

If **YES**:   How does the child usually communicate?   Tick ☑ one box

Speech ☐

Speech and other formal methods (e.g. signing) ☐

Formal systematised methods only ☐

Not communicating by speech or formal method ☐

COMMENTS: _____

	Yes	No	Uncertain

14. Has the child suffered from seizures in the past 12 months? Tick ☑ one box ☐ ☐ ☐

If yes - specify type(s) of seizure: _____

If no - has the child ever had seizures?   ☐ ☐ ☐
At what age? _____

COMMENTS: _____

_____

_____

_____

_____

_____

Financial support from the Medical Education and
Information Unit of The Spastics Society is gratefully
acknowledged.

7. Cerebral palsy: therapy management

M. Jones   V. Moffat   C.M. Mulcahy
C. Shumway Nicholls   G.T. McCarthy

This chapter is written by therapists and relates specifically to their aspect of work with children who have cerebral palsy. The need to work together as part of a wider multidisciplinary team must be recognised. The reader is referred to other chapters on Assessment, Postural Management, Orthotics, Scoliosis Management, Education, Augmentative Communication, and Rehabilitation Engineering for related information from other disciplines, as well as the chapter on Conductive Education describing a different approach to treatment and management.

CHARACTERISTICS OF TYPES

The varieties of cerebral palsy and their diagnostic signs have already been described. There is no defined treatment for any type of cerebral palsy and the diagnosis gives little indication of the child's ability. Each child must therefore be assessed individually, with specific plans made for treatment and management. There are, however, certain characteristics of specific types of cerebral palsy that should be borne in mind. These will help to define aims of treatment, expected prognosis, and priorities.

SPASTIC DIPLEGIA

Associated disorders of all types are common in spastic diplegia and can frequently be masked by relatively good hand function and speech. Included are: visual perception disorders, eye/hand coordination difficulties, dysarthria, and problems with incoordination of respiration and phonation, vision and learning.

The top half of the body (trunk, arms and head) is nearly always affected to some degree: a true paraplegia is rare in cerebral palsy. However, the top half is usually markedly more able than the lower half and most diplegics are very good at using their top half to make up for lack of ability in the lower half. This inhibits the development of motor abilities in two ways:

1. The lower half is not used for, and therefore does not develop, the abilities that are needed to contribute to various gross motor activities, e.g. stable sitting or walking.

2. As the top half is being used for the fundamental activity of balance, development of the finer activities using the hands, eyes and head is inhibited. In physical treatment and management, imagination is needed to devise ways of developing the abilities of the lower half itself.

Awareness of typical potential deformities is important so that measures can be instigated early enough to limit their development. What is usually seen is flexion, adduction and internal rotation at the hips, flexion at the knees, and equinovarus or -valgus deformity of the feet (Fig. 7.1). In planning management and treatment regimes it is important to determine *why* the deformities are developing, i.e. what their functional basis is. For example, flexion at the hips and knees is not necessarily due to being pulled down: it may be due to lack of ability to stay up.

Adduction and internal rotation at the hips is often related to lack of ability to shift and anchor weight through individual sides of the pelvis. Prolonged time with hips internally rotated, adducted and flexed, particularly when combined with lack of good, early weightbearing, is likely to lead to dislocation of one or both hips, the prevention of which is a prime aim. Equinus at the feet may be related to inability to bring the weight forward over the base of the feet using the anterior tibials, so 'launching' forward by plantarflexion is seen.

a
b

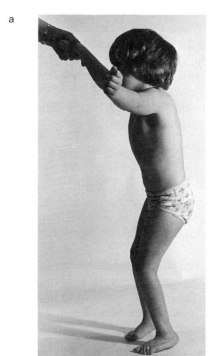
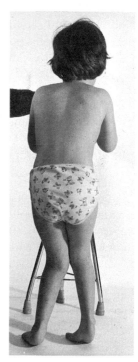

Fig. 7.1 Typical diplegic posture. **a.** Flexion of hips and knees. **b.** Adduction and internal rotation of hips, valgus deformity of feet.

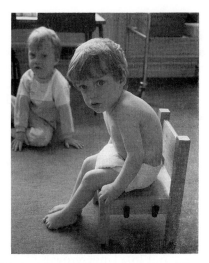

Fig. 7.2   Child with diplegia sitting with lumbar kyphosis, holding on precariously, unable to use hands except for balance at this stage.

Positioning for function is particularly important, even if the child is mobile. For example, fine hand function will be impaired if the child is struggling to maintain his sitting position (Fig. 7.2). Children with diplegia commonly sit with a lumbar kyphosis as a result of the hip extensor weakness. This may lead to scoliosis, particularly if asymmetry is present. A forward tilting seat may be tried to encourage a lumbar lordosis and greater spinal stability. Toilet training cannot progress if the child is not sitting stably, as increased extensor tone will inhibit relaxation of both anal and urinary sphincters leading to constipation and difficulty initiating micturition.

Also typical, and commonly seen around the early teens in conjunction with the growth spurt, is the problem of sinking, where a child previously able to walk becomes increasingly less able to hold himself up against gravity, and often ends up in a wheelchair. When considering surgery in diplegia it is important to note that lengthening (or over-lengthening) of the heel cords can facilitate sinking.

The school child may need help to keep up with his able-bodied peers by using a tricycle or powered wheelchair in the playground. Transport to and from school (however local) may be necessary in order to prevent fatigue.

HEMIPLEGIA

Diagnosis

Asymmetry is quickly noticed by parents, who may express this by saying that baby is strongly left or right handed. If this occurs in the first year suspicions of hemiplegia should be aroused. Another early sign is 'fisting' of the affected side. The leg is often said to be less affected than the arm. This is usually true in so far as the leg and foot have less precise functions than the arm and hand. Most hemiplegic children walk and use one hand well, but hand function varies enormously according to the severity of the brain lesion. They usually achieve independence and are not precluded from leading useful and satisfying lives by their handicap. Therefore, by comparison with many children considered in this book, their handicap is relatively mild. It is obviously helpful if the parents can be brought to a sense of perspective early. Bear in mind, however, that the hemiplegic child will probably attend mainstream school, and spasticity and frustration may increase when competing with able-bodied peers.

Associated disorders are common and include: sensory loss or inattention on the affected side (this may be suspected early if the function of the arm is worse than the degree of handicap would predict); hemianopia (loss of half the visual field on the affected side); squint; perceptual disorders; and epilepsy (see p. 176). Undergrowth of the affected limb may occur and correlates with the cortical sensory loss; both reflect parietal lobe involvement.

Management

In infancy symmetry is encouraged by using patterns of handling which elicit non-preferred postures and movements. It is essential to win the child's confidence before attempting positioning. Two-handed holding of feeding equipment and toys should be encouraged.

The main aims of therapeutic management are postural stability, symmetry of posture and movement, and body awareness, including the affected side. Thus, swimming, for example, is a valuable activity for children with hemiplegia.

Opportunities to improve the child's abilities occur during normal daily life and are elaborated in the sections on personal care (p. 140) and in Chapter 33. Dynamic postural work is necessary but should not be intensive, and considerable imagination and flexibility of attitude are required in order to gain cooperation.

Talking about the hemiplegic hand during washing, bathing and dressing, holding the toddler by the hemiplegic hand and using it in 'rough play' will help promote awareness in the early stages. A light opposition splint may occasionally assist a more functional position and encourage greater use of the affected hand. Encourage clothes that are easy to put on, so as to avoid conflict with the child during dressing. It is generally good practice to dress the affected side first, and undress it last. Later this helps the child to learn to dress himself.

Activities for the hemiplegic child should avoid extreme effort, hurry or frustration as these will increase hypertonus. The focus of treatment should change according to the results achieved. If a child treated early and adequately is still not using the hand by the age of 2 years, the function of the hand will always be very limited. Recognising this saves therapists, parents and not least the child from continuing frustration. However, work should continue to maintain symmetry and encourage optimum bilateral function for the individual child.

If the child cannot be stabilised, the object he is working with can be, e.g. rulers mounted on a magnet used with a metal sheet underneath the paper, and spring-loaded left or right handed scissors. Other aids for one-handed use are described in Chapter 33.

Deformities which may develop include flexion of the elbow, forearm pronation, flexion and ulnar deviation of the wrist, hip flexion, equinovarus or -valgus at the ankle, leg length discrepancy and scoliosis (Fig. 7.3).

Most hemiplegic children manage to reach developmental milestones at close to normal ages; treatment is therefore aimed at maintaining ranges of motion at the hip, knee and ankle so that the leg can be used as well as possible when the child does begin to walk. Individual leg lengths, as well as joint ranges, should be monitored so that the need for a shoe-raise can be recognised. Emphasis in treatment is also placed on improving ability to shift weight onto the affected side as it is often ignored and left to

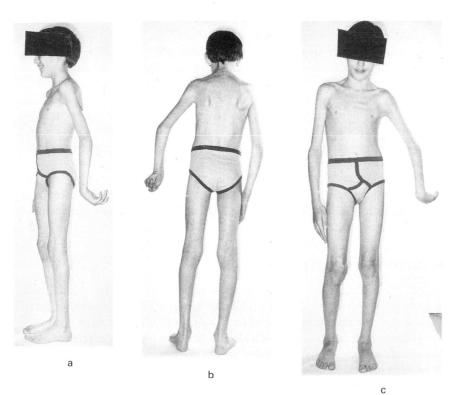

a

b

c

Fig. 7.3a, b and c. Typical hemiplegic pattern in early teen age.

lag behind. The use of plaster boots is particularly useful in hemiplegia in order to maintain the range of the tendo calcaneus, to facilitate weightbearing through the affected side, and to control genu recurvatum. This is demonstrated in the video *Camera Talks: Plaster boots* (see references).

As the child grows up, gradual introduction of ideas to encourage self-inhibition of spasm is valuable. In adolescence the desire to look 'normal' is very strong and can be capitalised upon. It is also a time when emotional support and counselling may be required to encourage self-esteem when peers may be rejecting or teasing.

SPASTIC QUADRIPLEGIA

As in diplegia, associated disorders are common, with an increased incidence of intellectual deficit in approximately 80% of cases, and a high incidence of visual problems and epilepsy (see p. 175).

The top half of the body is usually more involved than the lower half, and involvement is usually asymmetrical. The paucity of movement and asymmetry can lead to the following typical deformities: flexion deformities of the wrists and elbows; windswept deformities of the hips with related pelvic obliquity leading to scoliosis or kyphoscoliosis; knee flexion deformities; equinovarus or -valgus at the ankles (Fig. 7.4).

As children with quadriplegia are usually less able than those with diplegia, the functional contribution to the development of deformity is more likely to be related to an attempt to achieve and maintain some sort of balance in an effort to counteract the constant state of falling. For example, in lying supine, if most of the child's weight falls to the right with legs windswept to the right, the upper trunk and head may be rotated to the left in an attempt to keep from falling into side-lying, contributing to the development of asymmetrical deformity.

The inability to move purposefully in order to change position emphasises the need for positioning equipment to complement treatment and enable children to function (see. Ch. 25) and organisation of the environment (see p. 135).

DYSTONIC CHOREOATHETOSIS

It has been said that children with athetosis should be considered intelligent and deaf until proven otherwise. Hearing loss is now less common due to prevention of kernicterus, but continues to occur. The comment regarding intelligence still holds. These children often appear unintelligent due to their marked lack of physical ability and to the typical facial grimacing, but their eyes give them away.

In pure athetosis, where there is no diffuse cortical damage, but damage only to the basal ganglia, associated disorders are uncommon. Eye move-

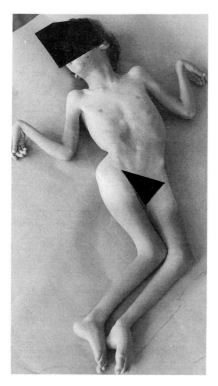

Fig. 7.4 Severe spastic quadriplegia with deformities of wrists, elbows, hips, knees and feet. Note asymmetry of hips—windswept position.

ments are usually normal and often provide one of the few means of accessing switches for the purpose of communication, mobility, etc. There may be perceptual disorders secondary to the lack of experience, and this is therefore an argument for providing these children with some form of mobility at an early stage of development.

Early signs (Fig. 7.5) include: fanning of fingers and toes; rhythmic/ writhing tongue with feeding difficulties; floppiness early on, except for a great ability to thrust backwards, often quite strongly. Rigidity and dystonia develop later within the first or second year.

Initially these children often appear much less able than children with spastic quadriplegia, but are frequently able to organise themselves posturally and achieve a higher level of function with maturity. This may partly be due to the lack of associated disorders. One must not be fooled by the extremes of movement into thinking that these children are not at risk of developing deformity. Deformity is likely if there is fixed posturing and rigidity, including scoliosis and kyphoscoliosis, and windswept hips with eventual dislocation. Flexion deformities of the hips and knees, with equinovarus or -valgus at the ankles is also common.

Provision of proximal stability and symmetry are the main therapeutic

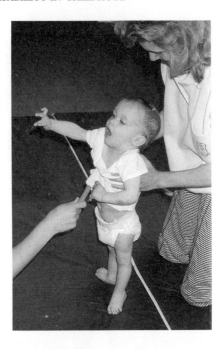

Fig. 7.5 Small child with early signs of fanning of fingers, associated movements of mouth and tongue, strong extensor thrust. Note the motivation and interest.

aims, enabling the child to develop as much control as possible within the limits of his neurological lesion. The importance of providing sufficient support for hand function and switch control is discussed on page 159.

ATAXIA

Ataxia is a relatively uncommon form of cerebral palsy and is frequently associated with other abnormalities. The hypotonic component of cerebellar involvement is the predominant feature in the early months, although in many instances this is also related to the learning difficulty. Early motor milestones are frequently delayed either because of, or in association with, the hypotonia, but the majority of children with ataxia alone acquire independence in walking as with other aspects of life.

There is as yet no specific technique of handling or drug therapy that inhibits the involuntary movements. Management consists of encouraging the child and parents through the normal sequences of development, and providing aids for stability as necessary. Confidence is all-important in gaining independence and children may finally walk without aids as late as 10 or 11 years.

Dysarthria may be severe and early speech therapy involvement is important. Augmentative communication may be required (see Ch. 26).

ASSESSMENT, MANAGEMENT AND TREATMENT

The disciplines must individually assess, identify abilities and problems, and specify aims. They must then jointly prioritise aims and identify possible means of achieving them. When treating a child, each individual member of the team should bear in mind the aims of the other team members and incorporate them into her work as appropriate. Conflicting aims and advice should be avoided. The situation where a child receives only specific sessions of individual therapy, with little interaction between the various therapists, teaching and care staff, and parents is felt to be counterproductive, although on paper or in reports home it is often seen as fulfilling the child's needs. The philosophy presented here is that a well planned and monitored regime of communication, handling and positioning should achieve the bulk of what is possible. This requires that a substantial percentage of the therapist's time is spent in educating parents, teachers, care staff and other therapists regarding each child's condition, possibilities, aims, prognosis and means (see Golding & Goldsmith 1986 for an organised approach). It may be that individual treatments should be carried on above and beyond this in order to tackle a specific problem, and that a conscious decision must be made regarding when to do this, with specific aims in mind.

The remainder of this chapter is divided into the overlapping areas of assessment, management, and individual treatment. There is little differentiation specified between various disciplines, as inevitably much overlap exists and, in a situation where people are really working together, whoever is most equipped to deal with an area will do so. In general, physiotherapists have responsibility for the realm of physical ability, occupational therapists for function (practical ability) and speech therapists for communication.

ASSESSMENT

Assessment is necessary in order to establish a baseline. Although it is often said that assessment in these children is ongoing and, indeed, specific tests of the daily effectiveness of treatment and management can be identified, periodic specified assessments are recommended. These serve not only to evaluate the effectiveness of the current regime, but also to bring everyone involved together on a regular basis. (See also Ch. 3.).

Assessment in any area should result in an understanding and, wherever possible, a quantification of the child's abilities and problems. Potential future problems are then identifiable. Aims and means can then be identified, taking into account the child as a whole, his situation, the family, the impact of intervention, as well as knowledge of available expertise and facilities. Decisions must be made as to what is significantly important to achieve, relative to the detrimental effect of intervention on the child and his family. Compromises are inevitable and acceptable. Referral to other centres or individuals for specific treatment or advice may well be considered necessary.

The various assessments can be divided into the areas of physical ability, practical ability and communication, with assessment of the child's situation common to all.

LEVEL OF PHYSICAL ABILITY

A good understanding of the basis of physical ability is crucial to understanding and influencing most other aspects, for example inhibition of deformity, decreasing influence of various reflexes, and improving independence. It also has a vital influence on other areas: communication, feeding, development of fine motor activity, and use of vision and hearing. Although it may be perceptual problems or lack of communication which are most disabling to a child in the end, successfully coping with the basic physical ability forms the foundation for dealing with these other problems. It is the background postural ability that results from the body's uncanny knowledge of mechanics and gravity which must be understood. In simple terms:

- For any object, the centre of gravity must fall within the area defined by its base of support or it will fall
- Conversely, for an area to act as a base of support, the centre of gravity must fall within it.

This has important implications for handling, positioning and treatment, as well as understanding the origin of impaired movements or reflexes. It also helps to explain the children's frequent fear and lack of willingness to move: many feel they are in a constant state of falling unless handled or supported correctly. The normal person is equipped with postural mechanisms whose main purpose is to maintain the centre of gravity within the base of support, i.e. to keep the body balanced (Traub et al 1980). When these mechanisms are impaired, movement is impaired.

DEVELOPMENT OF POSTURAL ABILITY

The basic postural abilities are sequentially acquired within the first 18 months of life in each of the positions of lying (supine, prone, side-lying), sitting (on the floor or a chair), and standing (leaning forward through hands, leaning back against a support, free-standing). The following classification of levels of ability has been found useful in defining both treatment aims and supportive equipment requirements, and can be applied to any position (personal work with N Hare 1977–1981, Mulcahy et al 1988).

1. Unable to be placed. This is a child whose body is totally disorganised as in Figure 7.4. When lifted and carried, his body does not come forward to conform to the body of the carrier, but extends away. He is often quite asymmetrical, bearing more weight on one side of his body than the other, with the related problems (or potential problems) of windswept hips, scoliosis, preferred head turning and preferred hand use. When placed in supine or prone, a symmetrical position is unattainable, and the child falls into partial side-lying, or takes up a 'corkscrew', ATNR posture, possibly in an attempt to find some point of control. He is generally 'top-heavy', unable to shift his weight down into the lower half of his body, and therefore unable to free his head and arms for use. On being pulled to sitting, he is unable to anchor his bottom, and it slides out from under him. Mere placement, with total support, in a reasonably organised sitting position can be nearly impossible. If the level of ability of these children is not improved and correct supportive equipment is not used, severe deformities will result. Treatment and handling are aimed at promoting active symmetry and flexion, as well as establishment of appropriate bases of support.

2. Able to be placed but not to maintain. In treatment and handling, it will be noted that the child has become 'placeable': his body is learning to accommodate to supporting surfaces, and he feels generally more organised. In lying, he is less 'top-heavy' and can momentarily lie fairly symmetrically, with hands by his sides, although they may still easily fly up beside his ears. When pulled to sitting, he is beginning to anchor his bottom but may do this asymmetrically—when pulled to sitting with one hand he comes up fairly straight, but with the other hand he spins. Improvement of the ability to shift and bear weight to each side via handling, positioning and treatment provides the basis for combatting the development of asymmetrical deformities.

3. Able to maintain but not function. This child can be placed in and can just maintain a position, but his own movement, or possibly any movement within his field of vision, causes him to fall. He is usually aware of this and, if not given appropriate additional support, he may either (sensibly) refuse to do anything, or he may stiffen his body in order to balance, making it impossible to function. The lower half of his body is still dependent on the top half for balance; improved abilities—to anchor through his base and shift weight fore and aft, and side to side—are needed before he can progress to the next level (see Fig. 7.2.).

4. Able to maintain and function within base of support. The child can now maintain a position and use his hands within the area defined by his base of support, but if he reaches or leans outside this base, he falls. He is beginning to split his body into two, enabling him to anchor his bottom half while his top half moves, but not well enough to allow it to move far or freely.

5. Able to maintain and function outside base. This child can reach well outside the area defined by his base of support, and movements are finer and more controlled. Increased dissociation between the top half of the body and the lower half, as evidenced by the development of the lumbar lordosis in sitting, allows this.

6. *Able to move out of position; able to attain position.* Children at these levels are relatively able and mobile. Moving out of a position may be a controlled fall, with improvement still needed in ability to shift weight into the lower end, and side to side and fore and aft. Even children who are independently mobile and able to attain positions independently will be seen to have deficits in shifting weight (probably to one side more than the other), in maintaining weight against gravity (the 'sinking diplegic'), and in dissociating the lower from the upper half of the body, and one side of the body from the other.

The postural abilities which allow one to attain a certain level of ability in any position can be further broken down as follows:

1. The ability to establish a base of support.
2. The ability to shift weight down into the lower half of the body (associated with the previous ability).
3. The ability to shift weight fore and aft, associated developmentally with shifting weight up and down the body—note rocking on all fours, and pivot prone where the child rocks and rotates on his tummy.
4. The ability to shift weight side to side—note the apparent progression of this ability, for example in sitting where the head and upper trunk may be shifted laterally but the ability to shift weight onto or down through one buttock may still be lacking.
5. The ability to maintain a base of support whilst the top part of the body moves: the development of dissociation and counterpoise.
6. The ability to maintain the body up against gravity.

Recognition of the presence or absence of these abilities results in definition of specific treatment aims. The performance of abilities 1–5 is centred in the *trunk* and, in handling and treatment, it is important to get the trunk to perform them. If the limbs are allowed to make up for the balance deficiencies of the trunk, the development of their use for other functional activities will be compromised.

Deformity

This is a major problem in cerebral palsy. Some deformities are particularly catastrophic, especially those of the spine and hips; if these are allowed to occur and progress, most abilities are compromised, as is ease of handling and comfort. Prevention of such deformities is therefore regarded as a priority.

Viewing deformity retrospectively, it is seen that most start off as 'postural' deformities—tendencies to spend most time in certain positions

(Fulford & Brown 1976, Robson 1968, Dunn 1976). They can then go on to become fixed deformities, where the non-bony structures become shortened or lengthened and then structural deformities, where there are actual bony changes. If deformity is to be prevented or inhibited, any tendency to deformity must be spotted early, while still only postural.

Their lack of postural ability makes people with cerebral palsy prime candidates for deformity in two ways:

- There is paucity of movement, with a few preferred positions and a lack of variety of positions
- There is excess activity in specific muscle groups in an effort to make up for lack of ability.

A child who feels threatened and unbalanced in any position will strive to find points of contact or balance; hence, the child who is unable to lie assumes a corkscrew/ATNR position in an effort to find some sort of security. This will eventually lead to deformity if not counteracted.

Other examples include:

1. The child who is unable to anchor his bottom adequately in sitting often flexes his knees strongly in an effort to 'hook' onto the chair, contributing to knee flexion deformity.

2. The child who is unable to bring his weight forward of his base to initiate walking in the normal way often launches himself forward using plantarflexion, contributing to equinus deformity.

3. The child having difficulty holding himself up against gravity may overuse extension activities, resulting in the thrusting/extending child with shortened hip extensors and difficulty handling and seating, or the walking child with overactive, shortened plantarflexors.

What must be particularly noted is the asymmetrical complex of deformity, which includes:

- Scoliosis
- Preferred head turning, possibly with related gaze defects
- Preferred hand use, due to more weight being taken on one side of the body, with the contralateral hand relatively freed for use. That hand will be more able, at least in the short term, but continued use of it will serve to reinforce the asymmetrical deformities
- Windswept hips, with the adducted hip in danger of dislocating posteriorly. Possibly more devastating is that the abductors of the opposite hip are in danger of becoming shortened, causing great difficulties with positioning in lying, sitting and standing, and with handling, and possibly leading to anterior dislocation of that hip (a difficult problem to deal with whether conservatively or surgically)
- Ankle and foot deformities.

In assessing deformity, measurement of joint ranges should be recorded and postural preferences/tendencies to deformity should be noted. Be particularly careful in measuring hip abduction, which must be done unilaterally and relative to the pelvis, not the other leg.

In attempting to prevent or inhibit the development of deformity one should:

a. Create a variety of 'corrected' positions for sustained periods, including sleeping positions (see Ch. 25)
b. Teach parents and care staff to do passive movements—their effectiveness might be queried, but they are often done and so should be taught correctly. Also, a parent's improved 'feel' for his child's range of motion and resistance to movement may be helpful in monitoring progression of deformity (see Tardieu 1988)
c. Attempt to improve those abilities that are lacking.

Weakness

Obviously weakness is an important issue in cerebral palsy: as certain movements, patterns, and groups of muscles are preferred, so other muscles will become weak. Recognition of weakness is important but cannot be taken at face value—it may be that the opposing muscle group is very strong or 'spastic', or that the postural mechanism which will allow the child to use certain muscles or movements is deficient. For example, one must differentiate between lack of antigravity mechanism and weakness of hip and knee extensors. The available range must be considered as well. Therefore treatment cannot consist solely of strengthening but must also include improvement of postural ability so that the child can actually use any improved strength and increased mobility.

ASSESSMENT OF PRACTICAL ABILITIES

The main factors which need to be taken into account during assessment of practical abilities are:

- Level of postural ability (as outlined above and in Ch. 25)
- The presentation of the task upon which the results of the assessment are based:
  — Is the response automatic or volitional? Is there a cognitive component to the result?
  — The complexity and composition of the instructions used: verbal (appropriate to comprehension level), demonstrations (bearing in mind any possible visual or hearing problems), modelling, single or multiple request.
  — Is the child able to concentrate: away from aural or visual distraction?
  — What is the child's emotional state during assessment? Fatigue, distress, playing to the crowd, hungry, constipated?

— Positioning: is the child in the best position for him to function?
— Is the task (or the reward) motivating for the child, particularly if he is asked to repeat it?

- Both the child and parent's attitude to (and level of understanding of) the disability. Consider also 'professional fatigue': Have they received conflicting or overwhelming advice in the past? What do they perceive are the major problems?
- What environmental and cultural considerations are there?

The occupational therapy approach to assessment should follow a specific model, e.g. Keilhofer (1985) and Mosey (1981). Standardised tests are becoming available (e.g. *BAOT Resource Book* (1990) and are increasingly used, particularly in the field of perceptual skills, but their limitations related to children with motor deficit, receptive/expressive language problems or a combination of handicaps must be considered. The problem-solving nature of the occupational therapy approach tends to diversify beyond the protocol of the standardised test to ensure that the child has the greatest opportunity to achieve. This may well affect the formal result of the test but gives positive indications for the means of remediation.

Commence the assessment with an overview of the child's postural abilities, evaluating any equipment used. Consider that, although the child at his best will be able to achieve a certain level, he cannot be expected to maintain this throughout the day, particularly when other skills are demanded of him. Thus the child who can sit on the floor (or even on a box) unsupported may require postural support in order to isolate the movement of his hand for writing. If correct postural support is not provided, the small amount of treatment time will be wasted.

Work through a checklist of appropriate practical skills, e.g. toileting, dressing, writing, cooking, eating, etc., ensuring that each task is presented in the most familiar place for the child (this may mean assessment of the same skill in school as well as home, for instance). It is important to know when it is not appropriate to assess, e.g. if the child is too embarrassed in front of peers or insecure with a strange therapist; reports from other members of staff in the team may need to be interpreted from the occupational therapy point of view. This may direct the therapist to specific areas requiring detailed assessment, and may indicate advice and goal planning through a third party more acceptable to the child.

Behavioural problems may be indicative of frustration, insecurity, social problems, sensory deficit, overcompensation and/or epilepsy and may need to be approached by use of non-threatening assessment activities, recognising that it is particularly important for these children to achieve.

The information gained from the assessment process should be interpreted and shared with all those concerned with the child. This will lead to appropriate goal planning (incorporated into the child's routine) and much work for the therapists in preparing the interdisciplinary treatment programme for practical abilities. Ideally work may be through one person whom the parents can relate to. This individual will not be providing all services but acting in a coordinating role, and is often identified unconsciously by the parents themselves.

The assessment process should result in an immediate, attainable goal for the child and family. This could be an aspect of good handling methods such as: holding the child in a good position which enables eye contact; encouraging the child to reach a toy, operate a computer or a powered chair; seeing his school work; facilitating eating, drinking, talking, etc.

ASSESSMENT OF ORAL COMPETENCE AND COMMUNICATIVE BEHAVIOUR

Assessment needs to incorporate general observations made of the child and family in familiar surroundings as well as direct assessment relating to oral competence and communication. Assessment will continue alongside therapeutic intervention as the child's responses to a treatment regime and his rate of progress will determine the profile that is being drawn up of his abilities and areas of weakness.

Assessment needs to highlight which learning systems are impaired whether they be sensory, cognitive, linguistic or emotional (see Ch. 1). Children with cerebral palsy may display both delay and disorder in learning, e.g. there may be a severe learning difficulty affecting the acquisition of language as well as a specific language disorder.

The child may demonstrate abnormal responses to sensory stimulation, i.e. touch, light, movement or noise. These should be noted and taken into account during assessment and in planning therapy intervention.

The child's response may be extremely slow and could be missed or misinterpreted as lack of comprehension or inability to perform a task. Conversely the child could be hypersensitive to stimuli, which would interfere with a correct response, e.g. the child is distracted from a task by his startle reaction following a sudden noise.

Observation must be made of the child's attentional levels. How distractable is he? Is he able to inhibit a physical response to sensory stimuli? The levels of attention are clearly described by Cooper et al (1978).

Finally assessment should determine *when* intervention is necessary, *what* method should be adopted, and *who* should be involved.

Assessment of oral competence

Considerable information of the child's potential for speech can be obtained from assessing the oral–motor skills required for eating and drinking. Brindley et al (1991) provide a detailed checklist examining the following seven areas of oral functioning by means of observation, examination and a series of performance tasks.

1. Posture

The key points of posture are examined as to how they affect oral control, e.g. seating in relation to the position of the head, chin, neck and stability of the hips, trunk and shoulder girdle. Posture directly influences the muscle tone required for eating, drinking and saliva control. There may be specific postures, which occur in isolation or as part of a pattern of movement, e.g. wide jaw opening and tongue thrusting associated with extension (see Ch. 8).

2. Reflexes/reactions

Children with cerebral palsy often display both retained and abnormal reflex patterns of movement (Table 7.1), which are sometimes excessively strong. These persistent abnormal reflexes prevent the older child from developing the more mature and controlled patterns of movement required for eating and drinking. For example, prolonged sucking or a strong bite reflex will hinder the development of a mature chewing pattern. The child may be hypersensitive in the mouth, which will produce an over-reaction to touch, or intolerance of food or feeding utensils. Conversely there may be a hyposensitivity problem where there is little or no awareness of food being in the mouth, even if there are strong flavours or extremes of temperature. The swallow reflex in this case may not have sufficient sensation to be triggered.

3 and 4. Respiration and phonation

It is important to determine the rate, depth and route of respiration, as well as the initiation, pitch, intonation and volume of voice. Look at the coordination of the diaphragm and abdominal muscles to see if they are working together or opposing each other. The incoordination of these muscles will cause difficulty with inspiration, directly affecting speech as well as swallowing.

Children with cerebral palsy often display rapid, shallow and dysrhythmic breathing patterns so that the child only manages one word per breath, or reverses breathing so that he speaks on an inhaled breath. The fluency of speech may be disrupted by irregular uncoordinated movements of breathing and phonation so that speech becomes scanning or the voice fades before the end of a phrase.

The importance of correct breathing, and how it affects swallowing, is stressed by Selley and his team from Exeter University (1990). They recognised an anticipatory stage in the swallowing process where exhalation

Table 7.1   Reflexes and reactions. Children with cerebral palsy often display both retained and abnormal reflex patterns of movement, which are sometimes excessively brisk or strong. These reflexes prevent children developing more mature and controlled patterns of movement.

Name	Description
Asymmetric tonic neck reflex (ATNR)	Head turned to one side causes limb to straighten on the same side. Bending arm to mouth causes head to turn away from that arm
Extensor thrust	The head is thrown back, spine arched, legs straight (sometimes scissored) and arms tight (in response to firm contact on the back of the head, trunk or soles of feet)
Startle reflex	Throws into extensor pattern on loud noise, sudden movement or unexpected event
Rooting reflex	Face turns to side where cheek is touched
Suckling and swallowing reflex	Lip, tongue, jaw, cheeks and pharyngeal muscles coordinate with breathing in an efficient suckle/swallow movement pattern. This is used primarily to draw liquid from a nipple/teat and occurs in response to sight, touch or taste of any stimulus approaching the mouth
Santmyer reflex	A puff of air on the face causes child to swallow
Primary chewing	Gnawing on object placed between gum ridges or side teeth
Bite reflex	Sudden jaw closure in response to front gums/teeth being touched
Cough reflex } Gag reflex }	Protective survival mechanisms, which stay throughout life

Effect on function

Posture—child can be difficult to position for feeding and has difficulty maintaining posture
Asisted/self feeding—child has difficulty looking at hand and bringing hand to mouth
Swallowing—head turned strongly to side prevents efficient swallow

Posture—hard to position the child for feeding
Assisted/self feeding is affected by posture and stiffness
Swallowing—chin thrust prevents efficient swallow and may cause choking
Oral control—jaw often thrusts preventing mouth closure and interferes with normal
  suckling or chewing movements

Posture—as above
Assisted/self feeding—sudden loss of the appropriate flexed posture may give feeling of
  insecurity
Swallowing—the fast intake of breath is likely to cause choking
Physiological response—due to release of adrenaline e.g. fast breathing, increased heart rate;
  sweating

Any stimulating to side of mouth or face takes child's head out of midline often with
  associated rounded lip posture or jaw thrusting

Interferes with:
1. Development of mature movements of lips, tongue and jaw
2. Chewing patterns
3. Development of breathing patterns; choking often occurs if solid foods are suckled

No apparent adverse effect and can be useful to prompt swallowing

Mature rotary chewing does not develop

Inability to open mouth and coordinate jaw movement whilst introducing food to mouth

Oversensitivity to food may cause frequent coughing. This overrides all other eating patterns
A brisk gag reflex retained at the front of the mouth reduces tolerance to food

always occurs as food approaches the mouth. If this stage is disrupted the whole swallowing process will be affected.

5. Orofacial structure and function

The structure and function of the head and face are examined to determine any cranio-facial abnormalities. The facial musculature will be observed for symmetry and expression. The habitual posture, tone and movement of jaw, lips and tongue are observed during eating and drinking. What oral patterns are used when dealing with food? What is the oral seal used when drinking? Is there nasal regurgitation of food?

Phonological analysis of the child's speech can be made by indirect methods of listening and recording sounds, or more directly from transcriptions of recorded speech and the use of standardised tests. The Renfrew Articulation Test provides a quick screening of the child's articulation.

The Frenchay Dysarthria Assessment (Enderby 1981) gives a reliable assessment in which the different features of the articulators are presented in bargraph form. It is easy to see from this the relative strengths and weaknesses of the child's speech, and structure therapy accordingly.

6. Dentition

The state of the teeth and gums is observed, and the alignment of the teeth is noted, e.g. an undershot jaw prevents oral seal.

7. Saliva control swallowing

The swallowing process is often severely affected in children with cerebral palsy and is manifested by (1) poor oral control of food and drink, resulting in poor growth and malnutrition; (2) drooling and (3) aspiration, which can cause chronic chest conditions.

It is therefore essential to determine which phase of this process is disrupted. This can be attempted by observation, examination or radiographic investigations, e.g. video fluoroscopy.

Following the suck–swallow reflex of early infancy (see Ch. 1) swallowing can be divided into four main phases:

1. The *pre-oral stage* or 'anticipatory' stage (Selley et al 1990), where the presentation of the food to the mouth stimulates and triggers various reactions, e.g. increased salivation, respiration, swallow reflex.

2. The *oral stage* (voluntary) where food is taken into the mouth and prepared into a bolus ready for swallowing. This stage involves movements of lips, tongue, jaw and cheeks to manipulate the food in the mouth to form a bolus, which is then transported by the tongue to the back of the mouth ready for swallowing.

3. The *pharyngeal stage*. The swallowing reflex is triggered when the bolus makes contact with the anterior faucial arches and the bolus is passed through the pharynx by peristalsis.

4. The *oesophageal stage* (involuntary). The bolus enters the oesophagus at the cricopharyngeal junction in a continuous peristaltic wave, and enters the stomach at the gastro-oesophageal junction.

It is important to ensure that there is no oesophageal or cricopharyngeal abnormality causing the dysphagia, gastric reflux or vomiting.

Assessment of communication

Assessment of communication will include non-verbal and social skills as well as verbal comprehension, expressive language and articulation.

There are a range of non-verbal behaviours which are used with intention or meaning. These include vocalisation, facial expression, eye-gaze, body posture and gesture. Although some of these normal modes may be affected in the child with cerebral palsy, these communicative behaviours need to be established wherever possible and parents/carers taught how to respond to and reinforce them (see Ch. 1).

Assessment of verbal comprehension and expressive language can be attempted using standardised tests for children who are able to manipulate objects or speak; but, for children who are unable to speak or use their hands, test material may have to be adapted—e.g. increasing size, re-organising layout—or carefully selected to utilise the child's ability to eye-point. It is often necessary to use a checklist or collection of items from different tests to gain a profile of the child's abilities (see Ch. 3).

Assessment will determine the child's oral motor skills and communicative behaviour, providing some prediction of his potential for using speech or whether he will require augmentative communication (see p. 451).

MANAGEMENT

ORGANISATION OF THE ENVIRONMENT

A consistent approach to the child's management throughout the day is essential so that intervention enhances other activities. It is necessary to recognise priorities and to ensure that the often numerous people involved understand the reasons for a particular course of action.

The therapists' roles in management are mainly advisory and cover all aspects of daily life. The following areas should be considered:

- Lifting and carrying
- Positioning
- Movement between positions
- Personal care

- Dressing (see Ch. 33)
- Sleeping
- Communication and language intervention
- Skills required for augmentative communication systems (see Ch. 26)
- Eating and drinking skills
- Accessing switches
- Mobility
- Education
- Transport
- Play and leisure.

These areas will now be examined in turn.

Lifting and carrying

Good lifting and carrying techniques encourage the child's ability and interaction with the environment, discourage deformity, and should be relatively easy and safe for the carrier. The child should be given enough support so that he is safe but not so much that he is passive.

Preparations must be made before lifting; one must decide how the child will be carried and where he will be placed. The child should be approached from the front and told what is about to happen. His body, particularly the limbs, should be organised so that both the child and the lifter feel secure. Safe lifting techniques should be employed as much as possible, i.e. use a wide base of support, bend the knees, keep the back straight and hold the child close.

Factors to be considered for the child include: level of ability, particularly of trunk and head; floppiness and general tendency to flex or extend; existing or potential deformity; the child's size. Other factors include the lifter's ability, size and strength; environmental factors such as how much space is available for lifting; how best to get the child out of his chair; and how far the child is to be carried.

Carrying methods (Fig. 7.6)

Curled in a ball. The carrier holds the child with one or both arms under the thighs, or even in front of the flexed knees. This provides maximal support and keeps the disorganised child gathered together, giving him a feeling of having a 'centre'. It inhibits extensor thrust. It is quite easy with a small child but more difficult with a larger one. A very floppy child may end up with his head buried, which is probably uncomfortable and provides no visual interaction with the carrier or the environment. Abducted legs can be kept adducted in this position but one must be wary of windswept deformity—a carrier often carries a child in the position he naturally adopts, therefore reinforcing a developing asymmetry.

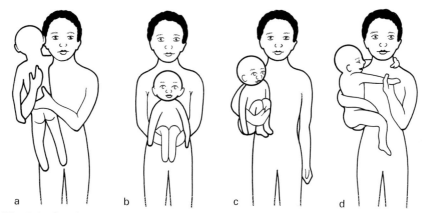

Fig. 7.6 Carrying methods. **a**. For flexed child. **b**. and **c**. For extending child. (The carrier's hands may be in front of or under the knees in either method of carrying.) **d**. For children with tight hip adductors, hemiplegia and more able children. The hemiplegic arm should be forward and held extended by the carrier.

Astride hips. This method is usually used for children with tight hip adductors and relatively good trunk and head control. Again there is a tendency to carry a child on one hip and to therefore reinforce asymmetry. A hemiplegic child should be carried so that the affected side is forward, and the carrier should hold the affected arm or hand; this encourages the child to look to his affected side, and to be aware of his affected arm; it also inhibits hip adductor tightness on that side. This position can be used with less able children provided they are given additional support, but be aware that they tend to fall or extend back away from the carrier.

Facing back over carrier's shoulder, or facing forward with hips and knees extended are positions used with very flexed children.

Positioning

For many children and adults with cerebral palsy, correct positioning is fundamental to any functional activity as well as to comfort and ease of handling. It is also vital in combating deformity where this is a potential or existing concern.

In defining positions to be used one may consider various positions relative to various activities and choose those which most nearly fulfill previously discussed criteria. These criteria may include:

- Function
- Correction or management of deformity
- Comfort
- Ease of use
- Feasibility in specified setting
- Ease of obtaining necessary equipment.

Obviously the weighting of criteria will vary according to the child, the activity, the setting and the carers involved.

For children unable to support themselves in certain positions and those at risk of developing deformity, there are specific fundamental positional needs for which recommendations and, where necessary, equipment must be provided and monitored as efficiently as possible, Bergen & Colangelo (1985) (see Ch. 25):

1. *Seating*—Whether on a lap for feeding a young child, on the floor for play, or requiring specialised supportive equipment.

2. *Standing.* Any child with cerebral palsy who is not standing well by the age of 12–18 months should be stood regularly, as correct, early weightbearing appears to be necessary for the correct formation of the acetabulum and femoral head and neck. The child should be stood with hips extended, slightly externally rotated, and abducted, and with knees straight and feet plantigrade. Care must be taken to avoid asymmetry as much as possible.

3. *Mobility.* Seating in a wheelchair or buggy may be needed, or advice for comfort and safety during transport.

4. *Deformity management* may dictate the need for certain positions both during the day and the night.

Movement between positions

Throughout the day a child will frequently be moved or will need assistance to move between positions, and these are appropriate times to reinforce and encourage ability. Also there are specific activities involving movement between positions, which are useful during individual and group treatments.

Rolling. The ability to roll depicts the ability to shift weight laterally in the lying position and, conversely, rolling may be used to improve this ability. A child who lies with more weight along one side of his body will generally roll more easily to that side, and asymmetries of posture and movement will be seen in other positions as well. These can often be alleviated by work in lying and rolling to the non-preferred side.

Lying to sitting. When pulling a child from supine to sitting, the ability to raise the head should be noted, but even more important is the ability to anchor the bottom in place. (When the newborn baby or the very unable cerebral palsied child is pulled to sitting, his bottom slides along the supporting surface. Once the normal baby is about 3 weeks old he gains the ability to anchor his bottom—an important precursor to later independent sitting.) This ability may be encouraged in handling and treatment, for example by pulling to sitting from part way up, by lying to supine from part way down, or by pulling up to sitting over one buttock. A more able child may have some ability to anchor, but not enough to allow independent sitting with function; his ability to anchor can be reinforced by having him push forward with his hands against resistance so that he must 'dig' his bottom into the supporting surface. This can be done unilaterally if there is asymmetry. The ability to get from lying to sitting independently can be encouraged by pulling the child partially up with one arm and waiting for the other arm to be used to push himself up the rest of the way (Fig. 7.7).

Creeping/crawling. All-fours is a difficult, complicated position, and movement within it is even more difficult. In order to be successful the child must learn to maintain himself up against gravity while balancing fore/aft (up/down) and side to side. The delicate line between being balanced and falling is often seen in this position. The child may shift his weight forward in order to move a leg but often goes too far and ends up on his nose. Many of the children remain top-heavy, with difficulty keeping some weight in their lower ends, and learn that in order to keep from falling onto their noses they must over-weigh their lower ends—hence the typ-

a

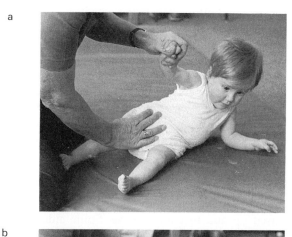

b

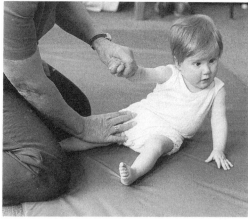

Fig. 7.7a and b.   Encouraging the development of support reactions.

ical bunny-hop position. As well as improving the above weight-shifting abilities, treatment in this position is helpful in loosening typically tight areas: rounded back and shoulders, posteriorly tilted pelvis, and tight proximal hip extensors.

Sitting to standing. In order to achieve this the normal person is able to bring the top half of his body well forward over his feet and then extend his legs to rise to standing. Those with cerebral palsy tend to either slide forward off the chair in a heap or, when trying to rise, they totally extend and fall backwards. In handling and treatment the cerebral palsied child should be encouraged to stretch or lean far forward while keeping his bottom in place, and then to rise without pushing his head back. For a child of the correct level of ability, frequent practice of rising from sitting to lean-standing, onto a table or walking sticks (do not allow pulling with hands), is very helpful. Most less able children have at least some ability to help with rising to standing if given appropriate support in the correct position. For these children this is an important ability to reinforce as it will be very helpful during transfers and other daily living activities as they grow.

Standing to walking. Rather than initiating walking by pulling his weight forward using ankle dorsiflexion, a cerebral palsied child is more likely to 'launch' himself by plantarflexing, thrust forward his abdomen, or poke his chin. It can be helpful to practice coming forward from leaning back against a wall in standing; use of leg gaiters can help to isolate activity at the ankles.

Assisted walking. In assisting a cerebral palsied child to walk, the helper should provide balance support and encourage the child to keep his weight forward. This is more easily done if the helper stands in front, facing the child and supporting him at the upper arms or hands (arm gaiters may be helpful when doing this). If the helper stands behind, the child is more likely to learn backwards. When providing aids it is better to use the least stable one that the child can manage: with this, he will be less able to use his arms to hold himself up and to counterpoise. Some aids now provide a variable amount of assistance with antigravity, and little balance so that the child must learn to balance himself (Fig. 7.8). For the less able child (often athetoid) who has some ability to hold himself up against gravity and to keep his weight forward over his base, but little or no balance, walkers such as the Cheyne walker may be useful; however, be aware that frequent use of such walkers may serve to reinforce any asymmetry if treatment, positioning and handling are not used well to counteract the detrimental effect (Fig. 7.9).

Personal care

Information on personal care is covered in Chapter 33 but there are some specific points relevant to cerebral palsy.

The way the child participates in his personal care can be used to improve his motor development; the more pieces of equipment or adaptations that are provided, the more complex and individual the child's environment

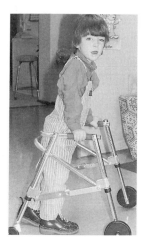

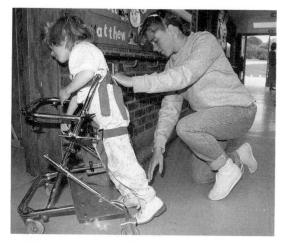

Fig. 7.8 Boy using the Kay Posture Walker, which encourages extension of the elbows and good trunk balance.

Fig. 7.9 Child with quadriplegia using a walker. She needs help to prevent increase in spasm and development of an abnormal pattern.

becomes in order for him to cope. Simple problem solving, such as support using the carer's body or a standard item of furniture, can be generalised to the child's environment as he matures.

The important principle is that the child feels secure, i.e. able to maintain a symmetrical posture balanced enough to move and participate in the required task, for example, reaching for socks and shoes. The task needs to be appropriate to the child's level of ability (see Ch. 25) bearing in mind the next achievable goal. In all aspects of personal care the child should take increasing responsibility for himself even where he is physically unable to perform unaided. It is important to create opportunities for independence, decision-making and self-assertion.

Sleeping

There are two main considerations when the child is sleeping:

1. *The posture of the child in the bed.* Maintaining a good position throughout the night will assist in prevention of deformity and will afford an opportunity for a long period of correct posture and stretch, ensuring that the child is in an optimal condition for the start of the new day. For the young child, improvisation using towels, sheets or nappies may be sufficient to maintain the child in abduction or side-lying (Finnie 1968, Millard 1984).

Older children or those with more severe involvement may require specialised equipment to maintain a correct position (see Ch. 25) throughout the night, i.e. splinting, personalised night boards and wedges (Fearn & Tutt 1989).

2. *The child's position in the room.* The decor of the room needs to provide adequate stimulation and ensure that the child is most likely to attend to stimuli on the more affected side if this is at all possible (Finnie 1968).

Communication

Early intervention is essential to establish the child's pre-verbal skills and to ensure communicative competence whether the child ultimately acquires speech or requires an augmentative system of communication (see Ch. 1).

The child with cerebral palsy may demonstrate all the prerequisites for verbal development, e.g. eye contact, listening, attentiveness, turn-taking and verbal comprehension, even though non-verbal interaction may be impaired, i.e. facial expression, eye movements, gesture.

It is necessary to develop the child's awareness of self and others in order that he can understand the function of language and its social use.

The child's attempts at communication, whether verbal or non-verbal, need to be continuously reinforced by parents and carers by encouragement to build vocabulary and develop expressive language through reinforcement and expansion of his own initiated attempts.

Language intervention

Language intervention can be organised individually or in groups, through language programmes or schemes. These may be:

- Topic-based—concentrating on developing listening skills, introducing language concepts, and expanding vocabulary and sentence building
- Developmentally structured—providing both assessment and remediation, e.g. the Derbyshire Language Scheme (Masidlover & Knowles 1979).

An integrated approach to language learning in the classroom can be achieved by teachers and therapists working together to adapt the requirements of the National Curriculum for children with learning difficulties.

Articulation

The motor delay and disorders associated with cerebral palsy also interfere with articulation, making speech dysarthric or dyspraxic.

These motor disorders include: abnormal muscle tone affecting posture and stability; abnormal postural and reflex behaviour; lack of movement or involuntary movements; problems with coordination of movements or breathing; and inadequate sensory awareness.

In addition these disorders are often compounded by cognitive deficits, which will affect the method and rate of learning of the precise skills necessary for articulation.

Wherever possible, therapy aims to facilitate normal function by use of specific techniques and treatment regimes. Intelligible speech should be the goal for the child who has the potential to speak. Intervention must occur at the optimum time to enable these skills to be learned and rehearsed in order that they become automatic and can be generalised into conversation.

The fine motor control required for speech production emerges during the second year of life and continues into early adolescence (Byers-Brown & Kenny 1989). The need for therapy will continue into adult life as, by the nature of cerebral palsy, functional control will fluctuate and change as the child grows.

The child with cerebral palsy has difficulty in coordinating respiration and phonation, imitating stress and intonation patterns and producing and sequencing speech sounds in the vowel and consonant patterns familiar to our language.

Therapy regimes can be introduced into the classroom, where listening and sound discrimination can be reinforced in language sessions and sound production can be tackled in small groups that focus on oral motor skills.

Speech techniques for relaxation and the coordination of breathing and phonation can be addressed during physiotherapy sessions, oral skills groups, and music or swimming lessons.

Breathing patterns

Breathing patterns can be improved by:

1. Good seating to ensure correct posture of head, neck and trunk, and to aid function of the diaphragm and abdominal muscles.

2. Practising voluntary control of inhalation and exhalation, e.g imitation of sighing and blowing, or vocalising on exhalation.

3. Exercises to promote phonation:

a. Breathing-in is associated with extension—the child's arms should be brought up and out during inhalation, and down and across the chest during exhalation.

b. Changing the child's position—movement stimulates phonation.

c. Vibration of the chest also stimulates phonation

d. Placing the floppy child into a weight-bearing position—vocalisation increases as tone increases

e. Encouraging laughing, coughing, crying.

Head and neck stability needs to be established so that lips, tongue and jaw can interact independently from the movements of the trunk and upper limbs.

Individual therapy will focus on the lip, tongue and jaw control needed for sound production, and the association of the sounds in words and their subsequent generalisation into speech.

Technology may help to overcome some speech difficulties that have not responded to intensive treatment by adolescence:

1. Electropalatography (EPG), which is a computer-based technique enabling detailed recordings of tongue movements to be stored and displayed on a computer screen, (Hardcastle et al 1989).

2. The Exeter Lip Sensor, which was developed to give an audio-feedback to children with an open mouth posture and poor lip closure, (Huskie et al 1981).

Oral skills

Feeding and speech are closely linked because the complex movements required for speech are superimposed on those patterns already acquired in breathing, eating and drinking.

Management will focus on reducing oral hypersensitivity by using de-sensitisation techniques and developing oral motor skills.

Oral desensitisation. The child with cerebral palsy is often hypersensitive around the head, face, and particularly the mouth. Desensitisation of lips, tongue and palate can be done indirectly through play, where the child learns to tolerate touch around the face and mouth. It can be achieved by using techniques such as touching, stroking, rubbing, tapping and brushing, and also by encouraging the child to mouth his own fingers and toys. The child should include brushing hair, washing face and cleaning teeth as part of his daily routine.

More direct methods, e.g. proprioceptive neuromuscular facilitation (PNF), use brushing and icing techniques and should only be attempted under the direction of a qualified person.

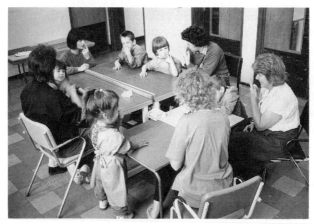

Fig. 7.10 Team approach to oral skills practice using the principles of conductive education.

Oral stimulation. It has been found that good oral motor skills can be established by daily practice. Ideally this can be organised in groups prior to mealtimes, so that not only are the movements reinforced during eating and drinking, but also the stimulation promotes improved oral competence for handling the food and liquid.

Children with cerebral palsy respond well to group participation, and the programmes can be devised using the principles of conductive education (Fig. 7.10). The areas covered by the programme include seating; posture; head position; jaw, lip and tongue control; and stimulation of swallowing.

Drooling

Drooling is a problem for a large number of children with cerebral palsy and is often the most offensive aspect of their disability.

Drooling interferes with eating, speech, self-image, and classroom and social activities; it can affect the ultimate placement of a child. It may also cause soreness of skin, infections, halitosis and, more seriously, aspiration.

Aspiration (entry of materials into the airway) can result from:

1. A disrupted oral phase before swallowing, usually due to poor tongue control. The saliva falls over the base of the tongue before the child is either aware or has time to initiate a swallow.

2. Delayed triggering of the swallowing reflex in the pharyngeal phase, allowing saliva to fall into the airway before the reflex is triggered.

3. Reduced pharyngeal peristalsis, which disrupts the transport of fluid to the oesophagus, leading to pooling of liquid in the pharyngeal recesses and subsequent spillage into the airway.

A multidisciplinary assessment is necessary and will include an ENT surgeon, paediatrician and speech therapist. Assessment includes:

a. Examination of the ear, nose and throat for infection or obstruction
b. Assessment of positioning and postural control
c. Assessment of intellectual capacity
d. Detailed analysis of oral motor skills.

Management of drooling. Traditionally, treatment has consisted of the use of drugs, surgery and intensive speech therapy. All have their limitations, and improvements are often not sustained:

1. *Drugs.* Glycopyrrolate and benztropine have been used successfully in reducing drooling, but there are sometimes side-effects and their long term use is not recommended.

2. *Surgery.* The operation found to be most successful is the transposition of the submandibular ducts to the tonsillar fossa. This may necessitate the removal of the tonsils if they are infected or enlarged. Further surgical intervention may require excision of the submandibular or sublingual glands.

3. *Intensive speech therapy.* Children may respond sufficiently well to an oral skills programme, and so obviate the need for surgery. It has also been found that the success of surgical intervention is enhanced by the children receiving oral skills training prior to surgery as well as postoperatively (Green, personal communication).

4. *Behaviour modification techniques* are used where children are trained to associate an auditory cue with swallowing. An electronic dribble-control device, which is a small box pinned to the child's clothing, emits a bleep at regular intervals, giving the child an auditory signal to swallow (or, if unable to swallow, to wipe the mouth).

5. *Palatal training appliances* are used if a sensory loss is indicated. The appliance can be fitted at any age and helps to prevent tongue humping, improves soft palate functioning and triggers reflex swallowing.

6. *The Exeter Lip Sensor* was developed to give audio-feedback to children with an open mouth posture and poor lip closure (Huskie et al 1981).

Evaluation of these procedures is necessary by detailed assessment of oral skills, taking base-line recordings of the amount of drooling prior to and following intervention.

Eating and drinking

However well positioned the child is, it may be difficult to control the shoulder girdle and head to maintain postural symmetry during the fine motor activity of eating and drinking. There are certain reflexes which affect oral function and independent feeding. These range from the asymmetric tonic neck reflex—difficulty in looking at the hand holding the spoon and in bringing the hand to the mouth in the midline, preventing efficient swallowing—to the bite reflex, where there is an inability to open the mouth and coordinate the movement while introducing food to the mouth (see Table 7.1, p. 132).

Mealtimes provide opportunities for the development of posture, head control and hand/eye coordination. Considerable language interaction occurs at mealtimes allowing vocabulary building, concept development and rules of social behaviour to be learnt.

Efficient eating is necessary to allow the child to receive an adequate and varied diet for health, growth and digestion. The patterns of movement of lips, tongue, jaw, breathing, etc., practised whilst eating, strongly influence the development of precise movements necessary for speech and control of saliva. Giving the child choice and control at mealtimes allows him to develop self-esteem, independence and his own identity. Integration into social eating is possible as the child's eating competence becomes more acceptable.

The preparation, i.e. management, of mealtimes is vitally important to ensure that the child receives maximum appetising nutrition content with minimum bulk food. There are many ways of doing this: group two or three small different courses (little and often), e.g. build up meals or snacks between meals; keep tastes separate, considering colour, texture and variety, allowing as much choice as possible. Vary the methods of feeding from spoon to finger feeding, and allow the child to participate in the food preparation itself.

The carer needs to have knowledge of how the food is going to behave—both on the plate and in the child's mouth; whether the food is going to be difficult or easy to manage. Advice from a speech therapist and dietician should be sought.

Accessing (Switch Use)

Use of switches can improve the range of opportunities for the child, e.g. play, powered mobility, communication aids, environmental controls and robotic devices.

Careful assessment and training is necessary to develop the skills required for effective switch use. The child has to have the necessary cognitive skills such as the ability to attend; an understanding of cause and effect; and consistent, reliable control of part of the body in order to operate the switch.

More control will be required if the child is to operate a powered chair; other skills such as the ability to scan may be necessary in order to use a communication device or environmental control system (see Ch. 24) (Thornett et al 1990). Switch use is a skill that requires careful introduction and training. A training programme should be planned for each child, with opportunity to practice progressing from play situations to use for mobility and communication purposes. The opportunities, such as mobility, that

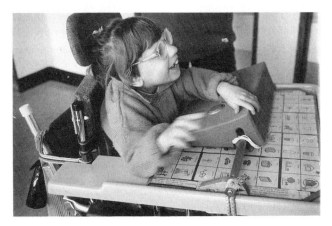

Fig. 7.11   Driving practice using a light touch switch with four buttons.

switches can offer can have a dramatic effect on the child's motivation and level of excitement, but may have an adverse effect on postural control, which therefore needs careful monitoring (Fig. 7.11).

Mobility

An adapted environment may be necessary to ensure that the child has access for independent mobility, (Goldsmith 1976). This is particularly pertinent when considering educational placement. Early mobility for the young child may be possible by provision of low-tech or high-tech equipment, e.g. adapted 'scooter boards' or peer-level powered mobility (Fig. 7.12) (Thornett 1990, Butler et al 1984). This early mobility gives the child a level of independence which helps to develop other skills such as cause–effect, problem-solving, assertiveness and perceptual skills.

a 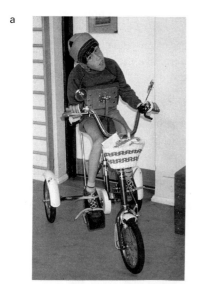 b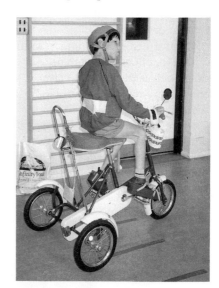

Fig. 7.12a and b. Athetoid boy riding a tricycle adapted to give chest support, with a wide saddle and fixed footplates. There is a fixed wheel mechanism to enable him to manoeuvre and brake. He is not able to walk independently.

Any equipment that is provided to assist independent mobility— e.g. orthotics, crutches, rollators, powered and manual wheelchairs, and their integral postural support—will all require frequent monitoring and rapid access for repair or replacement. Consistent use of the prescribed apparatus is essential to maintain, practise or improve skills, and avoid frustration.

Education

Within the special school, therapy for children with cerebral palsy can take place in groups or individual sessions. Both types of therapy are necessary as specific areas can be covered individually, supplementing the group programme. It is essential that group programmes and individual planning for the child should be undertaken by the multidisciplinary team in order to capitalise on the child's full potential, although only one or two members of the team may actually be involved with 'running' the group. Group work may not necessarily be class-based, but organised according to abilities such as hand function, language, augmentative communication, lying and sitting ability, and social and compensatory skills. The activity will be the same for the whole group, but individual targets and methods of achieving them will differ. Careful assessment for individual group members is necessary to establish appropriate goals for each child.

Emphasis is always placed on the education of the child but it is equally important to inform and ensure that all those involved with the child's programme are aware of the aims and the reasons behind treatment techniques and strategies.

In mainstream school, fatigue and pressures from keeping up physically with peers can be reduced by provision of independent mobility such as a bike in the playground and transport to school.

Transport

Any postural support that is normally required will need to be duplicated and probably increased in the upper trunk for the child's security and safety when using transport. Since vibration and jolting will affect postural and head control, the backrest will require an extension behind the head for safety and support.

Postural support used in the car, even when strapped in, will not necessarily be adequate as a safety seat (Department of Transport 1987, Standards Association of Australia 1987). Parents and carers should be aware of this. (See also Ch. 33.)

Children can spend long periods of time in transit to and from school, and require adequate postural support during this time. A long period spent in a poor position early in the day results in the child being tired and poorly organised physically for the rest of the day. Ensure that the feet are supported and that the child can see comfortably out of the window.

Play and Leisure

Early intervention is essential to develop the child's awareness of his surroundings and to achieve 'normal' auditory, visual and tactile experience. Since the child has a motor handicap he may need careful positioning in terms of posture and environment to enable him to explore and initiate play. An early example of this during the oral phase may be placing the small child in a position that encourages hand-to-mouth exploration (Wisbeach 1982, Enderby 1987). A child lacking head control may need to be supported in a symmetrical position that allows him to use his vision. Similarly, hearing can be affected by the child's position (Green 1987, O'Halleron, personal communication). Experiential play is important developmentally and the child should have the opportunity to play with all the normal play media. This should include messy play, mirrors and reflections, rough play and playground experience.

Opportunities for peer group interaction, and for observation and initiation of play and participation in sequential play, should be encouraged. Peers introduce spontaneity, motivation and direction, and adults should know when to withdraw attention. It can be a mutually beneficial experience if a child with a physical disability is part of the local toddler or playgroup.

Specialised play equipment may be necessary to encourage learning such as cause–effect, scanning, and spatial awareness. Such equipment is often available from toy libraries and local loaning facilities, which provide a variety and choice of toys (Fig. 7.13). There are specialised programmes that develop skills through a play format, e.g. the Derbyshire Language Scheme—which develops language through play and the Portage project. Individual programmes can be designed to use play to aid development—conversely, observation of play can guide assessment as to the level of the child's ability.

Play and leisure activities are essential for the child's growth, development and maturity. They allow the child the opportunity to interact with his peers and society but can also be therapeutic, e.g. the Halliwick swimming method (Ness & Bell 1989) can contribute to improved breath and voice control as well as physical ability. (For leisure activities such as riding, watching television and playing computer games, consider postural management including alternative positions and positioning within the room.)

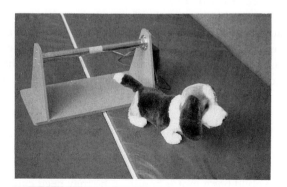

Fig. 7.13 A battery operated toy adapted for use with a bar switch.

INDIVIDUAL TREATMENT

GENERAL ACTIVITIES AND PRINCIPLES

There are numerous approaches to the treatment of children with cerebral palsy. An individual therapist will usually be particularly familiar with and/ or especially trained in one approach, and will use only that approach tempered with an understanding of others, plus some inevitable interpretations. One is more likely to be effective when using a method in which one is confident, knowledgeable and comfortable. However, it is important to recognise the contribution made by other approaches and to be aware of the sort of children, and families, for whom they may be indicated. It is also helpful to refer to, or collaborate with, other therapists skilled in different therapeutic methods.

It is well worth at least becoming acquainted with the general rationale of the better-known approaches: Bobath (neurodevelopmental therapy); Petö (conductive education, see p. 183); Vojta (which uses reflex locomotion as a working hypothesis); sensory-integrative therapy; and the Portage project. For a full account, see Scrutton 1984. Parents appreciate and need informed discussion, and should feel able to express their concerns and worries to their therapist, who is often their closest professional adviser in the early years.

Therapists must assess and define a child's abilities and inabilities, and their treatment aims. At the same time they must be aware of their own, and their facility's, strengths and weaknesses.

TIMES FOR INCREASED INDIVIDUAL THERAPY

In addition to an organised regime of management, handling, positioning and communication as previously described, there are certain problems, or certain times in a child's life, when individual treatment by the therapist or well trained parent or carer is required:

- At diagnosis
- During infancy
    - Posture management
    - Communicative competence
    - Oral skills/feeding
    - Potty training
- Preparation for school
- Introduction of switches for mobility and education
- Awareness of self and surroundings: coping with teasing
- Integration into mainstream education
- Adolescence
- Independent mobility
- Need for respite care

- Surgery
  — Preparation for surgery
  — Intensive postoperative intervention
- Preparation for school-leaving

Physical ability

The trunk

In the realm of physical ability the area often requiring individual treatment is the trunk. The trunk is the centre of balance and movement and when these abilities are deficient the child compensates by holding the trunk stiff and using the limbs to balance. There are many obvious examples of this: hooking an arm back over the handle of a wheelchair in order to stabilise the body; poking the head forward and rounding the trunk with protracted shoulders to keep weight forward over the base; hyperextending the neck and looking upwards in order to counterpoise a forward reach of the arm. The result is that the trunk becomes stiff, reinforcing the inabilities already apparent.

Use, or encouragement, of any balance abilities in the trunk becomes nearly impossible until the trunk is loosened. Note the great amount of subtle movement required around the trunk and pelvis in a normal person in order to allow and counterpoise functional activities: sitting using hands; rolling; rising to standing; walking; horse riding. (Also note the incapacity arising from a 'bad back'.)

Much of the stiffening and abnormal positioning of the limbs and even the eyes is secondary to the balance deficiencies and stiffness of the trunk; therefore these are often alleviated once the trunk is loosened and balance abilities are facilitated.

The 'unplaceable child'

Another specific difficulty requiring individual fairly intense input is with the child who is 'unplaceable' (see Fig. 7.4). As stated previously, if such a child's level of ability is not improved so that he becomes at least placeable, he is at risk of developing severe deformities and continuing to be very 'unable', uncomfortable, disorganised and difficult to handle.

Before and after surgery

Preparation for surgery and postoperative management are also times requiring intense individual input. Advice to parents regarding what to realistically expect from surgery in terms of various time spans, the child's discomfort, the sort of immobilisation in plaster that may be used, and any new handling and positioning that will be needed is essential prior to surgery (see p. 163).

Any special equipment or modification to current equipment that may be necessary postoperatively should be organised if possible, or arrangements made for it to be done as soon after surgery as possible. The occupational therapist may need to provide additional equipment at home to enable the family to cope with a temporarily immobile, and often heavy, child.

Parents, teachers and carers will all need additional advice and support from the team at this time.

INDIVIDUAL PHYSIOTHERAPY

Individual treatment should consist of a logical, effective sequence of activities, and each treatment should result in some change. Keeping a specific 'test' in mind to evaluate treatment effectiveness is helpful. For example, a child who sits asymmetrically with windswept hips due to inability to bring weight onto and anchor through one side of his body, may be treated in lying and standing but might be placed back into sitting to test the effect on his asymmetry.

The general sequence of activities during individual treatment often consists of the following.

Mobilisation activities

These are usually aimed at the shoulder/thoracic area, the low back, and the pelvic and hip area. Rather than rotating the trunk passively, it appears to be more effective to enlist active movement from the child in various weightbearing positions. Reference can be made to activities of the normal child: rocking on all-fours; going from side-sitting on one side to the other side; early rolling activities; raising the arms from the side; and reaching above the head in prone. All of these activities can be modified so that abnormal movements can be controlled and effort is used in the area where it is needed.

Activities to facilitate the postural abilities needed to be placed in or to maintain a position

These abilities include: establishment of a base of support and relating to a supporting surface; anchoring through the base; and shifting weight down into the lower half of the body. Activities similar to those mentioned above, but with a different emphasis, are effective. For example: rolling from supine to side-lying, particularly to the side that normally bears less weight, and emphasising the weight shift in the trunk; encouraging anchoring of the bottom during pull-to-sit, or sit-to-lie, or pull-to-sit with one hand to encourage anchoring of the contralateral buttock; having the child push forward against resistance in long or chair sitting to encourage the counterforce of bottom anchoring; and, in lean-standing (no pulling with the hands!), having the child rock forward and backward against resistance.

Activities to challenge a child's postural abilities once a position is established

These involve more complex weight-shifting abilities. Useful activities include: having the child reach outside his base in long or chair sitting—to the side, to the floor, above the head, forwards; in lean-standing, reaching for one or both knees, reaching forwards, coming to standing. More basic abilities for the disorganised, very unable child include: following an object in supine with eyes/head without the rest of the body becoming disorganised; turning head from side to side in prone, or in prone over a roll, while maintaining the organisation of the rest of the body; and freeing an arm from under the body in prone without disorganisation.

Activities to improve a child's ability to move from one position to another with control

Activities involving movement between positions (rolling, lying to sitting, sitting to lean-standing, lean-standing or wall-standing to walking) can be effective for both children who are, or are nearly, independent as well as much less able children, provided appropriate modifications to the activity and the support are made.

The sequence of activities during individual physiotherapy described above should not be considered as strict, but only as a guide. One must often work back and forth through the sequence to achieve one's aims. One activity can achieve a number of aims, although different aims may slightly alter the position, or the use and amount of resistance and external support, or the amount of 'abnormal' activity allowed. For example, the all-fours position can be used to mobilise the thoracic/shoulder areas and the low-back/pelvic areas, to encourage the ability to shift weight fore/aft, side to side, and up and down the body, or encourage the ability to move one part (head/eyes, arm, leg) without allowing disorganisation of the rest of the body. If, in this example, the main aim is to mobilise the low back, abnormal activity of the head, feet and other parts of the body may be allowed; but if the main aim is smooth, controlled movement, such abnormal activity would be undesirable.

INDIVIDUAL OCCUPATIONAL THERAPY

Having completed an assessment of all aspects of the child's practical abilities and readiness to acquire new skills, the occupational therapist will take a problem-solving approach to assist the child and family. This may involve working through/with others or working individually, but never in isolation from the multidisciplinary team. Treatment approaches may include:

1. *Perceptual training* to develop visual and sensory perceptual skills, particularly with regard to performance in the classroom, to aspects of body

image and to spatial awareness, e.g. learning to drive (manual or powered wheelchair), position of computer, environmental controls, paper/pencil skills. Time must be allowed for the child to gain experience of a variety of perceptual stimuli, both in gross and fine motor areas and feedback should be given in a practical way to enable the child to learn from the experiences.

2. *Work on gross and fine motor function,* ensuring that the child is in the optimum position in which to function. Management of posture can involve the maintenance of the child in positions that inhibit spasticity while facilitating normal function, or provision of postural equipment to provide the optimum position (Green et al 1991). Provision of a small grab rail for stabilisation of one or both hands during activity can assist in maintenance of postural stability and symmetry (see Ch. 25).

Work on fine motor function may be specific, e.g. working for active grasp and release, or opposition of fingers to thumb; or more general, e.g. working for bilateral hand function in the child with hemiplegia.

3. *Sensory stimulation,* particularly to the neglected side, to stimulate sensory acuity and reinforce body awareness.

4. *Activities of daily living*—work on practical skills (see Ch. 33). The need for close links with the Occupational Therapist working in the local area team office of the Social Services Department cannot be stressed too strongly.

5. *Assessment for provision of specialised equipment and adaptations.* Where the potential for acquisition of a practical skill appears exhausted, or impractical, the occupational therapist will assess and advise on suitable equipment to assist, e.g. computer/keyboard in the classroom, specialised switches for accessing technological devices, equipment to assist in personal care or domestic activities, and splints.

The equipment provided should allow the child to achieve something he/she previously could not achieve and should be provided with a review planned to ensure that the item is still being used correctly in the most therapeutic way. Some items may be used as a stepping stone to independent function, to be withdrawn as the child's practical skills improve.

At all times the occupational therapist should ensure that the treatment offered does not result in acquisition of 'splinter skills'; thus all activity should be able to be generalised into daily function.

REFERENCES

Ayres A J 1972 Sensory integration and learning disorders. Western Psychological Services, Los Angeles
Bergen A F, Colangelo C 1985 Positioning the client with central nervous system deficits. Valhalla Rehabilitation Publications, New York
Brindley C, Cave D, Crane S, Lees J, Moffat V 1991 Paediatric oral skills package (POSP). In preparation
British Association of Occupational Therapists 1990 Occupational therapists reference book. Park Sutton, Norwich, p 41
Butler C, Okamato G A, McKay T M 1984 Motorised wheelchair driving by disabled children. Archives of Physical Medicine and Rehabilitation 65: 95–97

Byers-Brown B, Kenny J 1989 A valuable friendship. Stockport Social Services Newsletter

Camera Talks: Plaster boots Available from 31 North Row, London, W1

Chailey Heritage 1991 Eating and drinking skills for the child with cerebral palsy.

Cooper J, Moodley M, Reynell J 1978 Helping language development, 3rd edn. Arnold, London

Department of Transport: Vehicle Standards and Engineering Division 1987 Code of Practice: The safety of passengers in wheelchairs on buses. London Department of Transport Publication VSE 87/1

Dunn P M 1976 Congenital postural deformities. British Medical Bulletin 32(1): 71–76

Enderby P 1981 Frenchay Dysarthria Assessment, 2nd edn. Frenchay Hospital, Bristol

Evans Morris S, Klein M D 1987 Pre-feeding skills. Winslow Press, Oxford

Fearn T, Tutt P 1990 Prone lying night wedge for postural control. Physiotherapy 76(6): 359–361

Finnie N R 1968 Handling the young cerebral palsied child at home. William Heinemann, London

Fulford G E, Brown J K 1976 Position as a cause of deformity in children with cerebral palsy. Developmental Medicine and Child Neurology 18: 305–314

Golding R, Goldsmith L 1986 The caring person's guide to handling the severely multiply handicapped. Macmillan Education, London

Goldsmith S 1976 Designing for the disabled. RIBA Publications, London

Green E M 1987 The effect of seating position on cognitive function in children with cerebral palsy. 59th Annual Meeting of the British Paediatric Association, Abstract G1 58, 108

Green E M, Mulcahy C M, Poutney T E 1991 An investigation into the development of postural control prior to sitting. In preparation

Hardcastle W J et al 1989 New developments in electropalatography. Clinical Linguistics and Phonetics, vol 3

Hare N 1977–1981 Personal communications

Howard I P, Templeton W B, 1966 Human spatial orientation. John Wiley, Toronto

Huskie C F, Ellis R E, Flack F C, Selley W G, Curle H J 1981 The Exeter Lip Sensor: a preliminary report. The College of Speech Therapy Bulletin, 35 and 36

Jolleff N, Moffat V 1987 Special needs of physically handicapped, severely speech impaired children, when considering a communications aid. In: Enderby P (ed) Assistive communication aids for the severely speech impaired. Churchill Livingstone, Edinburgh

Keilhofer G 1985 A model of human occupations. Williams and Wilkins, USA

Logemann J A 1983 Evaluation and treatment of swallowing disorders. Whorr Publishers Ltd, Turpin Transactions Ltd, Letchworth Herts

Masidlover M, Knowles W 1979 The Derbyshire Language Scheme. Educational Psychology Service, Ripley

Millard D M 1984 Daily living with a handicapped child. Croom Helm Special Education, London.

Mosey A C 1981 Occupational therapy: configuration of a profession. Raven Press, New York

Mulcahy C M, Poutney T E, Nelham R L, Green EM, Billington G D 1988 Adaptive seating for the motor handicapped: problems, a solution, assessment and prescription. Physiotherapy 74 (10): 531–536

Ness J C, Bell E J 1989 The Halliwick Swimming Method. Association of Paediatric Physiotherapists Newsletter 53, 3–6

O'Halloran J 1985 Personal communication

Portage guide to early education. NFER–Nelson, Windsor, Berkshire

Renfrew Articulation Attainment Test. Available from: North Place, Old Headington, Oxford

Robson P 1968 Persisting head turning in the early months: some effects in the early years. Developmental Medicine and Child Neurology 10: 82–92

Scrutton D 1984 Management of the motor disorders in cerebral palsy. Spastics International Medical, London

Selley W G, Flack F C, Ellis R E, Brooks W A 1990 The Exeter dysphagia assessment technique. Dysphagia, 4: 277–285

Standards Association of Australia 1987 Wheelchair occupant restraint assemblies for motor vehicles. Australian Standard 2942, Sydney, Australia

Tardieu C, Lespargot A, Tabary C, Bret M D, 1988 For how long must the soleus be stretched each day to prevent contracture? Developmental Medicine and Child Neurology 30: 3–10

Thornett C E E 1990 Mobility for very young handicapped children. Institute of Electrical Engineers Digest 1990/054

Thornett C E E, Langner M C, Brown A W S 1990 Disabled access to information technology—a portable, adaptable, multipurpose device. Journal of Biomedical Engineering 12: 205–208

Traub M M, Rothwell J C, Marsden C D 1980 Anticipatory postural reflexes in Parkinson's disease and other akinetic–rigid syndromes and in cerebellar ataxia. Brain 103: 393–412

Wisbeach A 1982 Positions for playing. Noah's Ark Publications, Potter's Bar

FURTHER READING

Levitt S 1982 Treatment of cerebral palsy and motor delay, 2nd edn. Blackwell Scientific, Oxford

8. Cerebral palsy: postural stabilisation

E.M. Green

Postural stabilisation is mentioned as a prerequisite for management of children with cerebral palsy in many places in this book. The basis for this has been investigated in various ways, and the benefits derived from postural stabilisation in sitting have been reported in the literature.

COMFORT

Electromyography of the lumbar muscles has been used to study sitting posture in the able-bodied population for years, particularly in relation to working and driving positions. Research suggests that an ideal posture has low myoelectric activity. Nwaobi et al (1983, 1985) have investigated the effects of various seating positions on the myoelectric activity of the major back muscles. As the orientation of the seat changed from upright to 30° reclined, the EMG activity increased. The reclined position is not one of relaxation in children with cerebral palsy who have not acquired sitting balance, as their postural mechanisms have not become automatic. Hundertmark (1985) suggests that the reclined position may elicit the tonic labyrinthine reflex, provoking a feeling of falling in these children. Discomfort has been shown to lower levels of performance in normal subjects (Bhatnager et al 1985).

FUNCTION

Adaptive seating has been shown to improve arm and hand function experimentally (Nwaobi 1985, 1986, 1987, Seeger et al 1982, 1984). Observational studies have also confirmed this (Wongsam 1985, Rang et al 1981, Motloch 1977).

McEwen & Karlan (1989) compared the effect of four adaptive positioning devices—a chair, stander, prone wedge, and side-lying board—on ability to access communication board locations.

Noronha et al (1989) did not find a difference in hand function when testing mildly handicapped children in adaptive seating and in a prone stander. Positioning may enable children with severe cerebral palsy to improve the gross motor movements of their arms.

POSTURAL DEFORMITY (see Ch. 25)

SOCIAL AND EMOTIONAL SKILLS

Correct positioning can enable children with a postural disability to use their environment and social structure more effectively. Hulme et al (1983) showed that subjects went to significantly more new places in the community following prescription of equipment *plus* a social skills training programme. In order for positioning equipment to have full impact, its prescription must be accompanied by advice on its application, and associated teaching of social skills. Reciprocal social behaviour and improved head control and eye contact may occur.

FEEDING AND ORAL SKILLS

Correct positioning of the child forms the basis of management of feeding difficulties (Treharne 1979). This has been confirmed by radiological studies (Siebens & Linden 1985). Hulme et al (1987) demonstrated the beneficial effects of positioning on eating and drinking. Speaking, swallowing and breathing involve common structures and nervous system pathways. Intelligibility of speech (Smith et al 1986) and respiratory function (Nwaobi & Smith 1986) have been shown to be increased by adaptive seating.

VISION

There is an obvious link between a child's head posture and visual field. A child with poor head control and insufficient support, such that the head hangs downwards, can only see his lap or the floor. Seating in a reclined position may only direct the eyes to the sky or ceiling. Correct positioning may increase a child's visual potential by allowing better scanning of the environment, promoting intellectual function and development of the visual system.

There has been a great deal of research into the development of the mammalian visual system. Visual stimulation during early infancy has been shown to be necessary for the full development of the visual cortex, Wiesel & Hubel (1963, 1965). In addition, in experiments where the eye movements of kittens were restricted after birth, some orientation columns in the visual cortex failed to develop (Gary-Bobo et al 1986, Milleret et al 1984).

Eye movement disorders, squints and visual perceptual difficulties are common in children with cerebral palsy. Correct positioning will encourage optimal visual stimulation.

COGNITIVE FUNCTION

Assessment of cognitive function can be exceedingly difficult in children with severe cerebral palsy, as most standardised tests rely on motor responses. Even methodologies such as measurement of attention require the child to be seated in a supportive chair. Computer technology has opened up a wider experience within the classroom for alternative methods of writing, learning to read and count, etc. Positioning for the functional operation of switches is essential.

Cognitive function itself may be impaired by poor positioning. Seven children with cerebral palsy aged 4–13 years were tested in three positions: upright seated; in the same seat tilted back 20°; and in an appropriate standard wheelchair without special support. Visual acuity and auditory discrimination were unaffected by the different seating positions. However, the children performed significantly better when seated upright, both individually and as a group, in tests involving visual discrimination and attention (a 'snap' card game), visual memory and digit span recall. Auditory acuity improved significantly in the upright seated position in two children.

There were differences in performance of the more complex tasks in the tilted seat positions and in the wheelchair with no support, but neither position was significantly better than the other.

It appears that tasks requiring simple perception are relatively unaffected, but more complex tasks involving cognitive function may be significantly affected by the seating system. The level of difficulty of the tasks was prescribed by the individual child's baseline function.

It seems that the task must be both complex and of sufficient difficulty before the effect of seating position is seen. This finding has implications for assessment and learning in children with cerebral palsy.

REFERENCES

Bhatnagar V, Drury C G, Schiro S G 1985 Posture, postural discomfort and performance. Human Factors 27(2): 189–199
Gary-Bobo E, Milleret C, Buisseret P 1986 Role of eye movements in developmental processes of orientation selectivity in the kitten's visual cortex. Vision Research 26: 557–567
Hulme J, Poor R, Schulein M, Pezzino J 1983 Perceived behavioural changes observed with adaptive seating. Devices and training programme for multi-handicapped, developmentally disabled individuals. Physical Therapy 63(2): 204–208
Hulme J, Shaver J, Acher S, Mullette L, Eggert C 1987 Effects of adaptive seating devices on the eating and drinking of children with multiple handicaps. American Journal of Occupational Therapy 41(2): 81–89
Hundertmark L H 1985 Evaluating the adult with cerebral palsy for specialised adaptive seating. Physical Therapy 65 (2): 209–212
Mc Ewen I R, Karlan G R 1989 Assessment of effects of position on communication-board access by individuals with cerebral palsy. Augmentative and Alternative Communication 235–241. Williams and Wilkins
Milleret C, Gary-Bobo E, Buisseret P 1984 The preferred orientation acquired by the kitten's visual cortical cells depends on the direction of eye movements during visual experience. Neuroscience (letter) 18: 574
Motloch W M 1977 Seating and positioning for the physically impaired. Orthotics and Prosthetics 31(2): 11–21

Noronha J, Bundy A, Groll J 1989 The effect of positioning on the hand function of boys with cerebral palsy. American Journal of Occupational Therapy 43: 507–512

Nwaobi O M 1986 Effects of body orientation in space on tonic muscle activity of patients with cerebral palsy. Developmental Medicine and Child Neurology 28: 41–44

Nwaobi O M 1987 Seating orientation and upper limb function in children with cerebral palsy. Physical Therapy 67: 1029–1212

Nwaobi O M, Brubaker C, Cusick B, Sussman M 1983 EMG investigations of extensor activity in cerebral palsied children in different seating positions. Developmental Medicine and Child Neurology 25: 175–183

Nwaobi O M, Hobson D, Trefler E 1985 Hip angle and upper extremity movement time in children with cerebral palsy. RESNA 8th Annual Conference, Memphis, Tennessee

Nwaobi O M, Smith P D 1986 Effect of adaptive seating on pulmonary function of children with cerebral palsy. Developmental Medicine and Child Neurology 28: 351–354

Rang M, Douglas G, Bennet G C, Koreska J 1981 Seating for children with cerebral palsy. Journal of Paediatric Orthopaedics 1: 279–287, Raven Press, New York

Seeger B R, Caudrey D J, O'Mara N A 1984 Hand function in cerebral palsy: the effect of hip flexion angle. Developmental Medicine and Child Neurology 26: 601–606

Seeger B R, Falkner P, Caudrey D 1982 Seating position and hand function in cerebral palsy. Australian Occupational Therapy Journal 29(4): 147–152

Siebens A A, Linden P 1985 Dynamic imaging for swallowing re-education. Gastrointestinal Radiology 10: 251–253

Smith P D, Holder L F, Nwaobi O M 1986 Effects of adaptive seating on speech intelligibility of children with cerebral palsy. Annual Meeting of AACPDM 1985, Developmental Medicine and Child Neurology Abstract 84: 119

Treharne D A 1979 Management of feeding difficulties. Nursing Times (18 Jan 1979): 108–109

Wiesel T N, Hubel T H 1963 Single cell responses in the striate cortex of kittens deprived of vision in one eye. Journal of Neurophysiology 26: 1003–1017

Wiesel T N, Hubel T H 1965 Extent of recovery from the effects of visual deprivation in kittens. Journal of Neurophysiology 28: 1060–1072

9. Cerebral palsy: orthopaedic management

J.A. Fixsen   G.T. McCarthy

Orthopaedic surgery can have profound effects on outcome in terms of mobility and comfort in children with cerebral palsy. In the past, children have been made worse by surgery carried out with the best intentions. In general, surgery should be considered as part of a team approach to the child with cerebral palsy. The surgeon should have experience in treating such children and be willing to listen to the other members of the team who know the child and family well. It is important that decisions concerning surgical management are made using accurate information of function, and gait analysis will in the future fulfil a role in clarifying some of the problems (see later). Regular review gives a longitudinal view of the child's evolving motor pattern.

Children and parents need to know what to expect from surgery and be prepared for both short and long term aims. In general, healing takes 3 weeks for soft tissues and 6–12 weeks for bone. Strengthening will take 6–8 weeks from the time of healing. Gait retraining takes a year or more.

There are many detailed books on orthopaedic management in cerebral palsy—only general principles will be discussed here.

MANAGEMENT OF THE HIPS

The early management of the hips in children with cerebral palsy has been the subject of much debate over the years. A review article by Scrutton (1989) sets out the problem in detail. Hips that are normal at birth but not subject to the normal forces of weightbearing, or perhaps bear weight in nonfunctional stereotyped postures, are at risk of impaired structural development. Judicious and early soft tissue surgery can prevent most dislocations. The tendency to dislocate seems to be directly related to the severity of impairment within certain postural groups, and increases directly with persistence of the posture, degree of adduction, imbalance between adductor and abductor activity, and (probably) lack of early weightbearing. Children who never achieve independent sitting are particularly at risk.

In a review of 184 children with four-limb cerebral palsy referred for orthopaedic follow-up (without dislocation when referred) Scrutton (1989) concluded that a number of lessons could be learned, in particular: radiographs

163

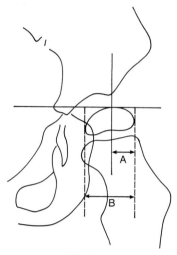

Fig. 9.1

should be taken at 1-year intervals, and reliance on clinical judgement of hip abduction can be deceptive.

The most important factor in hip stability was the age at pulling to stand. 130 of the 184 children had pulled to stand by 7½ years, and among those who had done so by 3 years, all but one (a child referred at 7 years) had a migration percentage (MP) of less than 50. The MP is the percentage of the femoral head uncovered by the acetabulum (Fig. 9.1). Among the children who had pulled to stand between 3 and 7½ years, four had an MP of more than 50, of which two had dislocated. No child learned to pull to stand after 7½ years. Thus among those who could pull to stand, less than 2% of hips were a continuing serious problem.

In contrast, among the children who never pulled to stand (20% of whom were diplegic), 26 hips (24%) of 17 children (31%) had an MP of more than 50. Of these 26 hips, 14 (13%) of 10 children (18.5%) were dislocated (6 of these children being referred between 5 and 8 years). This contrasts with overall figures of 3.8% of hips dislocated in 5.4% of all 184 children.

It seems clear that significant modelling of the acetabulum occurs in the first 3 or 4 years; this explains why soft tissue surgery is more effective if done in the early years, and also, perhaps, why children with acquired cerebral insults who have previously walked are much less likely to develop long-term dislocation problems. However, changes can occur up until maturity, especially during the adolescent growth spurt.

The importance of symmetrical positioning is discussed elsewhere (p. 126). Postoperative positioning is equally important following a period of postoperative fixation in a 'broomstick' plaster or hip abduction orthosis.

All four-limb cerebral palsy children, regardless of hip state, should be referred as young as possible to an orthopaedic surgeon with experience of young children with cerebral palsy. Early postural management by a physiotherapist is also essential (Scrutton 1989).

GAIT ANALYSIS

In the past decade gait analysis has been developed and refined, particularly in North America (Gage 1983, Sutherland et al 1988) but also in the UK (Patrick 1989). At present, gait laboratories are concentrated in a few centres but are likely to become increasingly available, providing impetus to better evaluation of gait problems and a more scientific approach to management. Gait analysis at its most sophisticated entails assessment using the following: videotape, linear measurements, kinematics, dynamic EMG, kinetics and energy assessment.

For some of us, videotape may be the only method available. It is useful in providing a sequential record, which can be repeatedly reviewed in slow motion and which permits some segregation of primary and secondary deviations. Primary deviations are the changes in gait caused by the neurological injury, and secondary deviations are those caused by the body's response to the deviant gait, e.g. trunk sway to compensate for hip weakness.

The aim of gait analysis is to assess the walking pattern in order to determine logical management, which may not necessarily be surgical. For example, the use of orthoses or footwear can be assessed.

The prerequisites of normal gait are: stance phase stability; swing phase foot clearance; appropriate pre-positioning of the foot in swing; an adequate step length; and energy conservation (Gage et al 1987).

It is likely that gait analysis will become more widely available and lead to gathering of information in cooperative research projects. The development of computer simulation of treatment may become possible via statistical pattern recognition and development of artificial intelligence and probability algorithms.

ORTHOPAEDIC MANAGEMENT OF DIPLEGIA

If contractures of the hips and knees have been acquired by the time weight-bearing and walking are established, they should probably be released. The timing of surgery depends on several factors; in general, it is better to wait until the gait reaches a plateau from the effects of maturation and growth. Patrick (1989) suggests that surgery should be delayed until after the age of 7 to allow for these effects.

Abduction can be improved by an open adductor tenotomy with anterior obturator neurectomy. This is obviously important if there is evidence of progressive subluxation of the hips as seen in serial radiographs (as discussed above). Simple valgus of the femoral neck and a break in Shenton's line are not in themselves indications for surgery, as any child with delay in weightbearing and limited walking will inevitably show these radiological features. Some surgeons prefer adductor transfer to simple release, particularly in the child with good walking potential. Iliopsoas release or recession should be considered if there is persistent fixed flexion at the hips after adductor release or transfer.

Many of the muscles of the thigh are acting on two joints. The *accelerators* provide the necessary power for movement; the *decelerators* are less important in cerebral palsy since these children walk slowly. *Stabilisers* are not usually involved in cerebral palsy unless they are overpowered by antagonists or have insufficient lever arm to work efficiently. Two-joint muscles probably never function appropriately in cerebral palsy but their function can often be enhanced if their action can be simplified or modified, e.g. transfer of the distal end of the rectus to sartorious (Gage et al 1987).

Persistent and disabling femoral anteversion may have to be dealt with by external rotation osteotomy, which involves a bony operation with internal fixation and usually 6 weeks in plaster. This should not normally be considered before the age of 10 years, otherwise recurrence is extremely common.

A tendency to flexion deformity at the knees may adequately be dealt with by serial plasters, gaiters or backslabs. In the presence of fixed flexion deformity, distal hamstring release is indicated. Occasionally, proximal hamstring release may be considered in the small group of patients who show very tight hamstrings, less than 30° straight leg raising, a short stride when walking, and less than 5° of fixed flexion at the knees with the hips extended.

It has been shown that persistent knee stiffness after hamstring lengthening may be caused by co-spasticity of rectus femoris; transfer may unlock the knee, improving the gait both cosmetically and in terms of energy conservation.

Management of equinus deformity

Dealing with flexion contractures at the hips and knees may be sufficient to correct equinus at the foot. The foot equinus may have been necessary, as the centre of gravity may be abnormally far forward due to the flexion of the trunk on the hips. In this situation, correction of the equinus by lengthening the tendo calcaneus makes walking more difficult and frequently impossible. Careful consideration of the child's necessity for various postural or fixed deformities for function, as well as assessment of alternative mechanisms, is required when contemplating surgery.

Valgus everted rocker-bottom foot

Once the equinus deformity has been overcome, the commonest foot deformity is the valgus everted rocker-bottom foot. The subtalar joint is always hypermobile in these children. The standard operation to stabilise the subtalar joint is the Grice subtalar arthrodesis, which can be carried out from the age of 4 years onwards. This is a bony operation and requires 2–3 months in plaster, often followed by support in an orthosis. Other options are discussed in the following section on hemiplegia.

Hallux valgus

In association with a pronated forefoot these children frequently develop increasingly troublesome hallux valgus. This can be corrected by osteotomy of the first metatarsal and release of the adductor hallucis from the base of the proximal phalanx of the big toe. This operation should probably be delayed until the age of 13 or 14 years unless absolutely necessary, otherwise recurrence with growth is likely to occur.

ORTHOPAEDIC MANAGEMENT OF HEMIPLEGIA

The greatest contribution of orthopaedics for the hemiplegic child is in the lower limb. In most cases the hip and knee deformities respond well to nonsurgical treatment and equinus remains the persistent problem. A below-knee plaster can be used very effectively to stretch the tendo calcaneus. The toes should be supported to prevent excessive flexion. The plaster is usually changed after 2–3 weeks and the child encouraged to stand and walk as much as possible. This can defer the need for surgery for some time and can be repeated with success. Once the contracture cannot be overcome under general anaesthetic, or recurs rapidly after plastering, then formal lengthening of the tendo calcaneus should be considered.

Elongation of the tendo calcaneus

Elongation of the tendo calcaneus by the slide method is the most commonly performed procedure. It is relatively simple, allows the child to stand and walk in the plasters 24–48 hours after operation, and only requires 4 weeks in plaster. Opinions vary about night splintage; in general, if there is good active dorsiflexion, prolonged night splintage is unnecessary, but if the dorsiflexors are weak then it is probably advisable.

Relief of equinus may be sufficient in itself to correct valgus or varus of the foot. If varus (the commoner deformity) persists and presents a functional difficulty, the tibialis posterior may be elongated or divided. Lateral transfer of the tibialis posterior is an attractive operation, but tends to lead to overcorrection of the foot with time, and should probably not be used. Recently, good results have been reported using a split tibialis posterior tendon transfer, which seems to avoid the problem of overcorrection seen with complete transfer. Valgus can be treated by elongating the peronei tendons and providing a medial arch support. If it persists a Grice-type extra-articular fusion of the subtalar joint can produce a stable and satisfactory result.

Compensation for shortening is always a consideration in the lower limb.

Traditionally 1.25 cm (½ inch) or less is ignored. More than this may be treated by raising the sole of the shoe. However, in a child who is using equinus deformity for support, this is merely a nuisance to be compensated for by further flexing the hip and knee. Raising the heel alone merely promotes equinus, but since this is often the most efficient posture for the hemiplegic child when 'abnormal' walking patterns are established, it might be accepted. Surgical lengthening is rarely if ever indicated.

Arm and hand

Proximal control as well as awareness of the hand should be present before any surgery is contemplated to hand or forearm.

Flexion/adduction deformities of the thumb may be prevented or deterred by the use of soft, firm plastic splints. Persistent abduction of the thumb can be corrected by releasing the thumb adductor from its origin on the metacarpals. Release of the permanently adducted thumb near or at maturity can be achieved by fusing the carpo-metacarpal joint.

Similarly, correction of fixed finger flexion contractures and forearm pronators can be achieved by mobilisation, release or transfer of appropriate muscles or tendons. This is usually a cosmetic procedure and is best performed after puberty. Release of persistent elbow flexion by a muscle slide is often also greatly appreciated from a cosmetic point of view.

Scoliosis may develop; its management is described in Chapter 22.

ORTHOPAEDIC MANAGEMENT OF SECONDARY STRUCTURAL DEFORMITY

Despite much handling and movement experience, secondary structural deformity, which may be damaging and painful, can develop (see Fig. 7.4) p. 121. It is here that the orthopaedic surgeon has most to offer. The major deformity in spastic quadriplegia involves the hips, which frequently take on the windswept position described as a result of the ATNR. The adducted hip is internally rotated and the abducted hip is externally rotated. The problem (if this position is maintained) is that the adducting hip becomes subluxed and then dislocated and painful. In addition the pelvis tilts up on the side of the adducting hip, leading to formation of a secondary scoliosis to the abducting side with further postural instability and pain. Early recognition and correction of an asymmetrical seating habit can postpone or even avoid surgery (see p. 426).

The adducted hip may be released with an open adductor tenotomy and anterior obturator neurectomy combined with release of the iliopsoas. If release of the iliopsoas is not performed, its flexed adducted position can produce increasing internal rotation and subluxation.

Persistent anteversion of the femoral neck occurs, probably as a result of lack of normal weightbearing, and supported standing should be encouraged from an early stage (see p. 138). Sometimes, if bony deformity has become too great, the severe anteversion of the femoral neck has to be corrected by external rotation osteotomy of the upper femur. Finally, if the hip is actually dislocated or is so severely subluxed that it cannot be relocated by soft tissue procedures, open reduction combined with femoral, and sometimes pelvic, osteotomy is necessary.

Early soft tissue surgery and the awareness of the dangers of leaving such a position may avoid this type of bony surgery. Some patients present with established dislocation and severe pain; if possible, the hip should be replaced in the socket, but sometimes the cartilage of the femoral head has been severely damaged and the socket is grossly dysplastic. In these patients it may be necessary to excise the upper end of the femur to below the level of the lesser trochanter, producing a flail hip, which is pain-free and can be positioned comfortably.

Rarely the surgeon is presented with a patient who has developed extreme extension and external rotation of the hips. This produces anterior subluxation of the hip with a characteristic bulge in the femoral triangle. These patients are in a parlous situation as they are usually unable to stand, and can only lie with their legs in the extended position. In such a case, excision of the upper end of the femur to below the lesser trochanter is probably the only way of getting mobile hips that allow the patient to sit up and be positioned in a chair. It is essential that at least the upper quarter of the femur is excised; otherwise, with time, the spasticity of the muscles will cause the femoral shaft to ride up, thus impinging on the pelvis and causing further problems with sitting and pain. Although this type of surgery may seem very major in often very severely handicapped children, results are extremely gratifying in terms of comfort for the patient and improvement in ease of management for the carers.

Flexion contractures of the knees are almost inevitable in children who spend most of their day sitting. Alternative positioning is important. They are not such a problem in a child who is not going to progress to standing and walking. However, sometimes the flexion contractures can become very gross with subluxation and distortion of the knee joints. If this cannot be controlled by conservative means, then excision of the hamstring tendons distally plus division of the two heads of the gastrocnemius muscle at the back of the knee is probably the only way of preventing recurrent flexion contractures at the knees.

Foot deformities in these patients do not usually require surgical correction unless the position of the foot is a great nuisance when the child is sitting in a chair.

REFERENCES

Gage J R 1983 Gait analysis for decision making in cerebral palsy. Bulletin Hospital for Joint Disease and Orthopaedics Institute 43: 147–163

Gage J R, Perry J, Hicks R R, Koop S, Werntz J R 1987 Rectus femoris transfer to improve knee function in children with cerebral palsy. Developmental Medicine and Child Neurology 29: 159–166

Patrick J 1989 Cerebral palsy diplegia: improvements for walking. British Medical Journal 299: 1115–1116

Scrutton D 1989 The early management of hips in cerebral palsy. Developmental Medicine and Child Neurology 31: 108–116

Sutherland D H, Olshen R A, Biden E N, Wyatt M P 1988 The development of mature walking. Clinics in Developmental Medicine 104/105. MacKeith Press, Blackwell Scientific, Oxford; J B Lippincott, Philadelphia

10. Cerebral palsy: medical problems and their management

G. T. McCarthy   R.D. Croft

SWALLOWING DIFFICULTIES

Swallowing difficulties and feeding problems are common early problems in cerebral palsy and may be the first indication of the diagnosis. If there is gross incoordination of swallowing, tube feeding may have to be instituted to prevent inhalation. Feeding may be very slow; it is important to give the mother help and support, especially if it is her first baby—otherwise this may be the first step in a cycle of failure. It is helpful to refer the baby to a speech therapist skilled in the management of feeding disorders at an early stage (see p. 27).

Gastro-oesophageal reflux is very common in infants with severe cerebral palsy. Its mechanism is not fully understood. Swallowing is normally coordinated with the motor activities of the oesophagus and the changes in tone of the oesophageal sphincter. A control centre in the medulla, with connections to the pons, cerebral cortex and brainstem motor nuclei, probably acts on the upper striated part of the oesophagus; the lower third is innervated via the autonomic nervous system. A recent study of the effects of cisapride, a drug which has been found to enhance gastric emptying and increase lower oesophageal sphincter pressure in neurologically normal subjects, showed a different response in children with cerebral palsy, suggesting that central mechanisms in such children are producing the uncoordinated sphincter mechanism (Brueton et al 1990).

Acid reflux may cause oesophagitis with ulceration and bleeding, which results in vomiting, pain and anaemia. Ulceration may be severe enough to cause perforation. The reflux may also be associated with silent reflex aspiration of stomach contents into the lungs, causing repeated pneumonia or nocturnal wheezing.

A sliding hiatus hernia may also develop and cause persistent problems unless diagnosed and treated. Investigations should include a barium swallow, chest radiograph and blood count.

Treatment. H_2-receptor blocking drugs such as cimetidine or ranitidine are indicated if there is oesophagitis or anaemia. The addition of an antacid containing alginates, e.g. *Gaviscon*, sometimes helps to protect against reflux oesophagitis. It is also important to treat the chronic anaemia and to carry out regular haemoglobin checks subsequently. It is rarely necessary to use anti-emetics. There is no ideal pharmacological treatment at present, but domperidone may be effective.

Surgical treatment is indicated in children with hiatus hernia who suffer chronic symptoms that are not influenced by adequate medical treatment. Fundal plication is carried out. This is major surgery involving the chest and abdomen, and should therefore not be undertaken lightly, but can be very helpful in carefully selected children.

The use of gastrostomy for children with severe swallowing problems is being increasingly advocated (see p. 175).

Sandifer syndrome is the association of hiatus hernia with torsion dystonia, and occurs in normal children. The movements disappear once the reflux is dealt with by antacids or surgery (Kinsbourne & Oxon 1964, Werlin et al 1980). Oesophageal reflux and hiatus hernia associated with athetosis may also increase the movement disorder.

CONSTIPATION

It is common for children with cerebral palsy to have problems with constipation (see Ch.15). This probably arises from a number of factors:

- Difficulty drinking sufficient volumes of fluid
- Loss of saliva from drooling
- Poor diet
- Abnormal posture, extension and muscle spasm making bowel emptying difficult
- There may also be central control areas, localised in the pons and acting on colonic and ano-rectal motility, which are damaged in children with cerebral palsy (Weber et al 1985).

Once established, the problem tends to be self-perpetuating unless measures are taken to reverse the vicious cycle. It is important for the child to be positioned correctly, sitting with the hips well flexed to prevent extension and associated spasm. The child must be well supported and feel secure, and be given privacy and time for bowel action.

Some children with severe spasticity have marked spasm of their anal sphincter, and suppositories may be needed to ensure a good bowel action. However, it is important to review management regularly as there is often change with maturity and the need for medication may become less.

BLADDER CONTROL

It is a common observation that children with spasticity may have difficulties with bladder control. This manifests itself in delayed acquisition of continence, urgency of micturition, giggle incontinence, difficulty initiating micturition on request, and sometimes urinary retention.

Urodynamic studies may show detrusor hyperreflexia, deficient vesico-urethral sensation or detrusor-sphincter dyssynergia (Drigo et al 1988). The mechanism of the problem may be central: a lesion in the cortico-pontine circuits results in deficit of voluntary control of the detrusor muscle with hyperreflexia—the disinhibited neurogenic bladder; a lower lesion at midbrain level is generally necessary for failure of coordination between the detrusor and external sphincter. It is suggested by the concomitant presence of signs of a brainstem lesion (absent pharyngeal and cough reflexes and difficulty in swallowing).

Usually a careful history of the problem, and explanation to parents is all that is required. They will then modify their management to cope with the difficulty. Occasionally the use of oxybutinin or other anticholinergic medication may be required to reduce the excess bladder activity. In children with episodes of urinary retention a muscle relaxant such as baclofen may be used to diminish perineal muscle tone.

NUTRITION AND GROWTH IN CEREBRAL PALSY

Children with cerebral palsy tend to be small. They are shorter, lighter and thinner than able-bodied children of the same age, and also than their able-bodied siblings. Many are underweight for their height. In infancy, linear growth is largely dependent upon nutrition, and children with cerebral palsy with feeding difficulty may fail to thrive. Height velocity after infancy is under growth hormone control. There is very little published data on the linear growth of children with cerebral palsy; in our experience they tend to have normal height velocities after infancy. Some of the the lighter, thinner children also have delayed puberty.

Stature and weight are related to degree of disability. Children with cerebral palsy who can walk independently tend to be shorter and lighter than able-bodied peers, but taller and heavier than those who are unable to walk independently. Children with severe motor disability are also more likely to be underweight for their height. At one extreme a child with a hemiplegia or diplegia may be below average or low normal in height, but well nourished. At the other end of the spectrum is the dependent spastic quadriplegic who is short but also underweight for his stature, emaciated, and with cold extremities, poorly developed musculature and short contracted limbs.

Obesity is uncommon in our experience but may occur in some non-ambulant children with good eating skills.

There appear to be two main factors affecting growth in cerebral palsy:

1. The degree of neurological involvement itself. Normal bone development partly depends on normal muscle tone and activity. It is not surprising therefore that children with severely impaired muscle tone and activity also have poorly developed bones with a corresponding reduction in length and weight of the body.

2. Poor food intake from a variety of causes. Children with impaired oral skills, little or no speech, and difficulty with chewing and swallowing are usually dependent upon care givers to choose and prepare food for them and put it into their mouths. They are unable to forage for snacks in the kitchen or the sweet shop and they rely upon their care-givers' skill and experience in interpreting their wishes and preferences.

The feeding difficulties may include poor lip closure, tongue thrust, or poor functional movements of the tongue. The child may find it difficult to form a bolus of food that is not spilled. The swallowing reflex is often delayed and pharyngeal peristalsis may be reduced. Gastro-oesophageal reflux or hiatus hernia may also be present (see p. 171). In severe cases children can take up to 20 times longer to eat a mouthful of food than a normal child. Perhaps for this reason children with cerebral palsy often have poor appetites, although some have voracious appetites that cannot be satisfied!

Another possible explanation for the poor nutritional state of some children with cerebral palsy is that they expend excessive amounts of energy either in athetoid movements or muscle spasm. It is certainly true that an activity such as walking is much more costly in terms of energy for children with cerebral palsy than for able-bodied children. It has also been shown that if their mechanical disadvantage is reduced by ortho-paedic surgery, the energy cost may be reduced. However, those who can walk are better nourished than those who cannot, doubtless because they can also eat well and are more able to meet their energy needs. Studies of oxygen consumption have not shown that children with cerebral palsy have a high metabolic rate. Basal metabolic rates were generally normal or low.

Management

Management of the nutritional problems in cerebral palsy should be directed towards treating gastro-oesophageal reflux, trying to improve oral skills, seating and diet.

Experience suggests that with time and effort oral skills will improve, and there is some research-based evidence to support this but there is a need for more information in this area.

There is evidence that adaptive seating improves some components of eating and drinking behaviour in cerebral palsy (see p. 160), such as head control, retention of food and drink in the mouth, and ability to eat solid food and drink from a cup. The social benefits of meals are also enhanced if children are well seated.

Improving dietary intake is more difficult. Intake is limited by mechanical factors already mentioned, but also by appetite. Food should be presented in an attractive way and served in a form that is easily eaten. Some children find mashed food much easier to eat than solid or lumpy food, and they are also less likely to cough and splutter whilst eating it. They need to be given sufficient mashed food to give them a reasonable calorie and protein intake. Much care, time and patience is required on the part of parents and caregivers, as a completely dependent child with poor oral skills may take an hour to finish a meal. It is important to keep it warm and palatable during that time.

We commonly recommend a protein/energy-dense dietary supplement, to be taken in milk, for children who have nutritional problems. This is best given at night to avoid depressing the appetite for main meals. It has been shown that it is possible to induce large weight gains in such children by nasogastric feeding for a few weeks (Patrick et al 1986). It is not clear, however, what the benefits of this are; for some children it can be an unpleasant and invasive procedure. Unless the weight gain represented functionally useful muscle it might be a disadvantage in terms of mobility.

There is also evidence to suggest that unless nutritional problems are tackled early, enteral feeding will not necessarily result in catch-up growth (Sanders et al 1990). Nevertheless there are some children who cannot eat or drink at all and they need to be fed by tube or gastrostomy. The recent introduction of a 'button gastrostomy', which can be introduced via an endoscope, may be a useful way of managing these children.

EPILEPSY IN CEREBRAL PALSY

Epilepsy occurs frequently in children with cerebral palsy. However, the various types of cerebral palsy are not equally associated with epilepsy; there is a higher incidence in children with quadriplegia and a lower incidence in those with dyskinesia and spastic diplegia, especially pre-term infants. Aicardi (1990) reviewed the subject in detail. Cerebral palsy associated with epilepsy is more likely to be accompanied by cognitive impairment and sensory handicaps.

Seizures that are prolonged and severe can cause further damage to the brain. However, the duration necessary to cause damage is not known.

Infantile spasms or salaam attacks

These are a form of generalised seizure which occur in babies and have a grave prognosis. 90% occur in the first year of life, and 60% in the first 6 months. The seizures follow a typical pattern of sudden flexion of the head and trunk with forward extension of the arms—as in a salaam. Less often the attacks are associated with extension. They usually occur in runs, often on waking or before sleep.

These seizures occur most often in babies with already damaged brains, particularly after anoxic–ischaemic encephalopathy, and are a further threat to development, as regression—particularly in visual and cognitive development—commonly occurs.

The EEG is diagnostic, showing hypsarrhythymia—'mountainous' waves. Treatment with ACTH or adrenal corticosteroids usually produces dramatic improvement, although recurrence often occurs after cessation of treatment. Benzodiazepine drugs—nitrazepam, clonazepam, and clobazam—are also effective. It is usual to start them at the same time as the steroids which are then tailed off. Sodium valproate also gives good results in some cases.

Infantile spasms tend to remission by the age of 2 years, but are often replaced by other forms of epilepsy.

Other types of seizures associated with cerebral palsy

Partial seizures are especially common in children with brain damage and often progress to secondary generalised seizures. Complex partial seizures also occur, with temporal lobe and psychomotor features.

Generalised seizures are not uncommon in cerebral palsy. Often with a focal onset, they may occur relatively infrequently, and a decision to start anticonvulsant medication needs full discussion with parents and other carers. For example, a child who has one seizure every 6 months may be managed with rectal diazepam as required.

Myoclonic seizures are a form of generalised epilepsy in which a sudden jerk of the whole body, or isolated muscle group, occurs. The attacks may be precipitated by a sharp or unexpected sound or flashing lights. The EEG shows atypical spike and wave discharges.

Focal myoclonus occurs in children with cortical dysplasia (Kuzniecky et al 1988).

Gelastic seizures occur with hamartomata of the third ventricle (Berkovic et al 1988).

Startle seizures are common in children with congenital hemiparesis due to cortical atrophy.

Partial continuous epilepsy may occur occasionally; one side of the body or one limb is involved and a progressive hemiplegia and 'shrinking cortex' may occur.

Petit mal absences are uncommon in children with cerebral palsy, though the term is often erroneously used to describe other types of brief attack. Loss of consciousness for a few seconds occurs without associated motor symptoms other than blinking of the eyes. The EEG is diagnostic: 3 Hz spike and wave discharges are seen over the frontal lobes. The attacks can often be induced by hyperventilating.

Management and therapeutic aspects

Aicardi (1990) states that three questions arise with respect to the influence of brain injury on management:

- Does the brain damage influence the manner of treating and the result of therapy?
- Does the treatment of seizures have any effect on the associated brain dysfunction?
- Does treatment prevent the occurrence of further brain damage?

Drug treatment for epilepsy

Drug treatment of epilepsy (Table 10.1) is usually very effective and not necessarily long term. Parents are often anxious about the side-effects of drugs and it is necessary to spend time discussing treatment and regularly reviewing drug dosage. It is important to understand that frequent seizures, even when they are relatively minor in nature, may have an effect on attention and learning.

Carbamazepine is the drug of first choice for partial and secondarily generalised seizures. It should be introduced slowly to prevent sedation and dizziness, giving a half dose in the evening for the first few days and gradually bringing the dose to a therapeutic level. Carbamazepine interacts with phenytoin, which causes the carbamazepine level to fall although its active metabolite remains unaltered. There is also interaction with the antibiotic erythromycin: the carbamazepine level rises and may move into the toxic range with a paradoxical increase in seizures. Carbamazepine levels can be checked meaningfully after 48 hours of changing dosage.

Phenytoin is a very effective anticonvulsant but has a more sedative effect than carbamazepine. The side-effects of gum hypertrophy, hirsutism, coarsening of the facies and reduction of plasma calcium make it less attractive for use in children. There is also a relatively narrow therapeutic window, and toxic effects of ataxia, nystagmus, slurred speech and blurred vision may be more difficult to detect in children who already have neurological problems. It is important to monitor drug levels at intervals and to

Table 10.1   Drugs for the treatment of epilepsy (from Aicardi 1988, with permission)

Epilepsy type	*Drugs*	
Partial seizures, primary or secondarily generalised tonic–clonic seizures	1st-line	— carbamazepine, phenytoin, phenobarbitone, primidone
	2nd-line	— sodium valproate/valproic acid, clonazepam, chlorazepate, acetazolamide
	3rd-line	— mephenytoin, phenacemide, ethoin, methsuximide, bromides
Absence seizures, juvenile myoclonic epilepsy, myclonic or atonic seizures	1st-line	— ethosuximide, sodium valproate/valproic acid
	2nd-line	— clonazepam, acetazolamide, methsuximide, primidone
	3rd-line	— trimethadione, nitrazepam, paramethadione
Infantile spasms	1st-line	— ACTH, corticosteroids
	2nd-line	— sodium valproate/valproic acid, nitrazepam, clobazam, clonazepam.

avoid multiple drugs if at all possible. Phenytoin takes 10–14 days to reach steady state levels after a change in dosage.

Sodium valproate is a very effective drug for myoclonic epilepsy and also generalised epilepsy. It may cause gastric irritation, an increase in appetite and occasionally hair loss. It has caused toxic effects in the liver in rare cases in young children who were also on other anticonvulsants. Blood drug levels are not very useful for valproate because of the short half-life and a wide range between the therapeutic and toxic dose.

Other useful drugs are listed in Table 10.1; there are also some new anticonvulsants being introduced, e.g. vigabatrin and lamotrigine, which may well have a place in the management of children with intractable seizures.

Rectal diazepam may be given to prevent prolongation of seizures to status epilepticus. The diazepam is absorbed rapidly from the rectal mucosa, giving a blood level similar to an intravenous injection. It should be given if a generalised seizure lasts longer than four to five minutes. The dose may safely be repeated once, if unsuccessful; or, if there are signs of respiratory depression, paraldehyde may be given by deep intramuscular injection. Phenytoin or chlomethiazole may be given intravenously if status epilepticus continues. It is important to monitor respirations and ventilate if necessary.

Prognosis for children with cerebral palsy and epilepsy

Brorson & Wranne (1987) showed that, after 12 years of observation, 63% of children with epilepsy and either cerebral palsy or mental retardation were seizure free, as were 37% of those with both conditions. However, failure of medical treatment is common among children with extensive brain damage and these are potential candidates for surgical treatment. Temporal lobectomy and hemispherectomy have been used successfully in such cases depending on the size, location of damage, and the presence or absence of hemiplegia. Longitudinal section of the corpus callosum is being used increasingly in the treatment of epilepsy associated with secondary generalised seizures and for the treatment of epilepsy associated with hemiplegia (Andermann et al 1988).

USE OF DRUGS IN CEREBRAL PALSY

The long-term use of drugs in cerebral palsy is rarely justified. However, in certain situations drugs can be helpful, e.g. on introduction of orthoses or for treatment of postoperative or nocturnal spasm.

Baclofen acts mainly as a gamma-aminobutyric acid (GABA) agonist (mimic) in the spinal cord, blocking the excitatory effects of the sensory input from limb muscles. It is most useful in the treatment of spinal spasticity but can also be used in cerebral palsy where there is very severe spasm. It may make children extremely hypotonic and less functional. It may also aggravate a tendency to urinary incontinence, cause headaches and confusion, and exacerbate epilepsy. In children the starting dose should be low: 5–10 mg in divided doses. It may be used at night for the relief of flexor spasms.

Diazepam Probably acts by enhancing the response to locally released GABA. Its action on the spinal cord is independent of any action in the brain, although doses that reduce muscle tone are often sedative. It has a longer action than baclofen, and the sedative effect can be overcome by giving a single daily dose at bedtime; it is particularly useful for night spasms.

Dantrolene acts directly on skeletal muscle, producing relaxation at the muscle fibre level. It is considered the drug of choice in adults with severe spasm. However, it is not licensed in the UK for use in children. Side-effects include drowsiness, weakness, fatigue and occasionally urinary or musculoskeletal disturbances.

SELECTIVE POSTERIOR RHIZOTOMY

Selective posterior rhizotomy is a neurosurgical procedure which was first used 100 years ago to reduce spasticity. It has become repopularised for patients with spastic cerebral palsy in North America due to refinements in technique. Peacock et al (1990) reviewed the state of the art. The rationale of treatment is the reduction of spasticity by selective division of posterior nerve rootlets from L2 to L5. The selection of abnormal rootlet responses is made by stimulating them electrically, and abnormal rootlets are divided.

Patients selected are those with spastic diplegia who can walk independently. Children with spastic quadriplegia in whom spasticity is interfering with positioning, function or care are also being considered. This procedure may be a useful addition to management but clearly needs to be carried out in centres equipped to evaluate and select children accurately, as in the wrong hands irreversible damage can result.

DOPA-RESPONSIVE DYSTONIA

It is important to be alert to the possibility of an alternative cause for a motor disorder labelled as cerebral palsy, especially in cases that appear to be progressive and where the onset of the gait disorder occurs after walking has been attained. Although this condition is rare it is one that is treatable. 86 cases have been reported in the literature (Boyd & Patterson 1989).

The classical features are:

- Normal development initially
- Onset of walking problem, often with asymmetrical signs
- Increasing dystonia—toe walking

- Clear diurnal fluctuation, worse in the evening, occurs in about one third of cases
- Loss of walking ability and progression to involving trunk and arms
- Dramatic, sustained response to levodopa
- Female preponderance.

The condition was first described by Segawa et al (1976). It is thought to be associated with a deficiency of biopterin (Fink et al 1988).

LESCH–NYHAN SYNDROME

Another rare disorder commonly misdiagnosed in the early stages is the Lesch–Nyhan Syndrome. It is an X-linked condition caused by an inborn error of purine metabolism. There is usually no evidence of perinatal insult and the first signs are of motor developmental delay with marked hypotonia which evolves into athetoid cerebral palsy. The classical sign of compulsive self-mutilation does not usually manifest itself until around the age of 2 years. The other sign of 'sand in the diaper' was described by Lesch & Nyhan (1964). This is caused by the precipitation of crystals in the urine, which are usually a mixture of urates and other purine metabolites.

The enzyme defect results in a failure of the normal chain reaction that should occur in the metabolism of protein. There is a build up of uric acid in the blood, and also xanthine and hypoxanthine. These are excreted in the urine and may cause renal damage, producing renal calculi. It is possible to lower the concentration of uric acid in the blood by giving allopurinol, a drug that is also used in gout. However, it is important to give the correct dosage, as the metabolite of allopurinol—oxipurinol—may also precipitate out in the urine and cause calculi and renal damage.

REFERENCES

Aicardi J 1988 Clinical approach to the management of intractable epilepsy. Developmental Medicine and Child Neurology 30: 429–440
Aicardi J 1990 Epilepsy in brain injured children. Developmental Medicine and Child Neurology 32: 191–202
Andermann F, Olivier A, Gotman J, Sergent J 1988 Callosotomy for the treatment of patients with intractable epilepsy and the Lennox–Gastaut syndrome. In: Niedermeyer E, Degen R (eds) The Lennox–Gastaut Syndrome. Alan R Liss, New York, p. 361–376
Berkovic S F, Andermann F, Melanson D et al 1988 Hypothalamic hamartomas and ictal laughter: evolution of a characteristic epileptic syndrome and diagnostic value of magnetic resonance. Annals of Neurology 23: 429–439
Boyd K, Patterson V 1989 Dopa responsive dystonia: a treatable condition misdiagnosed as cerebral palsy. British Medical Journal 298: 1019–1020
Brorson L 0, Wranne L 1987 Long term prognosis in childhood epilepsy: survival and seizure prognosis. Epilepsia 28: 324–330
Brueton M J, Clarke G S, Sandhu B K 1990 The effects of cisapride on gastro-oesophageal reflux in children with and without neurological disorders. Developmental Medicine and Child Neurology 32(7): 629–633
Drigo P, Seren F, Artibani W, Laverda A M, Battestella P A, Zacchello G 1988 Neurogenic

vesico-urethral dysfunction in children with cerebral palsy. Italian Journal of Neurological Science 9: 151–154

Fink J M, Barton N, Cohen W, Lovenberg W, Burns R S, Hallet M 1988 Dystonia with marked diurnal variation associated with biopterin deficiency. Neurology 38: 707–711

Gisel E, Patrick J 1988 Identification of children with cerebral palsy unable to maintain a normal nutritional state. Lancet 1: 283–285

Kinsbourne M, Oxon D M 1964 Hiatus hernia with contortions of the neck. Lancet 1: 1058–1061

Kuzniecky R, Berkovic S, Andermann F, Melanson D, Olivier A, Robitaille Y 1988 Focal cortical myoclonus and Rolandic cortical dysplasia: clarification by magnetic resonance imaging. Annals of Neurology 23: 317–325

Lesch M, Nyhan W L 1964 A familial disorder of uric acid metabolism and central nervous system function. American Journal of Medicine 36: 561–570

Mathisen B, Skuse D, Wolke D, Reilly S 1989 Oral motor dysfunction and failure to thrive among inner-city infants. Developmental Medicine and Child Neurology 31: 293–302

Patrick J, Boland M P, Murray G E et al 1986 Rapid correction of wasting in children with cerebral palsy. Developmental Medicine and Child Neurology 28: 724–739

Peacock W J, Staudt L A et al 1990 Spasticity in cerebral palsy and the selective posterior rhizotomy procedure. Journal of Child Neurology 5: 179–185

Sanders K D, Cox K, Cannon R, Blanchard D, Pitcher J, Papathakis P, Varella L, Maughan R 1990 Growth response to enteral feeding by children with cerebral palsy. Journal of Parenteral and Enteral Nutrition 14(1): 23–26

Segawa M, Hosaka A, Miyagawa F, Nomura Y, Imai H 1976 Hereditary progressive dystonia with marked diurnal fluctuation. Advances in Neurology 14: 215–233

Segawa M, Nomura Y, Kase M 1988 Diurnally fluctuating hereditary progressive dystonia. In: Vinken P J, Bruyn G W, Klawaris H L (eds) Handbook of neurology. Amsterdam Elseveir Science, vol. 5, p. 529–539

Weber J, Denis P, Mihout B, Muller J M, Blanquart F, Galmiche J P, Simon P, Pasquis P 1985 Effect of brain-stem lesion on colonic and ano-rectal motility. Digestive Diseases and Sciences 30(5): 419–425

Werlin S L, D'Souza B J, Hogan W J, Dodds W J, Arndorfer R C 1980 Sandifer syndrome: an unappreciated clinical entity. Developmental Medicine and Child Neurology 22: 374

11. Conductive education

G.T. McCarthy   M. F. Martin

Conductive education (CE) was developed by Professor András Petö in Hungary after the Second World War. He had worked in rehabilitation and psychiatry, and after the war he requested facilities to work with motor disordered children (Cottam & Sutton 1986). He lived and worked with small groups of children developing a programme of education which included teaching motor skills as an integral part of the educational process. To avoid the division of disciplines he created a new professional—the *conductor*; to create the best milieu for learning, repetition and reinforcement he organised the children into homogeneous groups; and to enable the children to learn the movements and skills necessary for daily living he originated a specific learning method—'rhythmical intention' (Cotton 1965–1974).

The National Motor Therapy Institute opened in Budapest in 1952. After much hard work the method was finally accepted by the Ministry of Education in 1963, and a system of conductor training was officially established.

On Professor Petö's death, his assistant Dr Mária Hári became Director of the Institute. The new András Petö Institute for Motor Disorders was opened in Budapest in 1985.

A great deal of misunderstanding has arisen about conductive education since it was given publicity by the news media in the mid 1980s. This has led to considerable anguish for some families who feel they must follow every possible avenue of treatment for their child. Nevertheless it does have a number of unique aspects and is an excellent method of overcoming motor disorder for those children who have sufficient potential to do so. The major difficulty is in defining the early signs that give us that information.

Perhaps more important to professionals working with motor disordered children is the philosophy of expectation and enthusiasm, hard work and centralisation of effort through one person, which has much to recommend it. Its other important philosophy, which should be adopted for all children with motor disorders, however severe, is to make the child responsible for his own movement in order to function; the motto of the Institute is 'Not because, but in order to'.

KEY ELEMENTS OF CONDUCTIVE EDUCATION

Early intervention

The School for Parents is available for all motor disordered children in Hungary who are referred to the Institute for assessment. There is a selection process carried out by the conductors within the school for parents unless the child is thought to be unsuitable according to a number of stated criteria, such as orthopaedic deformity, or profound mental handicap with seizure disorder. The principle of early work with families is clear.

Mothers are taught how to handle their child by being shown how to carry out the programme practically. They are encouraged to carry out the programme daily for 2 or 3 hours. The mothers and children are admitted for 2–3 week sessions at regular intervals, or attend daily if they live in Budapest. The conductor decides whether babies are suitable for CE by a process called conductive observation. This seems to be an assessment of the child's willingness to learn, attention, persistence, and 'contact', i.e. eye contact and level of alertness. *Early intervention is thought to develop body image, self-concept and spatial awareness, leading to a concept of mobility.* In Budapest the children are admitted to the kindergarten at the age of about 3 years.

The conductor

The conductor is a professional person who has undergone a 4 year training encompassing (among other subjects) education, child development, physical therapy, neurology, psychology, speech therapy and music. The training is both theoretical and practical: the students work in the Institute alongside trained conductors for half of each day. The conductor's certificate is considered equivalent to a university degree.

The group

Group work is used to encourage the children, who develop a very strong group identity. The motivation provided by the group is almost tangible: the children form strong attachments to their friends and the conductors working with them. The group works as a family for the children in some respects, and when they return home for holidays they may exhibit behavioural problems not seen in the Institute.

The children are not grouped according to the type of cerebral palsy they have. The essence of the group is the strength of the emotional bond that is forged between the children themselves and with the conductors. To work well the group must be balanced so that the children have something to aim for, both physical and intellectual. The members of a the group share the same educational aims and work towards common goals. They work towards these in a series of small steps within a task series. The task series

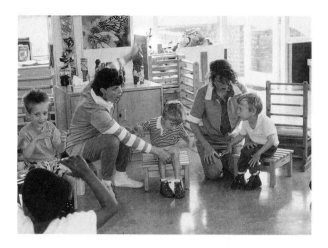

Fig.11.1   Group activity with young children encourages participation.

provides the framework for problem-solving for the individual child. It encourages the child to take the initiative, to be active, and to be encouraged by small successes to inch forward (Fig. 11.1).

The daily programme is worked out for the group and the individual child. The day is planned so that the group moves from one activity to the next. The individual programme encompasses short and long term aims from waking to sleeping, and each child's individual needs should be met in the programme and integrated in the group. Always the aim is to hand over responsibility to the child.

Rhythmical intention

Speech is used to guide action, at first spoken aloud and later internalised. The use of speech to direct function and behaviour is a distinctive feature of conductive education. Speech has an important role in the 'stage theory' of human development proposed by Vygotsky and further tested by Luria and others (Jernqvist 1985, Luria 1979, Luria & Yudovich 1959). Both motor and semantic aspects of speech are used for self regulation. Motor regulation precedes semantic regulation and external speech is followed by inner speech.

The task series

The task series may be looked on as a pyramid: at the base are the functions already achieved, and at the apex are the goals almost achieved. The child builds upon his achievements. The importance of having immediate results is stressed.

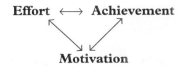

Effort ⟷ **Achievement**

Motivation

Each part of the day is used for learning, in the complex programme that shapes the daily routine. Common goals are shared, although individual methods of achieving the goal will vary. The programme directs all the conductors within the group on methods of facilitation required by specific children and in specific situations. This assures consistency and continuity of teaching (Todd 1990).

Orthofunction

This is a concept of completeness of the person despite continuing disability. It combines physical, psychological and social aspects. Orthofunction is the determination to succeed, which equips the person with the physical and mental capacity to live and blend into the home, school or work environment. It is the general capacity for adaptation or learning (Hári & Akós 1971).

THE BASIC MOTOR PATTERN

The notion of the basic motor pattern was first explained by Cotton (1980) and grew out of her intimate knowledge of normal development and motor dysfunction, and later her encounter with Petö. However, the basic motor pattern must not be confused with conductive education, which is a much more comprehensive approach to neurological dysfunction.

The basic motor pattern can be defined as the minimum physical requirement to perform all tasks. A motor pattern is a series of movements—which develop through trial, error and practice—used to perform a task. The movements are performed in a coordinated harmonious manner. Motor patterns flow smoothly from one to another, and so an individual's movement or task performance is known as 'kinetic melody' (Bernstein 1967). The brain is not aware of separate muscle actions, but only of the goal; therefore it follows that each individual's motor patterns will vary according to size, shape, age, etc. although the goal remains the same.

The basic motor pattern in normal development

By 5 months a normal baby will be content to lie in supine and play with his hands and feet in the midline. He can reach and grasp, stretch his arms, bend his hips, and fix one part while moving another. As the baby matures a similar combination of movements can be seen in sitting, when he supports himself on extended arms or plays. The process of becoming a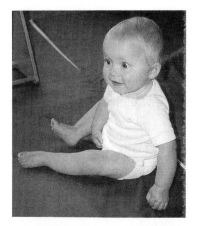

b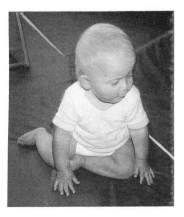

c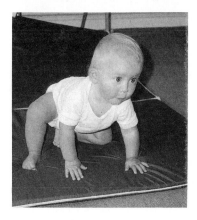

Fig. 11.2a, b and c. A normal baby at 10 months demonstrating the ease of movement, which allows acquisition and generalisation of motor skills.

upright means the hand is used again to reach and grasp, and the extended arm to prop before the hips extend from 90° too upright. The baby will practise the basic motor pattern endlessly at all levels, thus acquiring and generalising the skill (Fig. 11.2).

The development of the baby with cerebral palsy is interrupted by abnormalities of tone and persistent nonfunctional reflexes. He has ineffective grasp and lacks fixation, so is unable to move one part while keeping the other still. He cannot extend his elbows and flex his hips, nor is he able to keep his head in the midline and sustain his gaze.

Observation and analysis of any simple function—grasp and release, fixation, midline orientation, extension of the arms with hip mobility—will reinforce the need for the basic motor pattern. Each part of the basic motor pattern has an influence on another. When active extension of the elbows is learned, hip mobility will follow. If grasp and release can be learned, then fixation, midline orientation, mobility and a change in the motor pattern can be achieved.

To move in a coordinated fashion it is necessary to fix one part while moving another. The finer the movement required, the greater the fixation, e.g. threading a needle is more successful with the elbows bent and held by the sides than with elbows extended. In studying motor patterns it becomes clear that there must be a minimum requirement for simple tasks of daily living. This requirement comprises the abilities to:

- Flex one joint while extending another—with hip flexion and elbow extension paramount
- Grasp and release
- Fix one part while moving another
- Maintain symmetry in the midline
- Look and sustain gaze.

Children achieve a basic motor pattern through normal development, which can roughly be divided into three stages:

1. Asymmetry—reflex, life-saving, nonfunctional
2. Symmetry—functional
3. Asymmetry—functional

However, the child with cerebal palsy must be taught and learn the basic motor pattern in order to achieve not only physical but academic goals.

REFERENCES

Bernstein N A 1967 The co-ordination and regulation of movement. Pergamon Press, Oxford.
Cottam P J, Sutton A 1986 Conductive education: A system for overcoming motor disorder. Croom Helm, London
Cotton E 1965–1974 Conductive education and cerebral palsy. Spastics Society, London
Cotton E 1980 The basic motor pattern. Spastics Society, London
Hári M, Akós K 1971 Conductive education. English translation published by Routledge 1988
Hári M 1975 Scientific studies on conductive pedagogy. Conductor's College, Budapest
Jernqvist L 1985 Speech regulation of motor acts as used by cerebral palsied children. Götebourg Studies in Educational Sciences 54
Luria A R 1979 The making of mind. Edited by Cole M & Cole S, Harvard University Press
Luria A R, Yudovich F A 1959 Speech and development of the mental processes of the child. Staples Press, London
Robinson R O R, McCarthy G T, Little T M 1989 Conductive education at the Petö Institute, Budapest. British Medical Journal 1145–1149
Todd J E 1990 Conductive education: The continuing challenge. Physiotherapy 76(1): 13–16

FURTHER READING

Cotton E The hand as a guide to learning. Spastics Society, London
Read J 1988 Come wind, come weather. A study of the difficulties faced by British families taking children to the Petö Institute in Budapest. Warwick Department of Applied Social Studies, University of Warwick

12. Spina bifida

G.T. McCarthy   R. Cartwright   M. Jones   J.A. Fixsen

Spina bifida is a developmental defect caused by failure of fusion of the neural tube early in embryological life, around the 28th day. It is one of the conditions known as neural tube defects, which are among the commonest handicapping conditions of childhood. Hydrocephalus develops in about 80% of children with spina bifida (see Ch.13).

The prevalence of neural tube defects began to decline in England and Wales after 1972. From 1972 to 1981 to 1989 the national notification rate fell from 1.47 per 1000 live and stillbirths to 0.39 to 0.05 for anencephaly, and from 1.88 to 1.04 to 0.2 per 1000 for spina bifida (Leck 1983, OPCS 1991). Prenatal diagnosis and terminations of pregnancy have had some effect on prevalence. However, the number of legal terminations of pregnancy for fetal malformations of the central nervous system have also fallen. In 1985 Cuckle et al (1989) estimated that the decline in prevalence was 32% after the effect of screening was taken into account. 15 years ago Great Britain had the second highest birth prevalence of neural tube defects in the world. Now it has one of the lowest rates.

GENETICS

There is known to be a genetic element, which is multifactorial with a risk of a second affected child being 1 in 20, and with a similar risk of the affected person passing the defect on. After two affected children the risk rises to 1 in 10, and after three as high as 1 in 4. Multi-centre trials using multivitamins and folic acid (e.g. Pregnavite Forte F) suggested that prevention of neural tube defects is possible (Smithells et al 1981, 1983, 1989). Final confirmation that folic acid is the protective agent was obtained in a multicentre trial reported in *The Lancet* by Wald et al (1991): *'Folic acid supplementation starting before pregnancy can now be firmly recommended for all women who have had an affected pregnancy.'*

The neural tube may be affected anywhere along its length. If the forebrain fails to develop, anencephaly ensues and this is not compatible with life. Failure of fusion of the neural tube is associated with defective closure of the vertebral canal and often with other defects of the base of the brain, classified as the Arnold–Chiari malformation, in which there is herniation of the medulla and often cerebellar herniation through the foramen magnum (see Fig. 13.1, p. 214).

The commonest position of a spina bifida lesion is the thoracolumbar region, followed by the lumbosacral, thoracic and cervical regions. Spina bifida occulta describes a lesion which is hidden from view. Skin covers the vertebral defect, which is usually a simple failure of fusion of one or more of the posterior vertebral arches in the lumbosacral region. A defect limited to a single vertebra, usually L5 or S1, can be regarded as a normal variant (Laurence 1969). If there is an associated lipomatous mass or a hairy patch or naevus, or skin dimple, then the underlying spinal cord may be abnormal, and occult spinal dysraphism may be present.

SPINA BIFIDA CYSTICA (APERTA)

Meningocoele (Fig. 12.1a). The meninges form a sac lined by arachnoid membrane and dura containing cerebrospinal fluid (CSF) and, rarely, a small amount of nervous tissue. It is relatively uncommon (4% of cases of

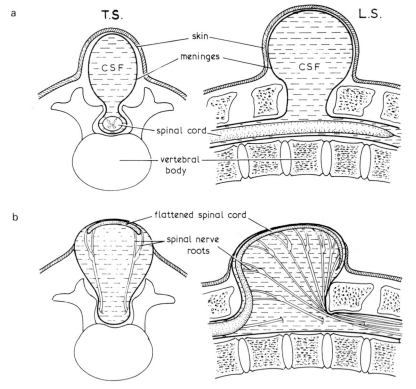

Fig. 12.1a. Meningocoele **b.** Myelomeningocoele.

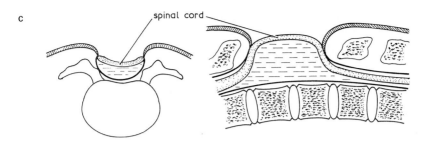

Fig. 12.1c. Rachischisis.

spina bifida cystica) and may be associated with cutaneous lesions. The skin over the sac is usually intact.

Myelomeningocoele (Fig. 12.1b). The neural tube is closed and covered by a membrane centrally and skin peripherally, but the spinal cord and all the nerve roots are outside the vertebral canal. In many cases there are associated anomalies of the cord with dilatation of the central canal, lipomata and other associated neural defects such as split cord or tethering of nerve roots.

In *rachischisis* there is no sac, and the spinal cord is flattened and lies wide open on the surface (Fig. 12.1c).

ASSESSMENT OF THE NEONATE WITH SPINA BIFIDA APERTA

Whether or not a policy of selection is carried out, all babies with spina bifida should be examined by a paediatrician or paediatric surgeon with experience in assessing such babies and in their long-term management.

Neurological examination

The purpose of the examination is to determine, as far as possible, the level at which normal cord function ceases, and to assess the presence and degree of hydrocephalus.

Skull

The skull should be examined and the sutures and fontanelle palpated for evidence of distension and increased pressure. Measurement of the occipito frontal circumference (OFC) should be carried out, and eye movements noted by stimulation of the optokinetic responses.

Cranial nerves

The cranial nerves should be assessed:

1. Observe the movements of the eyes; visual responses to the face, a brightly coloured ball and light; pupil reactions and optic fundi. Optic

nerve damage and oculomotor (particularly 6th nerve) palsies can occur if the intracranial pressure is high.

2. Observe facial movements and those of the tongue and palate; watch the baby suck. Occasionally, bulbar problems can arise in the newborn period, especially immediately after back closure if hydrocephalus begins to develop more rapidly and there is pressure on the Arnold–Chiari malformation.

Spine

The spine should be palpated along its length as sometimes there are multiple lesions that are not all obvious. The length and width of the lesion should be measured and the position on the spine noted.

Limbs

The presence of active movements of the limbs should be looked for by stimulating the legs and eliciting neonatal reflexes. The power of the muscles may be assessed by making them operate both with and without gravity and with and without resistance, and it is useful to make a muscle chart. Deformities such as talipes and congenital dislocation of the hip should be looked for.

Bowel and bladder

Sphincter tone and bladder function should be assessed and the anal reflex tested by stroking with an orange stick. A patulous anus and dribbling incontinence are associated with a lesion at the level of sacral S2–4. Retention of urine is associated with a lesion at S1.

Sensory level

This is taken as the first dermatome of normal sensation above the area of anaesthesia. It may be difficult to elicit a sensory level in a baby, but easier in the newborn than later. If the baby is asleep, or awake and quiet, it is possible to produce a level by stimulation with a pin, starting at the lower sacral territory—perianal region, buttocks, thighs and legs—and moving upwards over successive dermatomes of the anterior surface and on to the abdomen. The level at which general arousal occurs is noted. The sensory level may give important information on future prognosis. Hunt (1990), in a long-term study of unselected cases of open spina bifida, showed that the sensory level was the best predictor of long-term outcome provided no serious complications occurred later. Occasionally there is asymmetry between the two sides of the body.

Radiological examination of the skull, spine and hips should be carried out, and bacteriological swabs taken from the sac and umbilicus.

Types of lesion

At birth, two types of lesion are recognisable (Stark and Baker 1967):

Type 1 (one-third of patients). There is complete loss of the spinal cord function below a certain segmental level, which results in sensory loss and absent reflexes. These infants have characteristic deformities of muscle imbalance, the deformity depending on the level of the lesion.

Type 2 (two-thirds of patients). Associated with interruption of the corticospinal tracts. There is preservation of purely reflex activity in isolated distal segments.

There are three subgroups:

Subgroup A. Below the level of spinal cord involvement there is a segment with flaccid paralysis and sensory and reflex loss and, below this, isolated cord function with reflex activity and spasticity. Toe clonus may be striking (Fig. 12.2).

Subgroup B. A flaccid segment is almost absent and, therefore, there is virtually complete spinal cord transection with only reflex activity below the level of the lesion (Stark and Drummond 1971) (Fig. 12.3).

Subgroup C. Incomplete transection of the long tracts occurs, so the child has a spastic paraplegia with some preservation of voluntary movements and sensation. There is also a small group of patients (5%) with a hemi-myelomeningocoele, in whom one leg is more or less normal, but the other leg is affected by a Type 1 or 2 lesion.

On the basis of evidence of clinical and electrodiagnostic studies, it

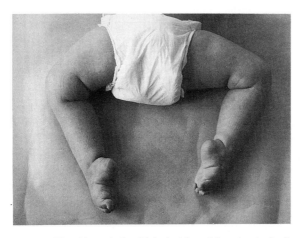

Fig. 12.2   Flaccid paralysis with isolated cord function in the feet.

a

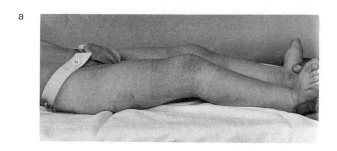

b

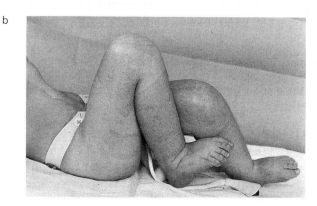

Fig. 12.3   Marked reflex flexor activity: **a.** Legs held. **b.** Legs released. No active muscle power.

is likely that paralysis in myelomeningocoele is due to a lesion of the upper motor neurone (UMN) rather than the lower motor neurone (LMN). In high lesions the UMN lesion tends to occur above the plaque. In low lesions it may occur elsewhere, e.g. within the plaque itself. The UMN lesion may be a primary developmental anomaly, but is more likely to be related to secondary changes occuring before, during or shortly after birth.

SELECTION FOR TREATMENT

The early management of spina bifida cystica has been the subject of debate and changing policies over the last 30 years. In the 1960s early back closure was advocated as a matter of urgency and the insertion of ventriculo-atrial shunts for control of hydrocephalus. This was followed by numerous operations to straighten limbs and relocate dislocated hips. This policy was reviewed in the early 1970s when a number of papers were published, starting with Lorber (1971), advocating the need for selection of cases for early treatment. Major adverse criteria were defined relating to later predictable physical handicaps:

1. *The degree of paralysis.* The greater the paralysis, the worse the

prognosis—not only in terms of mobility, but also IQ, associated spinal deformity, and severe renal complications.

2. *Excessive head circumference.* If the infant's head circumference is at or over the 90th centile at birth and disproportionate to weight, the degree of hydrocephalus is usually gross, with poor prognosis in terms of IQ.

3. *Kyphosis.* Kyphosis present at birth has a very poor outlook in terms of later severe deformity, paralysis and incontinence.

4. *Associated gross congenital anomalies* such as heart disease and severe birth injury are of the gravest prognostic significance.

It is now clear that there are different survival rates, which can in large part be related to the severity of the neurological lesion (Hunt 1990). It is also evident that the criteria being applied for selection relate not to mortality, but to morbidity, whether they are primarily physical or intellectual (Evans et al 1985). Since the urgency of back closure has not been established, a rational approach is to select those children for early closure who, on established criteria, are likely to be minimally handicapped.

Children with more severe lesions can be treated more conservatively; this allows time for proper evaluation of the baby and discussion with the parents who will bear the burden of care (Guthkelch 1986). The back lesion is dressed and hydrocephalus treated if it becomes necessary, or at 3–4 months when the back lesion epithelialises. The back can then be closed to make nursing easier (Rosenbloom & Cudmore 1985). Thereafter acute and chronic problems should be managed in the same way as the earlier treated children.

MANAGEMENT OF ANAESTHETIC SKIN

From birth the parents have to be vigilant in the care of anaesthetic skin. Friction from crawling, hot liquids, and pressure from shoes and appliances may cause problems. Poor skin and tissue cover over a prominent kyphos may easily be damaged by pressure and lead to ulceration. Regular inspection of the anaesthetic areas must be carried out while the child is young, and as soon as the child is able to take responsibility he must learn to examine himself, using a mirror for the back and bottom. Changing time and bathtime are good for this.

PRESSURE SORES

Pressure sores almost inevitably develop in some children. The factors involved are:

- Excessive pressure localised to a small area, caused by deformity and asymmetrical posture
- Poor circulation of both blood and lymph

- Optimum microclimate—wet skin, contaminated with urine or faeces
- Abnormal skeletal structures, e.g. prominent kyphosis, scar tissue over excess callus formation following orthopaedic surgery
- Scar tissue associated with poor subcutaneous tissue following closure of back lesion.

All of these factors are exacerbated by the absence of sensation which normally stimulates alteration of posture before tissue necrosis occurs.

Prevention

Buttocks. Good basic hygiene with a daily bath, combined with control of incontinence, is the first consideration. The sitting posture is also of great importance, as is the use of a cushion carefully chosen to minimise the danger of excessive pressure localised to a small area (see p. 439). In addition the child should be encouraged to lift the pelvis off the seat several times each hour.

Lower limbs. Great care should be taken in the fitting of orthoses and in providing extra padding for postoperative plasters. Paralytic toes should be uncurled before the shoe is laced up. Extra padding is needed under plasters after surgery, or for serial plasters. It is essential to maintain good circulation in the lower limbs as oedema aggravates the tendency to pressure sores. If a limb is elevated to improve circulation, the change in pressure under the buttocks must be re-assessed. The seat of the wheelchair must be checked to ensure that venous return is not being impeded behind the knees and the feet should be supported on footrests and covered with warm footwear (see p. 445).

In the past lumbar sympathectomy has been carried out in some children with very poor circulation, but this may cause pooling of venous blood in older subjects.

Spine. Pressure areas related to spinal deformities can be protected by the use of Stomahesive applied directly to the skin. Cushions with cut-out areas may be required.

Management (Fig. 12.4)

Conservative management. It is essential to provide effective relief of pressure. In the buttock area this can sometimes be achieved by the use of a chip-foam cushion with a cut-out area over the vital point (p. 441) but it will often be necessary to avoid sitting until sound healing has occurred; the use of a self-propelled prone trolley can be a useful aid in such circumstances. For the legs, plaster of Paris or Baycast splints, changed weekly, can be a most effective aid in relieving pressure. Once the ulcer is well healed, careful massage with grease can mobilise adherent scars, so reducing the risk of recurrence.

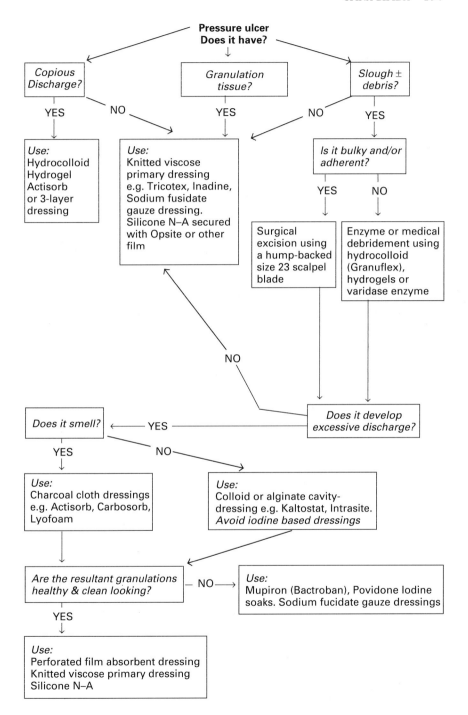

Fig. 12.4   Management of pressure ulcers. (Provided by D'A Matlhoko.)

Minor surgery. The healing process can be accelerated by the excision of necrotic tissue and fibrotic areas. Traumatising the edge of an indolent ulcer will stimulate the inflammatory reaction and so promote healing.

Plastic surgery. While most pressure sores arise from without, others are due to shearing forces. The latter can cause a deep breakdown of tissue, with the formation of bursae that can be very extensive. Final ulceration through the skin will then lead to communication into the bursa. Surgical excision of the bursa, combined with a rotation flap, is then required. This can be a very extensive procedure, which alters the blood supply to the skin, and so may not be repeatable in any given area.

ORTHOPAEDIC MANAGEMENT

Myelomeningocoele produces a bewildering variety of orthopaedic problems in the lower limbs. It has also become clear that in the majority of spina bifida patients the neurological deficit can progress and alter with increasing age. As a result early operations based on the principles used in poliomyelitis are likely to fail or need revision.

Originally orthopaedic surgeons advised early surgery to correct the limb deformities before the age of 18 months to 2 years, when the child would be ready to walk. This doctrine resulted in a large number of operations being performed that later proved to be ineffective and of no benefit to the child. The present approach is best summarised by the title of the Casey Holter Memorial Lecture given by Menelaus in 1976—'A plea for realistic goals to be achieved by the minimum of surgery'.

The patient should be seen and assessed from the orthopaedic point of view as soon as possible after birth. A muscle chart at this stage is useful to provide a baseline. However, it is essential to realise that some or all of the movement observed in the lower limbs may be involuntary or reflex (see p. 193). Such movement, far from being of use to the children, is often a handicap and a major deforming force that may require both conservative and surgical treatment.

Until the general condition and prognosis of the child can be accurately assessed, the lower limb deformities should be treated by passive stretching and careful splintage. Surgery is rarely indicated until it is clear the child is going to be capable of standing and walking. Sometimes a simple tenotomy of the adductors at the hip or a specific deforming tendon around the ankle or knee is worthwhile to allow effective conservative treatment to continue and prevent gross progressive deformity. Major operations should rarely be done until it is clear that the child is going to be a useful walker, or a deformity prevents satisfactory positioning in a wheelchair.

The foot

The whole range of foot deformities may be seen in spina bifida patients. The deformity is frequently quite different in each limb.

Talipes equinovarus (TEV)

It is important not to think that the neurological talipes equinovarus seen in spina bifida will behave in the same way as the so-called idiopathic congenital talipes equinovarus (CTEV). Initial treatment is the same in the two conditions: careful stretching and strapping or serial plasters. Great care should be taken to avoid pressure sores due to the disturbance of skin sensation in these patients. Early operation is rarely indicated unless the deformity is completely incorrigible, when a simple tenotomy of the deforming tendon will usually allow further effective correction by conservative means to continue.

Sometimes an arthrogrypotic type of limb is encountered in spina bifida. In these patients early radical surgery may be necessary, but must be followed by diligent and continuous splintage for many years. The problem of anaesthetic skin can make this difficult to achieve. Once the child shows his potential to walk or is already standing on his deformed feet, then definitive surgery can be undertaken, if possible in combination with any other surgery necessary in the limbs. Surgery should be done in as short a time as possible to avoid long periods of immobilisation in plaster, which results in disuse osteoporosis and frequent fractures when the child starts to mobilise again.

Calcaneovalgus foot

The calcaneovalgus foot is also common. A mild degree causes little disability. If the deformity is severe, division of the overacting dorsiflexors is worthwhile. Gross valgus instability of the subtalar joint is sometimes controllable by transferring the tendon of peroneus brevis into tibialis posterior. A below-knee orthosis and boot, usually combined with an inside 'T' strap, will also support the calcaneovalgus foot very successfully. If necessary the subtalar joint can be fused by the Grice-type subtalar arthrodesis once the bones have reached a reasonable size.

In the older child with a calcaneovalgus deformity it is very important to assess the ankle joint. Much of the valgus of the foot may be due to a valgus tilt at the ankle joint itself. This can be corrected by a supramalleolar medially-based wedge osteotomy at maturity.

Triple arthrodesis can be considered at maturity. However, this produces a rigid foot, which can be cosmetically pleasing, but its rigidity may lead to sores and problems with walking. Arthrodesis at the ankle joint is not recommended, as this usually fails and forms a mobile pseudarthrosis or Charcot joint.

Clawing of the toes and pes cavus deformity

Clawing of the toes and pes cavus deformity can be a considerable problem in a good walker. The resulting high pressure areas on the sole and toes predispose to sores. It is vital to keep the foot plantigrade, if possible, to avoid intractable skin ulceration. For this reason, surgical correction is often necessary in older children who remain good walkers.

The knee

At the knee, flexion is the chief problem although hyperextension can also occur. In the first 1–2 years passive stretching and splinting should be used to try and mobilise the knee and get as a good a passive range of movement as possible. When the child wants to walk, and particularly if he needs an orthosis, significant knee flexion should be corrected. It is difficult to fit a satisfactory orthosis with a knee flexion deformity of 25° or more. Correction by posterior soft tissue release at the knee is the simplest and best operation. Transfer of the hamstrings to the quadriceps apparatus is rarely indicated and may result in stiff, extended knees. This is fine when the child is small and can sit down with his legs straight out, but is of no help to the older child who has to spend most of the day sitting in a wheelchair. Similarly, patients born with stiff, extended legs manage very well until about the age of 8–10 years, when their inability to flex becomes an increasing nuisance and quadricepsplasty may be necessary.

Supracondylar osteotomy of the femur to correct flexion deformity should be avoided in the early years, as it can produce a very awkward anterior angular deformity with growth. At maturity, however, it can be a very useful and successful method of correcting persistent and recurrent flexion deformity of the knee, plus any varus or valgus deformity.

The hip

Dislocation, subluxation and dysplasia of the hip are extremely common. Nowhere has the attitude to orthopaedic treatment changed so much in the last few years. It is vital to remember that the dislocation is neurological in origin and not a congenital dislocation of the hip (CDH). In the 1960s an aggressive approach to reducing and stabilising the hips by surgery in the first 2 years of life was strongly advocated. However, this led to large numbers of stiff and sometimes painful hips that were of no benefit, or even a positive disadvantage, to the children.

Nowadays, if both hips are dislocated, they should nearly always be left alone unless the child has a pure lower motor neurone lesion and is going to be an active community walker, probably without any aids at all. A single dislocated hip should be replaced if the child is going to be a good walker, but not otherwise. Splintage in the traditional frog position can lead to severe contracture in this position. If a child has a dislocated hip at birth that is not reducible, it should be left alone until it is clear that he is going to be a good walker. If it is then causing problems, operative reduction can be considered. If a hip is dislocated but reducible at birth, a simple abduction broomstick-type splint can be used, as advocated by McKibbin.

If the hip adductors are tight and tending to cause subluxation or dislocation, then closed adductor tenotomy is all that is necessary, followed by passive stretching. The iliopsoas tendon transfer which was widely used in the past is now rarely indicated. The anterior iliopsoas transfer can be of use in those children who have a true lower motor lesion, a powerful iliopsoas and who walk with a Trendelenburg lurch, i.e. the same type of patient who responded well to this operation when it was described by Mustard for use in poliomyelitis.

Many of these children have an upper motor neurone lesion and spasticity of the adductor muscles. This can lead to progressive subluxation, and open adductor tenotomy (as in cerebral palsy) will be necessary. Hip dysplasia is very common in spina bifida and may require treatment by operation on the acetabulum if the child remains a good walker, but otherwise surgery is unnecessary. Flexion deformity at the hip is also common. If this fails to respond to the conservative stretching, surgical flexor release may be indicated to allow the hip to extend so that the child can stand in an orthosis. Abduction deformity can occur, but is usually correctible by passive stretching and physiotherapy. However, if this fails, soft tissue release at the hip can be used.

Orthoses

Orthoses of some kind will be necessary for the majority of patients. In general, a pelvic band is often necessary to start with; if a child continues to require thoracic support, he is very unlikely to use orthoses as an adult. Although there are some notable exceptions, these patients will almost invariably prefer to use a wheelchair as adults. It is most important to be realistic about the aims in these children. Once it is clear that elaborate orthoses are not going to be used as an independent means of locomotion as an adult, then time and effort should not be wasted on further training with them, but should be directed towards encouraging independence in a wheelchair. Patients who are independent in knee–ankle–foot orthoses (KAFOs) or ankle–foot orthoses (AFOs) normally continue to use these as adults if walking does not become too laborious and exhausting.

The aim of orthopaedic surgery is to allow the child to be as independent as possible within his limitations at maturity. This should be achieved by the minimum of surgery, backed up by regular physiotherapy done by the parents under the supervision and guidance of the physiotherapist.

PHYSIOTHERAPY AND OCCUPATIONAL THERAPY MANAGEMENT

THE PRESCHOOL CHILD

The aim in the first year of life is to help the baby to develop as normally as possible within the limitations of his neurological problems and to attain the normal developmental milestones of head control, grasp, sitting balance, rolling and pulling to sitting and movement on the floor, and either shuffling or 'commando' crawling. The anaesthetic legs may be in danger of friction damage if not covered, and sheepskin bootees can be made to protect the feet.

Different positions for play will encourage spatial awareness; a suitable highchair with a tray or table at the correct height and with knees and feet supported at right-angles is important for play. Obviously the level of the spinal lesion will affect the degree of sitting balance; for some children sitting balance is not possible without using arm support, and therefore support of the back will enable them to use their hands properly in play. Even babies with low lesions (L5–S1) have problems with hip stability and need more support than usual.

Babies with hydrocephalus may have the added problem of ataxia, which interferes with their balance and makes them anxious about sitting and standing with support. It is important to progress at the pace of the child and to decide for the individual when to stand and begin the process of learning to walk with support. For the toddler stage, the Chailey chariot enables the child to move around rapidly at his own level. The Oswestry swivel walker may be helpful in giving the toddler the experience of standing and moving in an upright position (see Fig. 12.12, p. 208).

At first the general care of the baby may be frightening for the parents and they may need advice, or just the support, of a professional who understands the condition. The repaired area of the back may need protection. The skin must be regularly inspected for poor circulation and signs of pressure sores. A good time to do this is at bathtime. The parents need to be aware that these problems can occur however carefully the baby is handled. If the baby is very immobile, changes of posture are necessary.

Toileting

Even though the baby may be expected to be doubly incontinent and need to wear nappies, it is important to establish a regular routine for bowel evacuation at around the age of 2 years to try to produce a pattern of bowel management. A potty chair with a bar across the front will give the child confidence and allow him to lean forward and push, either to empty the bowel or bladder (see p. 556). There are large nappies and a variety of protective pants on the market. The pants need to be well-fitting around the thighs, but not so tight as to restrict the blood supply.

Bathing and dressing

As the child gets older and heavier, a shallow bath insert can be used to lessen the strain on mother's back (see Ch. 33). The empty surface of the insert makes a convenient site for drying and dressing the child. It can be hung on the wall above the bath when not in use. When the child has learnt to transfer from one surface to another, he can begin to get in and out of the bath by himself. Great care is needed to ensure that the temperature of the bath water is not too hot and the hot water tap is fully closed, as a dripping tap can easily scald a toe.

Undressing is usually achieved before dressing, and the clothing is more easily discarded from the top half of the body, particularly if the child wears high orthoses.

A joint home visit by the occupational therapist and social services department needs to be arranged, so problems of access in the home can be assessed and plans for future adapations and additions to the house can be started.

Ambulation

When the child is ready to stand, usually between 18 months and 2 years, an assessment needs to be made of the degree of support required from the orthosis. At first, more support may be necessary and can be removed gradually as the child becomes stronger and more confident. Table 12.1 shows the usual degree of support needed according to the neurological level of the lesion, and Figure 12.5 shows the segmental nerve supply to the legs.

Orthoses (Figs 12.6–12.9)

If they are to be used successfully, orthoses must become as much part of the child's daily living routine as his clothing. It has been clearly shown that children who require orthoses with pelvic support or higher are very

Table 12.1   Ambulation support according to neurological level

Level of paralysis	Equipment required
Above L1	Thoraco-lumbo-sacral orthosis (TLSO) with knee-ankle-foot orthoses (KAFOs) Hip-guidance orthosis (HGO) (Rose et al 1981)
Below L2	TLSO with KAFOs Lumbar-sacral orthosis (LSO) LSO with KAFOs
Below L3–4	LSO with KAFOs KAFOs alone
Below L5	KAFOs or AFOs
Below S1	AFOs

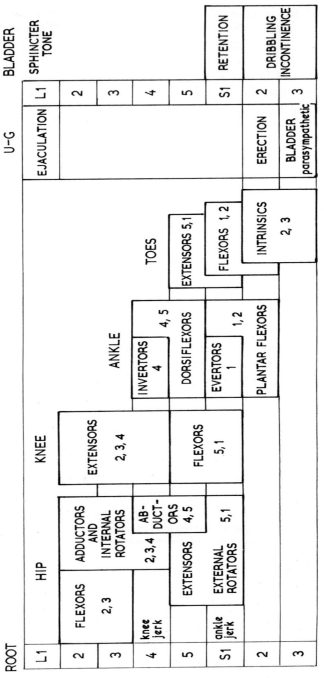

Fig. 12.5 Segmental nerve supply to the legs.

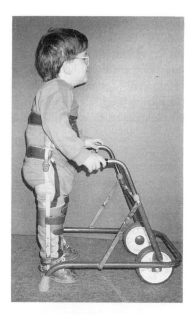

Fig. 12.6   TLSO with KAFOs—
child using a rollator walker.

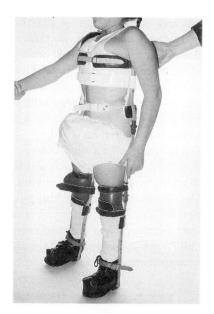

Fig. 12.7   TLSO with KAFOs
and separate LSO.

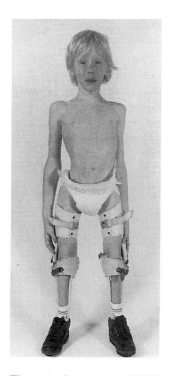

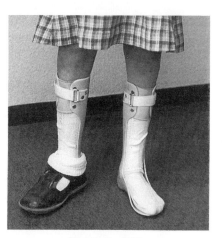

Fig. 12.9   AFOs.

Fig. 12.8   Polypropylene KAFOs.

unlikely to use them as adults. They almost invariably prefer to use a wheelchair, and it is important to be realistic about the aims in these children. There are, however, positive gains to standing and walking in childhood, even for a short time. Circulation is improved as the child starts to move, and kidney function is also facilitated. A change of posture is important so that standing, even without walking, is worthwhile in a small child, and a standing table may be used for him to play on or as a desk in the schoolroom when he is older.

The child with a high lesion requires a pelvic or thoracic band for support, and he usually needs a rollator walker initially (Fig. 12.6); he learns to move by a swivel movement, changing weight from one leg to the other. He may then go on to a 'jump-to' gait, either using the Rollator walker or parallel bars. The length of time taken to progress to using quadripod sticks, independent sticks or crutches varies tremendously according to the child's self-confidence and personality, and also to the enthusiasm and encouragement given to the child by the parents. A swing-through gait using

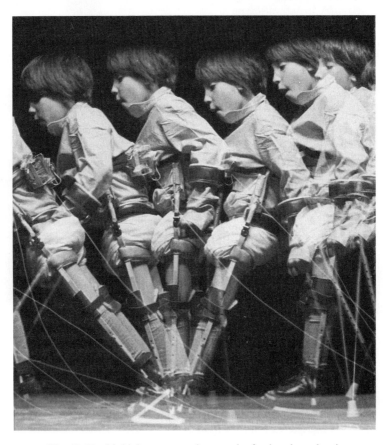

Fig. 12.10   Multiple exposure photograph of swing-through gait.

crutches (Fig. 12.10) allows for rapid movement and is achieved by many children, even with high lesions. Some very active children may damage their ankle and knee joints by overenthusiastic walking, especially using a swing-through gait. Parents need to be informed and realistic about the aims of walking and the use of orthoses, and encourage the child to continue at home under the supervision of a physiotherapist.

The hip guidance orthosis (HGO) was developed for children with high lesions with a relatively poor prognosis for long-term walking (Rose et al 1981). It permits low-energy-cost ambulation at a reasonable speed. The brace incorporates:

- Hip articulation during ambulation, which is mechanically satisfactory
- Very rigid body-brace and leg-brace
- Fixed adduction angle of 5° at hip level
- Limitation of flexion at hips (from 5–10°)
- Lateral rocking with a shoe rocker.

Swivel walking plates (Fig. 12.12) may allow the child to move in an upright position before walking is possible.

In the more severely handicapped child a wheelchair will be used and seating must be looked at regularly as the child grows (Ch. 25). Transfers and lift-ups must be practised daily and the child taught to transfer from one position to another when on his feet or in a wheelchair.

Before starting primary education, the therapists and the parents will need to visit the chosen school to look at access to toilets, classroom and playground, and talk to the teachers and school helpers. A supportive role is then established so that when difficulties arise the therapists will be contacted.

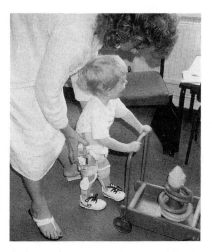

Fig. 12.11   Small child being assisted to walk with a new type of hip guidance orthosis (J. Florence)

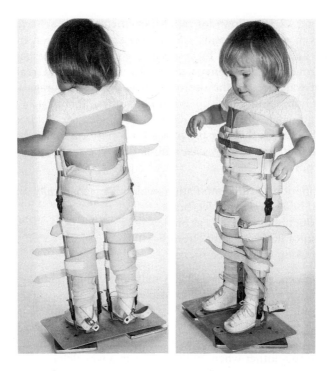

Fig. 12.12 Swivel walking plates attached to TLSO with KAFOs and LSO

Parents need advice and encouragement in the management of orthoses. For example:

1. Toes may become curled inside a boot and produce pressure sores
2. A regular check of boot size needs to be made
3. Orthoses, jackets and boots can rub sores very quickly and regular inspection of the anaesthetic areas must become a routine. Red areas will develop and need to be distinguished from true pressure sores
4. Clothing must be pulled down to prevent pressure under the orthosis
5. Nappies are difficult to apply, especially when the child is wearing a thoraco-lumbo-sacral orthosis (TLSO), and nappies need to be well out of the way of orthoses.

THE SCHOOL CHILD FROM 5–11 YEARS

Occupational Therapy

Learning to dress is a continuing process, and parents and children need encouragement to persist in gaining independence in this skill. The rush of getting the child ready for school in the mornings makes this difficult during the week, but should be practised at weekends when the family is more relaxed. The aim should be complete dressing in 20 minutes, including orthoses and boots. The choice of clothing is important. Socks without heels, preferably of wool, help to avoid pressure sores and keep the child's legs warm. Open-to-toe boots are desirable so that the position of the feet can be checked easily. High equipment must be put on next. At first the mother will need to support the child's legs as he transfers into the orthosis, and to check that the spurs are fitted into the sockets of the boots and that ankle, knee and thigh straps are at the correct tension. Help will be required to position polypropylene equipment. Protective underpants will then need to go on over the orthosis, together with a pair of loosely fitting trousers. The trouser fly may need to be lengthened down to the crutch seam, so that it will be easier to empty the urine bag, and the waist band may need enlarging to accommodate the equipment.

Special care needs to be given to the type of clothing to be worn as some materials cause friction, which can produce pressure sores. There needs to be a compromise between suitable clothing that the child can put on himself, and fashion (see Ch. 33).

Children with hydrocephalus often have perceptual problems and these may be highlighted by their difficulty in learning daily living activities like dressing and teeth cleaning, as well as learning to move about, either walking or in a wheelchair. Body image is impaired when vision is excluded and is complicated by lack of sensation in the legs and trunk. Basic work on body image can be incorporated into practice of activities of daily living such as dressing and bathing.

It is very important to develop problem-solving concepts and manipulative skills at primary school age as a foundation upon which further new skills can be built. If a child does not develop a work method of his own he will be unable to relate any new task to previous experience; each new skill should be seen as an isolated task, needing to be broken down into small stages and gradually built up. Many teachers in primary schools are unfamiliar with the hidden disability, and the occupational therapist may have an important role in working with the child on this type of splinter-skill training, and building of self-esteem as well as abilities (Ayres 1972).

Physiotherapy

Where a child is attending a normal school, it may be easier for staff to manage him in a wheelchair but it is important that his walking ability is not neglected; therefore he is encouraged to spend at least part of the day on his feet. This can be achieved by using a standing chair, thus eliminating the necessity of manipulating hip locks. If small wheels are attached to a standing chair it can be transported between classrooms by the school helper, the child walking if possible.

A great deal of encouragement is needed to keep the more severely handicapped child on his feet. It is worthwhile in the early years, particularly in keeping weight down and strengthening arms and shoulders.

Equipment will need to be checked regularly at least at 6-monthly intervals; the physiotherapist needs to see the child and encourage the parents to work with him on walking, transferring from one position to another, getting up from sitting to standing, and from standing to the floor, managing steps and stairs.

Independence from a wheelchair is also important, and advice needs to be given to allow the child to participate in gym lessons, swimming and games. The individual problems of the child can be pointed out at a school visit. The problems of spastic arms, anaesthetic skin, fractures, friction and pressure sores must be brought to the attention of teaching staff. Out-of-school activities with able-bodied children of their own age can include participation in PHAB clubs (Physically Handicapped and Able-Bodied), swimming, archery, riding for the disabled, Brownies and Cubs.

ADOLESCENCE

Towards the end of primary education, consideration of the next type of school requires consultation between the parents and the team. This is often the point at which a child can no longer manage in a normal school because of problems of access, frequent changes of classroom and, occasionally, educational problems. It may also be the time when the family decide that a boarding school might be appropriate. It is vital that therapists pass on relevant information about the children.

At this stage of the child's development it is easier to see what permanent alterations to the home are necessary, and the requirements of the family need to be discussed with the social services so that suitable alterations to the house can be organised.

Independence in dressing, bathing and toileting need to be stressed at this stage with the emphasis on personal hygiene. Many of the youngsters are unaware of their body odour, and the occupational therapist can help to overcome this by pointing out its social unacceptability.

From the age of 14 it can be useful to assess the independence of the teenagers when not being prompted by their family or care staff, and in a suitably adapted environment. Short stays, when they can look after themselves in a bungalow or flat with an occupational therapist as an observer, can often pinpoint the areas of independence on which most work needs to be done. At Chailey Heritage, independence training is carried out in pairs and the youngsters are responsible for themselves in every stage of the procedure; packing, menu planning, shopping, cooking, housework and taking of medications are among the expected activities. At the end of the 2 or 3 day session the occupational therapist prepares a report on each child which can be used by the family, care staff and teaching staff as a basis for continued activity. The Association for Spina Bifida and Hydrocephalus also organises holidays with the aim of encouraging independence.

Physiotherapy and the adolescent

The onset of puberty is often early in children with spina bifida and this aggravates the problems of adolescence because of the associated social and emotional immaturity. Parents need even more patience and tolerance in dealing with their child at this stage of development. It is often a time when a decision needs to be made about continued walking. The less severely handicapped need to be encouraged to overcome problems in order to stay on their feet.

During the growth spurt of adolescence, spinal deformities increase and this may interfere with balance, both in sitting and standing (see Ch. 22). It may also be necessary to support the spine with a polypropylene jacket (TLSO) and, if there is instability in sitting, a flanged jacket or one fixed to the back of the wheelchair may be used (see p. 377). Both these types of jacket are bulky, and clothing may need to be adapted, but with careful planning and some dressmaking this can be overcome. It is possible to attach the straightforward polypropylene TLSO to KAFOs (Fig. 12.7), or it may be easier to fit the equipment over the TLSO. However, as the child becomes older, walking with high equipment may be found to be impractical and a decision to use a wheelchair may be taken. At this stage the physiotherapist's role is supervisory, and the parents need to continue to encourage their child if he is able to maintain mobility.

THE ADULT WITH SPINA BIFIDA AND HYDROCEPHALUS

The population of children with spina bifida treated in the 1960s is now adult, and they have proved to be a very vulnerable group of disabled people. Their multiple medical problems which were treated under the umbrella of paediatric care have been referred to specialists in adult surgery and medicine with variable success. Several studies have highlighted the need for continued care in an adult setting (Thomas et al 1990, Rickwood et al 1984).

Personal experience (McCarthy 1986) in setting up a clinic for young people with spina bifida and hydrocephalus has produced a disturbing catalogue of medical problems. Particular areas of concern are renal failure, shunt malfunction, and severe ulceration of the skin—often associated with obesity. Provision of orthoses can become a problem in some cases.

No less concerning are the social and emotional problems, in particular the need for independence and daytime occupation. The plight of young adults with spina bifida has served to highlight the need for clinics for all young people with physical disabilities.

REFERENCES

Ayres A J 1972 Sensory integration and learning disorders. Western Psychological Services, Los Angeles.

Cuckle H S, Wald N J, Cuckle P M 1989 Prenatal screening and diagnosis of neural tube defects in England and Wales in 1985. Prenatal Diagnosis 9: 393–400

Evans R C, Tew B, Thomas M D, Ford J 1985 Selective surgical management of neural tube malformation. Archives of Disease in Childhood 60: 415–519

Guthkelch A N 1986 Aspects of the surgical management of meningomyelocele: a review. Developmental Medicine and Child Neurology 28: 525–532

Hunt G M 1990 Open spina bifida: outcome for a complete cohort treated unselectively and followed into adulthood. Developmental Medicine and Child Neurology 322: 108–119

Laurence K M 1969 The recurrence risk in spina bifida cystica and anencephaly. Developmental Medicine and Child Neurology 11(20): 23.

Leck I 1983 Epidemiological clues to the causation of neural tube defects. In: Dobbing J (ed) Prevention of spina bifida and other neural tube defects. Academic Press, London.

Lorber J 1971 Results of treatment of myelomeningocoele. An analysis of 524 unselected cases. Developmental Medicine and Child Neurology 13: 279

Lorber J 1972 Spina bifida cystica. Results of treatment of 270 consecutive cases with criteria for selection for the future. Archives of Disease in Childhood 47: 854

Lorber J, Salfield S A W 1981 Results of selective treatment of spina bifida cystica. Archives of Disease in Childhood 56: 822–30

Mawdsley T, Rickham P O, Roberts J R 1967 Long term results of early operation of open myelomeningocele and encephalocele. British Medical Journal 1: 663

McCarthy G T 1986 A clinic for young adults with spina bifida and hydrocephalus. Association of Paediatric Physiotherapists Newsletter 41: 11–15

Menelaus M B 1976 Orthopaedic management of children with myelomeningocele: a plea for realistic goals. Developmental Medicine and Child Neurology 18 (37): 3–11

OPCS (Office of Population Censuses and Surveys) 1990 Congenital malformation statistics notifications. HMSO, London

Rickwood A M K, Hodgson J, Lonton A P, Thomas D G 1984 Medical and surgical complications in adolescent and young adult patients with spina bifida and hydrocephalus. Health Trends 16: 91–93

Rose G K, Stallard J, Sankarankutty M 1981 Clinical evaluation of spina bifida patients using hip-guidance orthoses. Developmental Medicine and Child Neurology 23: 30–40

Rosenbloom L, Cudmore R E 1985 Spina bifida: do we have the right policies? Archives of Disease in Childhood 60: 401–404

Smithells R W et al 1981 Apparent prevention of neural tube defects by periconceptual vitamin supplementation. Archives of Disease in Childhood 56: 911–918

Smithells R W, Nevin N C, Seller M C 1983 Further experience of vitamin supplementation for prevention of neural tube defect recurrences. Lancet 1: 1027–1031

Smithells R W, Sheppard S, Wild J, Schorah C J 1989 Prevention of neural tube defect recurrences in Yorkshire: final report. Lancet 2: 498–499

Stark G D, Baker C W 1967 The neurological involvement of the lower limbs in myelomeningocoele. Developmental Medicine and Child Neurology 9: 732

Stark G D, Drummond M 1971 The spinal cord lesion in myelomeningocele. Developmental Medicine and Child Neurology 13 (25): 1

Thomas A P, Bax M C O, Smyth D P L 1990 The health and social needs of young adults with physical disabilities. Clinics in Developmental Medicine 106. Blackwell Scientific, Oxford

Wald N, Sneddon J, Dewsem J, Frost C, Stone R 1991 Prevention of neural tube defects: results of the Medical Research Council Vitamin Study. Lancet 338: 131–137

FURTHER READING

Anderson E M, Spain B 1977 The child with spina bifida. Methuen, London

Delight E, Goodall J 1990 Love and loss. Conversations with parents of babies with spina bifida managed without surgery. Developmental Medicine and Child Neurology 61 (32): 8

Seller M J 1982 Paediatric research: a genetic approach. In: Neural tube defects: cause and prevention Spastics International Medical Publications, William Heinemann, London

13. Hydrocephalus

G.T. McCarthy   R. Land

Hydrocephalus, literally 'water in the head', is the abnormal accumulation of cerebrospinal fluid (CSF) in the ventricular systems of the brain, caused by obstruction to normal circulation, excessive production or failure of absorption of CSF. It is usually associated with a rise in intracranial pressure and rapid enlargement of the head.

COMMON CAUSES OF HYDROCEPHALUS

- *In association with neural tube defects.* Hydrocephalus occurs in about 80% of children with spina bifida. It may be of the *obstructive* type, at the aqueduct; or caused by malabsorption or overproduction of CSF, where it is termed *communicating* hydrocephalus. In many cases the hydrocephalus is caused by a mixture of these factors. The Type III Arnold–Chiari malformation is common; it consists of prolongation of the cerebellar vermis and the fourth ventricle into the cervical spinal canal, and kinking of the inferiorly placed medulla. This may produce obstruction of the fourth ventricle. Figure 13.1 shows the mechanism of production of syringomyelia in Type III Arnold–Chiari malformation
- *Congenital narrowing or obstruction of the aqueduct.* This is occasionally genetically determined in X-linked hydrocephalus. Examine the hands of boys for flexion deformities of the thumbs, which may be present in this condition. Mental handicap is usually present
- *Cerebral or ventricular haemorrhage.* An increasing number of premature babies who suffer cerebral or ventricular haemorrhages also develop hydrocephalus. The common cause is blockage of the arachnoid granulations by debris and blood in the CSF. Debris may also block the aqueduct.
- *Intrauterine infection,* e.g. toxoplasmosis
- *Malformation of the posterior fossa*—the Dandy–Walker syndrome
- *Tumours or cysts causing obstruction* of aqueduct
- *Tumour of the choroid plexus* causing increased CSF production
- *Meningitis,* particularly in the perinatal period
- *In association with malformations in the CNS* or elsewhere (there are over 100 syndromes described).

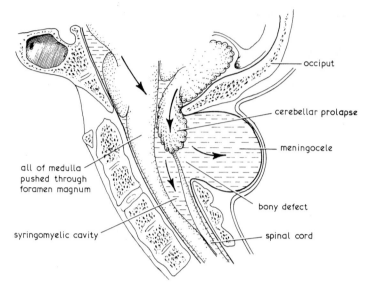

occiput

cerebellar prolapse

meningocele

all of medulla
pushed through
foramen magnum

bony defect

syringomyelic cavity

spinal cord

Fig. 13.1   Type III Arnold–Chiari malformation.

PRESENTATION AND EARLY MANAGEMENT

Hydrocephalus may be present at birth in babies with spina bifida, or become overt on closure of the back lesion, when the head circumference rapidly increases. Babies with congenital hydrocephalus may also present at birth or there may be a more insidious rise in pressure with gradual abnormal increase in head circumference.

In the baby presenting early the anterior fontanelle becomes tense and may even bulge under the pressure, and the skull sutures separate. There may be associated feeding problems, vomiting and swallowing difficulties. The eyes may also show the 'setting sun' sign or a squint may develop.

Older children presenting with hydrocephalus often do not complain of headache. Early morning vomiting may occur. Visual signs include chronic papilloedema, 6th nerve palsies with limited abduction of the eyes, and occasionaly nystagmus. Ataxia may be marked.

In most cases it is necessary to insert a *shunt* to carry the excess CSF from the ventricles of the brain into the peritoneal sac or circulation. Different types of shunt are used (Fig. 13.2). They have in common a one-way valve system, which opens under pressure to allow the passage of CSF from the dilated ventricles into the bloodstream or peritoneal sac, where it is absorbed. The earliest valve, the Spitz-Holter, is still used. More modern systems have additional functions, e.g. an on-off mechanism or a reservoir, which allows the insertion of antibiotics or measurement of intraventricular pressure. The opening pressure of the valve can be chosen to try to prevent rapid changes in ventricular size with development of subdural collections.

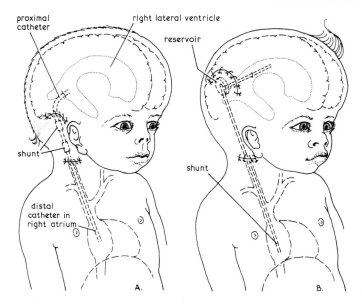

Fig. 13.2   Shunt systems for the treatment of hydrocephalus. **a.** Spitz–Holter. **b.** Pudenz.

In theory the shunt system allows the brain to grow at a normal rate by normalising the pressure in the ventricles. In practice it is often difficult to estimate the correct shunt pressure, so the ventricles may collapse down to narrow slits, which may become unduly stiff and vulnerable to small changes of pressure; or conversely the ventricular size may not alter markedly and the pressure within the system may remain high.

Ultrasound in the first 18 months and computerised axial tomography (CAT or CT scan) demonstrate ventricular size accurately. It is important to carry out imaging following shunt surgery so that a baseline of ventricular size is available. It is now common practice to carry out a scan if there is doubt about shunt function. Radiographs of the shunts, which are usually radio-opaque, will also give information on the integrity of the system. It is not uncommon for shunts to become disconnected; occasionally the material disintegrates after many years of service.

SHUNT COMPLICATIONS

The common complications arising from shunts are *obstruction and infection*. General assessment shall be considered first, followed by details specific to obstruction and infection.

ASSESSMENT

Obtain case notes and previous radiographs. Need to know:

1. Type of shunt: VA, VP, reservoir or on–off facility

2. Previous shunt problems: revisions, infection, blockage
3. Other medical problems: urinary tract, previous infections, ? on prophylactic antibiotics
4. Previous assessments of blood pressure, optic fundi
5. Previous ventricular size.

History of present illness

- *Headache:* Worse at night? on lying down? on coughing? wakes in the morning with it?
- *Vomiting:* Only in the morning or worse in the morning? nausea present or absent? effortless? worse on lying down? other family members affected? diarrhoea present?
- Change in level of consciousness, irritability, increase in epileptic fits or onset of epilepsy which is often difficult to control
- Slowing of performance, often noticed by teachers. Personality changes
- Visual problems: increase in squint or diplopia
- Weakness of the arms or loss of dexterity
- Swallowing difficulties and intractable bronchitis.

Examination

- *Fever:* think of URTI, UTI
  — Pneumonia: feeding difficulties, reflux vomiting—aspiration?
  — Infected shunt: V-P ? peritonitis, examine abdomen carefully. V-A ? septicaemia
- *Level of consciousness:* pupillary reactions. Assess and record formally
- *Pulse, blood pressure:* slowing pulse with increasing BP is a sign of raised intracranial pressure. The trend is important, so monitor frequently. Irregularities of the pulse may also indicate a rise in ICP
- *Neck pain and stiffness:* Look for local causes, e.g. tonsillitis, cervical lymphadenopathy
- *Optic fundi:* papilloedema, haemorrhages—*Always significant.* Papilloedema is often absent in the presence of shunt malfunction. The onset of visual deterioration may be very insidious and should always be investigated. Optic atrophy (pale discs) is *not* a sign of *acute* intracranial problem, but may mask papilloedema
- *Examine shunt system:* resistance to emptying suggests distal block; if empties readily but fails to refill, or refills very slowly, suggests proximal block (this can be misleading)
- *Examine track of catheter,* and insertion wound, for localised areas of swelling, erythema or tenderness.

Investigations

1. For infection: throat swab; urgent urine microscopy; urine culture and

sensitivities; FBC with differential WBC; blood cultures; CXR; C-reactive protein; consider CSF from shunt—always discuss with the neurosurgeons first

2. If vomiting marked: electrolytes, urea, creatinine
3. X-ray entire shunt system
4. Consider CT scan if shunt system intact on X-ray but clinical evidence of raised intracranial pressure.

SHUNT OBSTRUCTION

Upper end block

The choroid plexus of blood vessels may become wrapped around the ventricular catheter, or the catheter may simply become submerged in the brain tissue due to changes in ventricular size. The shunt may fail to refill or do so very slowly.

Lower end block

- *Ventriculo-atrial shunt (VA)*: This may simply be caused by withdrawal of the atrial catheter from the fast moving blood flow by growth. Once in the great veins the irritant effect of the CSF on the wall of the vein will lead to inflammation and thrombosis, at first partial and finally complete
- *Ventriculo-peritoneal shunt (VP)*: The peritoneal catheter may be wrapped around by the surrounding tissue, usually omentum, and become enclosed in a pocket of CSF, causing slowly rising pressure.

Management

Any child suspected of having a blocked shunt should be transferred to a neurosurgical unit for observation and possible treatment. Some shunt blockages right themselves, but others do not, and it is impossible to say how much time can be safely allowed for observation.

If the clinical assessment suggests a severe rise of pressure, emergency aspiration of CSF via the shunt or reservoir or ventricle may be a life-saving measure before transfer to a neurosurgical centre. In some centres it is regular practice to insert a separate reservoir through an anterior burr hole in order to be able to carry out a ventricular pressure check whenever there is doubt about possible shunt malfunction.

In the absence of a reservoir, if the child is rapidly deteriorating a lumbar puncture needle may be passed along the side of the ventricular catheter. Aspiration of the valve reservoir may also be indicated, using a fine hypodermic needle and full antiseptic precautions. Sudden death can occur in children with hydrocephalus and shunt systems. The wide range of symptoms, from subtle behavioural changes to sudden death, indicates a need to follow closely every child who has a shunt. Hayden et al (1983) recorded five sudden deaths in their longitudinal study of 360 patients with hydrocephalus.

Preventive surgery. Many surgeons prefer to lengthen the distal atrial or peritoneal catheter at intervals as the child grows, to prevent the complications of lower end block. This may prevent exposure of the child to episodes of uncontrolled raised intracranial pressure.

SHUNT INFECTION

In those systems which drain into the circulation, the tip of the distal catheter acquires a coating of fibrin and blood clot, which provides an ideal culture medium for circulating bacteria. An episode of bacteraemia can thus infect the tip of the catheter, and infection may spread up into the valve and the cerebral ventricles. Infection may be introduced at the time of operation and commonly is associated with bacteria that normally inhabit the skin. The presence of these organisms in the circulation may also produce a sensitivity reaction, resulting in the development of nephritis or nephrotic syndrome. Occasionally, embolic phenomena occur, with the development of bacterial endocarditis and patchy areas of pneumonia.

The catheters draining into the peritoneal cavity can also become infected if the catheter tip lies in close proximity to the wall of the bowel for any length of time. The irritant effect of the CSF may produce inflammation in the wall of the bowel, which allows the passage of bowel organisms into the peritoneal cavity. Infection of the distal catheter and eventually the whole valve system and brain may follow.

Clinical presentation of shunt infection

Pyrexia: caused by escape of organisms into the circulation. The pyrexia may take the form of isolated spikes of temperature, a continuous swinging temperature, or a low-grade pyrexia associated with failure to thrive and chronic anaemia. In rare cases infection may be complicated by bacterial endocarditis: a systolic murmur may be heard, with patchy consolidation of the lungs, enlargement of the spleen, and finger clubbing.

Meningism. Headache, vomiting, drowsiness and neck stiffness may occur.

Shunt nephritis. Oedema, proteinuria, haematuria and hypertension may occur. Unrelieved, this will ultimately lead to chronic renal failure.

Investigations

- Blood cultures should be carried out at intervals, preferably at the time of pyrexia, and a positive culture will usually be obtained

- Blood counts typically show anaemia with some degree of leukocytosis
- CSF aspirated from the valve will culture the organism, but there will be no cellular response in the CSF until the ventricles become infected
- The C-reactive protein level taken at intervals can be helpful in children with low grade infection, which is difficult to confirm.

Treatment

Successful treatment almost invariably involves the removal of the entire shunt system and the insertion of a new one, once the infection has been overcome by means of systemic and intrathecal antibiotics (the latter only being required in ventriculitis).

Preventive treatment. In those shunts that drain into the circulation, prophylactic antibiotics should be given to cover any procedure, such as a dental extraction, that may provoke a bacteraemia.

OTHER SHUNT COMPLICATIONS

1. Overdrainage of the ventricles with overlapping of the sutures and craniosynostosis in babies. In older children a low pressure syndrome may occur with headaches characteristically developing in mid to late morning, and improving on lying down. Shunt studies reveal patent shunts with low or negative pressures relative to the reservoir. Insertion of a higher pressure valve system relieves the symptoms.

2. Intermittent shunt function has been shown to occur sometimes in association with a fibrous track, which develops after disconnection of the catheter.

3. Peritoneal loculation can also present with symptoms of intermittent block. Occasional localised peritonitis without meningitis has been reported (Hayden et al 1983).

4. Occasionally the catheter perforates the heart or abdominal viscera or becomes detached from the valve, causing pulmonary embolism. Skin necrosis over the shunt can also occur.

5. Insidious visual deterioration occurs in the presence of a slow rise in intracranial pressure in some patients.

INTELLECTUAL DEVELOPMENT OF CHILDREN WITH HYDROCEPHALUS

General intelligence

Surveys have shown that children with hydrocephalus have lower IQs than their brothers and sisters. They are also interesting differences between spina bifida children with and without shunts. Table 13.1 shows the results of assessment using the Wechsler Intelligence Scales for Children (WISC) at age 11 years in the Greater London Council (GLC) survey.

Table 13.1   WISC mean IQs at 11 years (standard deviations in parentheses). (From Halliwell et al 1980)

	Number	Full Scale IQ	Verbal Scale	Performance Scale
Controls	45	112.0(11.9)	110.4(11.5)	111.3(13.0)
Shunt	67	80.0(17.4)	84.3(18.8)	77.4(16.5)
No shunt	30	100.1(16.1)	98.8(15.0)	100.4(17.1)

The distribution of intelligence within the whole group is slanted towards the lower end of the IQ range, and intelligence is particularly affected in the shunt-treated group, who also had average performance scale scores lower than verbal scale scores. This is particularly true for low-ability children. The presence of a shunt indicates an initial degree of hydrocephalus though some children without shunts may have some degree of hydrocephalus. A large survey by Lonton (1979) relating intellectual skills and CT scans in children with spina bifida and hydrocephalus showed that even large degrees of hydrocephalus had insignificant effects on the verbal IQ, but there was a small but statistically significant effect upon performance scale IQ on the WISC. The abilities most affected were motor and perceptuo-motor skills.

Children with shunts were only found to be substantially inferior in skills to those without if their ventricles were very large or abnormally small. The highest proportion of children with shunts was found in the group with small ventricles.

Visual perception

Several studies show a general trend towards inferior functioning in visual perception in children with hydrocephalus. The type of task the children find difficult is the embedded figure test, where a simple figure like a triangle or a star has to be picked out from a group of overlapping shapes (Miller & Sethi 1971, Tew 1973).

Scanning ability

Hydrocephalic children may have difficulty in rapidly surveying a visual array before responding. Tasks like working from left to right, looking between their work and a key, or finding their place on a page may be particularly difficult for them.

On tasks combining perceptual and motor skills hydrocephalic children may have marked difficulties from an early age. Impaired hand function may also be present as a result of cerebellar involvement in the Arnold–Chiari malformation (Fig. 13.1). Children with lower cognitive ability (IQ less than 80) are more likely to have difficulty learning to read. Sometimes they learn to read fluently, but their reading comprehension is poor.

Verbal ability

Most children with spina bifida give the impression of having normal verbal ability by being 'chatty' and using quite complex language structures, but on the other hand there can be an apparent lack of understanding. Several studies show that spina bifida children have normal verbal memory and development of vocabulary.

Hyperverbal ('cocktail party') behaviour is an extreme form of fluent speech coupled with poor understanding. Not all children show it although the label can get widely applied. Tew and Lawrence (1972) found evidence of hyperverbal behaviour in 28% of their sample. In the GLC survey, 40% of the children at 6 years were rated clinically as hyperverbal, although only 20% showed it to a marked degree.

Mathematical ability

Restricted mobility and impaired hand control may impoverish the child's preschool experience and lead to delay in the acquisition of number concepts. If this is associated with perceptual, sequencing and organisational problems, the child may have difficulty carrying out the operations required for number work. Assessment of the child's difficulties and careful teaching is necessary to overcome these problems.

Children with hydrocephalus in association with perinatal cerebral haemorrhage will have the associated learning problems encountered in cerebral palsy (see Ch. 27).

REFERENCES

Halliwell M D, Carr J G, Pearson A M 1980 The intellectual and educational functioning of children with neural tube defects. Zeitschrift für Kinderchirurgie 31: 4
Hayden P W, Shurtleff D B, Stuntz T J 1983 A longitudinal study of shunt function in 360 patients with hydrocephalus. Developmental Medicine and Child Neurology 25: 334–337
Lonton A P1979 The relationship between intellectual skills and CAT scans of children with spina bifida and hydrocephalus. Zeitschrift für Kinderchirurgie 28: 4
Miller E, Sethi L 1971 The effect of hydrocephalus on perception. Developmental Medicine and Child Neurology 13 (25): 77–81
Tew B J 1973 Some psychological consequences of spina bifida and hydrocephalus and its complications. In: Proceedings of the 31st Biennial Conference, ASBAH (Association for Spina Bifida and Hydrocephalus, London).
Tew B J, Lawrence K M 1972 The ability and attainments of spina bifida patients born in South Wales between 1965–72. Developmental Medicine and Child Neurology 27: 124–31

FURTHER READING

Minns R A 1991 Problems of intracranial pressure in childhood. Clinics in Developmental Medicine Nos 113/114. MacKeith Press, Blackwell Scientific, Oxford

14. The neuropathic bladder

M. Borzyskowski   D. Nurse

INTRODUCTION

There are many causes of neuropathic vesico-urethral dysfunction in childhood, spina bifida (open and closed) being the commonest. Other causes include spinal cord tumour and trauma; transverse myelitis; sacral agenesis and a small group in whom a cause is not found. Some of these children have only a minor neurological deficit and the bladder dysfunction is their major handicap. Defective innervation of the bladder and urethra results in inefficient bladder emptying, raised intravesical pressure, incontinence and recurrent urinary tract infections, with the risk of impairment of renal function. The aims of management of these children are firstly and most importantly preservation of renal function; secondly continence; and thirdly social integration. However, there must be a realistic approach to management and the methods used must be acceptable to both the child and those looking after him.

ASSESSMENT

Any child or infant in whom a neuropathic bladder is suspected should have a full assessment of bladder and renal function. In a baby with spina bifida, bladder and renal function should be assessed early. Renal ultrasonography can be carried out at the same time as the ventricles are being scanned for evidence of hydrocephalus, and can be repeated each time this is carried out. In addition it is important to observe the baby during micturition to see whether he is able to pass urine in a stream, whether he is incontinent on crying, and whether the bladder is palpable.

ASSESSMENT OF RENAL FUNCTION

This includes measurement of plasma creatinine, urea and electrolytes; glomerular filtration rate; renal ultrasound; and an intravenous urogram. In children under 1 year of age, a dimercaptosuccinic acid (DMSA) nuclear scan provides better images of the kidneys. If renal function is impaired or there is evidence of upper tract dilatation, more detailed investigations using radionucleotide scanning techniques such as DMSA scan or diethylenetriamine penta-acetic acid (DTPA) scan may be required. The advent of renal ultrasonography performed by an experienced radiologist has made a tremendous difference to the management of these children and those particularly at risk for renal damage can be monitored closely by this means. Thus problems can be detected early and dealt with. In addition it has cut down vastly the amount of X-ray irradiation these children receive. Naturally the urine should be checked regularly for evidence of infection.

ASSESSMENT OF BLADDER AND URETHRAL FUNCTION

The advent of the videourodynamic study (VDU) has greatly increased our understanding of the pathophysiology of this condition, which in turn has improved management. Analysis of the results of these investigations has revealed that in the vast majority of children the entire lower urinary tract is involved and, in many, urethral dysfunction is more important than bladder dysfunction; thus it is more accurate to describe the dysfunction as one of neuropathic vesico-urethral dysfunction rather than neuropathic bladder alone.

The study itself consists of a filling and voiding cystometrogram combined with a micturating cysto-urethrogram (MCU) (Bates et al 1970, Whiteside 1972). The two are displayed side by side on a television screen and can be recorded onto videotape for playback at a later date, so that events occurring in the bladder and urethra can be correlated with pressure changes and vice versa. The study provides information on: bladder size, shape and capacity; residual urine; the presence or absence of vesico-ureteric reflux (VUR); detrusor pressure at rest, during filling and detrusor contraction; and the behaviour of the bladder neck and distal urethral sphincter during filling and during a detrusor contraction.

If treatment is going to be selective for each individual patient, a VDU is mandatory. It should be performed as soon as possible after the diagnosis has been made, and—in babies born with spina bifida—as soon as feasible after closure of the spinal defect. In this situation, if it is not possible to carry out a VDU, an MCU should be performed to look for reflux and to assess the ability of the bladder to empty.

ABNORMALITIES OF THE BLADDER AND URETHRA IN NEUROPATHY

The majority of these children have congenital spinal cord lesions that are incomplete, and therefore classification based on the type and extent of the lesion would be very complex. We therefore use a classification system based on the urodynamic findings (Rickwood et al 1982) and the overall ability of the bladder to hold and void urine (Raezer et al 1977).

Bladder behaviour is defined as contractile, intermediate or acontractile (see p. 226), depending on its ability to contract and to give a useful degree of bladder emptying. Detrusor sphincter dyssynergia (DSD), which causes outflow obstruction at the level of the distal urethral sphincter, is now recognised as the single commonest cause of impaired renal function in children with congenital cord problems (Mundy et al 1982). DSD occurs when the distal urethral sphincter contracts instead of relaxing when the bladder muscle (detrusor) contracts, resulting in an obstruction to urine flow and raised intravesical pressure. If reflux is present in this situation the kidneys are particularly at risk, especially if the child develops a urinary tract infection. It is thus important to identify these children and a VDU study is the best way to do so.

In 1985 Mundy et al reported their findings in 402 VDU studies carried out over a 5 year period in 207 children with spina bifida, aged 1 month to 16 years. Detrusor behaviour was classified as above, and bladder neck and distal sphincter behaviour was assessed during filling and during detrusor contractions. The conclusions were that, with the possible exception of a few children with spinal cord lesions, urethral dysfunction was almost universal. In the 73 children with contractile detrusor dysfunction, the bladder neck was incompetent in 50% and the distal sphincter dynamically obstructive (i.e. DSD) in 95%. In the 82 children with intermediate and 52 with acontractile bladder dysfunction, the bladder neck was incompetent in all at their usual bladder volumes, although it sometimes appeared competent when the residual urine was completely removed. The distal sphincter mechanism in these two groups was both obstructive and incompetent due to a more or less fixed distal sphincter resistance. This obstruction was static in nature and led to leakage in the intermediate group at a critical detrusor pressure level and at a critical volume in the atonic group. This study confirms the importance of urethral dysfunction in children with congenital cord lesions. (See Figs 14.1–14.3.)

Naturally our increased understanding of the pathophysiology of this condition has influenced our management, particularly as we are now aware that the dysfunction changes with time. Reflux, which can be present at birth, is often not apparent until 18 months to 3 years of age. DSD may not appear until 5 years of age. DSD, reduced compliance and sphincter weakness tend to worsen with time and particularly in the late teens. Thus there may be deterioration in continence or renal function or both. The most vulnerable times for renal function are the first 5 years of life and the late teens, but changes can occur at any time. It is clear that life-long follow-up and regular reassessment are mandatory. Some children, particularly those with reflux and DSD, require very close supervision, commonly (particularly in infancy) having monthly ultrasonography so that upper tract changes can be picked up early and management modified.

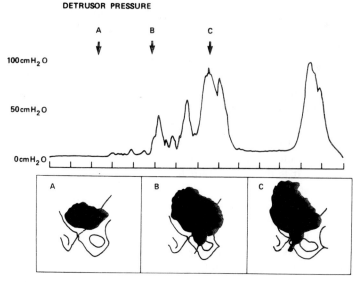

Fig. 14.1 Contractile dysfunction–video-urodynamic features. (In this and in Figs 14.2 and 14.3 only the detrusor pressure trace is shown, although in an actual urodynamic trace, total bladder pressure, abdominal pressure, flow rate and filling volume would also be shown. The detrusor pressure is the most important parameter and is electronically derived from total bladder pressure minus abdominal pressure, which are measured by catheters in the bladder and rectum respectively.) Detrusor pressure trace shows high-amplitude swings in detrusor pressure (detrusor hyperreflexia). Synchronous video-MCUG shows initial bladder neck competence and trabeculation (A); opening of the bladder neck with a detrusor contraction (B); but failure of opening of the distal sphincter mechanism (C) due to detrusor–sphincter dyssynergia.

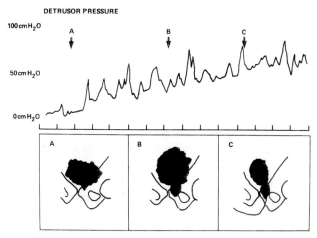

Fig. 14.2 Intermediate dysfunction. Detrusor pressure trace shows a steady rise in baseline pressure (low compliance) and constant detrusor activity of varying amplitude. However, as distinct from Fig. 14.1, this activity is poorly sustained and is therefore ineffective—it is sufficient to restrict filling but insufficient to produce voiding. Synchronous video-MCUG shows bladder neck incompetence (A), which gets progressively worse (B) with detrusor–sphincter dyssynergia during detrusor contractions (C).

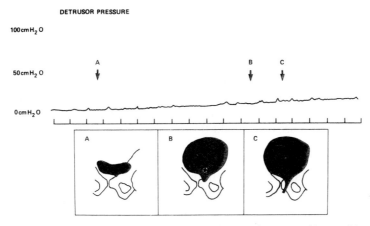

Fig. 14.3 Acontractile dysfunction. Detrusor pressure trace shows no evidence of detrusor contractility. Synchronous video-MCUG shows bladder neck incompetence with early 'beaking' of the bladder neck (A), which becomes more marked with filling (B). On coughing (or attempted voiding by straining) sphincter weakness incontinence occurs (C), but the urethra in the region of the distal sphincter mechanism fails to open adequately because of static distal sphincter obstruction. (Figs 14.1–3 are reproduced, with permission, from Mundy A R (1986) Neuropathic bladder. In: Postlethwaite R J (ed) Clinical paediatric nephrology. Wright, Bristol.)

CONTROL OF INFECTION

This is obviously important, particularly if reflux is present. All children should have regular urine cultures and this may need to be carried out monthly in those most at risk. Clearly any symptomatic urinary tract infection must be treated with an adequate course of the appropriate antibiotic. Asymptomatic urine infections (i.e. those detected by urine culture) do not all require treatment; indeed some children on clean intermittent catheterisation (CIC) or with an indwelling catheter will nearly always harbour organisms in the urine. If vesico-ureteric reflux is present all infections should be treated.

In addition all children with reflux and those with recurrent infections should be on prophylactic antibiotics given as a single dose at night. Cotrimoxazole, trimethoprim or nitrofurantoin are the usual drugs given.

Adequate bladder drainage is fundamental in the prevention of urinary tract infections, and is at the heart of the problem.

MANAGEMENT

Continence and preservation of renal function are the aims. However, any scheme of management must take into account the child's motivation, manipulative skills, neurological deficit, skeletal deformity and intellectual level.

Commonly these children have a combination of problems, neuropathic bladder dysfunction being only one of them. It is therefore important that the specialists involved work closely and see the children in joint clinics whenever possible. In addition an integral and invaluable member of the team managing these children is a home liaison nurse, who not only sees the children when they attend hospital but also visits them at home or at school. She is responsible for liaison between the hospital and community and will advise on various forms of nappies, pads and incontinence appliances. She also teaches and advises the children and their carers on techniques such as clean intermittent catheterisation. We find that the children and their parents are best taught this technique at home.

The key factors in management are:

- An understanding of the pathophysiology of bladder and urethral dysfunction
- VDU assessment
- A realistic approach to management.

The key factors to achieve continence are:

- A reasonable bladder capacity
- A reasonable degree of outflow obstruction
- A means of emptying the bladder.

In general, although drugs may improve bladder capacity indirectly by reducing detrusor overactivity, medical management aims to improve bladder capacity by improving bladder emptying and so increasing the interval between voids. The limiting factor for achieving continence is severe sphincter weakness.

The adverse factors for renal function are:

- DSD
- Reflux
- Raised intravesical pressure
- Reduced bladder compliance
- Recurrent infections.

Any scheme of management must take into account any of these adverse factors that are present so that the risks related to them can be reduced as much as possible.

MEDICAL MANAGEMENT

BLADDER EMPTYING

Effective bladder emptying can be achieved by:

1. Bladder expression
2. Bladder straining
3. Clean intermittent catheterisation
4. Continuous catheterisation.

Bladder expression

The Credé manoeuvre has be used extensively over the years. However, it is often disliked by children and is difficult to perform well. In the presence of DSD, bladder emptying is unlikely even though great pressure is applied. Expression is not recommended in the presence of reflux, particularly if distal urethral obstruction is present. Bladder expression can be a useful way of emptying an acontractile bladder and may result in a reasonable degree of continence if sphincter weakness is not severe. Alpha-adrenergic drugs can be used to increase outflow resistance and thus continence if bladder neck weakness is mild.

In some children reflex emptying of the bladder occurs if the skin over the lumbosacral area is tapped or the skin of the lower abdomen or thigh is pinched.

Bladder straining

This can be an effective means of bladder emptying in the older, motivated child in whom the innervation of the abdominal wall musculature is preserved. However, any sphincter weakness will have to be dealt with, either pharmacologically or surgically.

Clean intermittent catheterisation (CIC)

This has undoubtedly made a tremendous difference to the management of these children since it was first introduced by Lapides et al in 1972. Since that time there have been numerous reports showing improvement in continence, renal function and infection rates (Lapides et al 1972, 1974, Borzyskowski et al 1982, Diokno et al 1983). Indirectly it has been responsible for the marked decrease in the number of urinary diversions performed (Lyon et al 1975, Crooks & Enrile 1983). It is purely a means of emptying the bladder when expression or straining are ineffective or when there is distal urethral obstruction. It is particularly useful in those with DSD, as both bladder emptying and thus protection of the upper tracts is achieved. It is also this group that has the best chance of achieving continence with this method of management. If detrusor hyperreflexia is a problem and causes leakage between catheterisations, adjuvant anticholinergic agents are often beneficial by reducing detrusor hyperreflexia and thus increasing bladder capacity. Mild degrees of bladder neck incompetence usually respond to alpha-adrenergic drugs.

CIC can be used in both sexes, and self-catheterisation should be encouraged from the age of 6 years. The parents of some severely handicapped children prefer this form of management if continence is achieved, even though they accept that self-catheterisation will never be possible. However, Robinson et al (1985) found that in 24 severely handicapped children who learned to catheterise themselves, complete or nearly complete continence was achieved in 21, and was sustained successfully in 14, showing that severe handicap does not preclude this form of management.

Although CIC undoubtedly plays a major role in the management of these children, it is not the answer for all. Children who have very small capacity bladders or marked hyperreflexia that does not respond to anticholinergic agents, or those who have marked sphincter weakness, will not become dry. In this group of children surgical intervention will usually be necessary, either on the bladder to increase its capacity and to reduce the intravesical pressure or on the urethra to correct sphincter weakness, or both. The timing of such intervention is usually determined by the renal function or the age and motivation of the child. It should be remembered that bladder and urethral dysfunction deteriorates in the late teens with the result that CIC and pharmacological agents may no longer achieve satisfactory continence, in which case management will have to be modified.

Method

Prior to catheterisation the hands are washed and the child should be encouraged to pass urine if this is possible. When the bladder is empty the catheter is slowly withdrawn and washed in soapy water. It can be kept in a plastic or polythene container; it does not need to be kept in an antiseptic solution.

Catheterisation in an ordinary toilet is the aim. We recommend that the catheter is changed weekly.

Continuous catheterisation

This is mandatory for at least 4 to 6 weeks in the child who presents with dilated upper tracts secondary to obstruction to urinary outflow. The effect of this can be assessed using ultrasonography, and further management can be planned when the upper tracts are decompressed. In addition this may be the only way to achieve continence in a severely handicapped wheelchair-bound girl. This method of management is usually disliked by the mobile child and the complication rate can be as high as 25% (Minns et al 1980).

INCONTINENCE APPLIANCES AND PHARMACOLOGICAL AGENTS

Penile appliances

In boys these can be used instead of an indwelling catheter if there is no obstruction to urinary overflow. In young boys it is often very difficult to achieve a good fit, and leakage often occurs in mobile boys. It is easier to achieve a watertight fit in adolescents and adults. The child should be encouraged to empty the bladder regularly and, if distal urethral obstruction is present, endoscopic sphincterotomy may be necessary to ensure bladder emptying and thus reduce the risk of infection and upper tract problems.

Pads

In the past few years a number of manufacturers have cooperated in trials to produce more effective products of differing sizes, and also different types, for the two sexes.

Pharmacological agents (Table 14.1)

Three groups of drugs are currently used:

1. *Anticholinergic agents.* These have proved to be most beneficial. They reduce detrusor hyperreflexia and indirectly increase bladder capacity. They can be used on their own or in combination with other forms of management, particularly CIC. If they are used on their own in the presence of DSD, regular bladder emptying must be ensured to prevent back-pressure effects on the kidneys.

Propantheline and oxybutynin have been used most commonly. In our experience oxybutynin is more effective.

2. *Alpha-adrenergic agents* act by increasing the tone in the bladder neck region. Ephedrine is used most commonly but this will not prevent stress incontinence if there is marked bladder neck weakness. This drug can be used on its own or with CIC. Regular bladder emptying is important.

3. *Cholinergic agents* have a very limited place in the management of these children. They act by increasing bladder contraction where this is reduced, but have not been shown to be very useful (Finkbeiner 1985).

Table 14.1 Pharmacological agents used in neuropathic vesico-urethral dysfunction

Drug	Type	Dose
Propantheline	Anticholinergic	1 month–12 years: 1 mg/kg/day in 3 doses Over 12 yrs: 15 mg 8-hrly
Oxybutynin	Anticholinergic	Over 5 yrs: 2.5 mg bd increasing to 5 mg tds
Dicyclomine*	Anticholinergic	6 months – 12 years: 2 mg/kg/day in 4 doses Over 12 yrs: 60 mg daily in 4 doses
Bethanechol	Parasympathomimetic	0.6 mg/kg/day in 3 doses
Ephedrine	Alpha-adrenergic	1 month – 12 years: 2.5 mg/kg/day in 3 doses Over 12 yrs: 30 mg 8-hrly

* Dicyclomine is the only anticholinergic available as a liquid.

Alpha-adrenergic agents are rarely indicated, as bladder neck obstruction is extremely rare in congenital vesico-urethral dysfunction (Mundy et al 1985). Indeed there is currently no recommended alpha-adrenergic agent for use in children; phenoxybenzamine is no longer recommended since it was found to be carcinogenic in rats when used continuously for 2 years in high doses.

If, despite all these measures, the child is unacceptably wet, or renal function shows signs of deterioration, or both, then serious consideration has to be given to surgical intervention.

SURGICAL MANAGEMENT

Surgery is the last treatment option and is considered in the presence of deteriorating renal function or intractable urinary incontinence. In the presence of upper tract deterioration there is little choice in the timing of the procedure, but surgery for urinary incontinence is preferably delayed until it is clear that the child is capable of understanding what needs to be done and is motivated to cooperate with the treatment and after-care.

In the neuropathic patient a deterioration in renal function is due to outflow obstruction, which occurs at the distal sphincter mechanism. The renal damage may be compounded by reflux and high pressure detrusor contractions. Reflux may be dealt with by ureteric reimplantation but if the other problems of outflow obstruction and high pressure detrusor contractions are dealt with this may not be necessary.

It is worth restating that all these children require full investigation prior to surgery. They will need an intravenous urogram (IVU) to assess anatomy of the urinary tract, videourodynamic study (VDU) to assess the lower tract function, and GFR to assess renal function. The IVU gives information pertinent to the operative procedure, the VDU gives the information on which the operative treatment is based, and the GFR gives a baseline measurement of renal function.

The VDU will enable the child to be classified into one of the following three groups with regard to vesico-urethral function.

1. Acontractile

The bladder neck is incompetent; the distal sphincter presents a static obstruction to flow but remains partially open, thus allowing sphincter weakness incontinence; and the detrusor does not contract to facilitate complete bladder emptying.

In this group intractable incontinence may be treated by implantation of an Artificial Urinary Sphincter (AUS), or by reconstruction of the bladder neck, or possibly by bladder neck elevation—a colposuspension-type procedure.

It should be noted that, in a number of these patients treated with an AUS, the provision of an adequate outflow obstruction has unmasked hyperreflexic detrusor activity requiring treatment in its own right.

2. Contractile

The bladder neck is competent in 50%, the distal sphincter is dyssynergic in most, and the detrusor contractions generate high pressures. Incontinence occurs with the high pressure contractions, but voiding is incomplete, the bladder is thick walled and the capacity is often reduced.

Sphincterotomy may be required to treat the outflow obstruction. Hyperreflexia and reduced capacity require a cystoplasty (bladder reconstruction procedure) and continence may be achieved using an AUS.

3. Intermediate

The bladder neck is incompetent; the distal sphincter is a static obstruction resulting in incomplete voiding and sphincter weakness incontinence; and the detrusor is thick and contracted resulting in poor compliance and a small capacity with an actively contracting detrusor. This combination results in continuous incontinence.

Sphincterotomy may be necessary to treat the outflow obstruction. Continence can be achieved with an AUS and the detrusor will need to be replaced by cystoplasty.

As previously stated, the key factors in achieving continence are:

- Reasonable bladder capacity
- Reasonable degree of outflow obstruction
- Satisfactory bladder emptying.

A further requirement is a low pressure bladder.

DEALING WITH OUTFLOW OBSTRUCTION

In cases where distal sphincter obstruction is causing a deterioration in renal function, the aim of treatment is obviously to relieve the obstruction. This can be achieved by an indwelling catheter, or by cutting the sphincter muscle (sphincterotomy) resulting in sphincter weakness incontinence. In some of these patients the outflow obstruction is utilised to provide continence, and voiding is achieved by intermittent self-catheterisation. This is only applicable where the upper tracts are not subjected to high pressures, i.e. where the detrusor hyperreflexia is controlled with anticholinergics.

In boys, sphincterotomy will result in total incontinence if the bladder neck is incompetent; this must be managed using pads, external appliances, an indwelling catheter or, surgically, by implantation of an AUS.

In 50% of those boys with contractile bladders the bladder neck is competent and in this group sphincterotomy may result in improved bladder emptying with reasonable continence, thus achieving the 'balanced bladder'.

In girls, an indwelling catheter is preferred, as external appliances are impractical; sphincterotomy offers little chance of preserving any continence and may damage the urethra to an extent that later corrective procedures, such as the insertion of an AUS, are interfered with.

Sphincterotomy is an endoscopic procedure, and is somewhat imprecise as there are no reliable landmarks dictating the length or depth of the incision. Therefore it should be understood that when cautious sphincterotomy is undertaken, with the intention of achieving a 'balanced' bladder, relief of obstruction may be incomplete and the procedure may well need to be repeated.

Sphincterotomy is necessary to protect upper tracts from damage due to incomplete bladder emptying. It is not an essential procedure if other treatments are being employed, for example if high pressure detrusor contractions are abolished by cystoplasty and the detrusor sphincter dyssynergia provides continence; voiding may then be achieved with clean intermittent self-catheterisation (CISC) thus avoiding the destruction of the sphincter and the use of an AUS.

ACHIEVING A REASONABLE BLADDER CAPACITY

A reduction in bladder capacity may be due to a number of factors:

1. Small functional capacity due to a large residual volume because of outflow obstruction and unbalanced voiding. This may be dealt with by instituting a regime of intermittent self-catheterisation, or by dealing with any outflow obstruction as described above.
2. Small, contracted, poorly compliant, thick-walled bladder.
3. Reduced functional capacity because of hyperreflexic detrusor activity leading to incontinence.

The small contracted bladder and that with reduced capacity due to hyperreflexia can be treated surgically by a 'cystoplasty' operation, where the bladder may be enlarged or replaced—the so-called 'augmentation' and 'substitution' cystoplasties respectively.

Augmentation cystoplasty

The bladder is split open in the coronal plane, and a piece of the patient's own bowel—usually ileum—is used as a patch and sutured into the gap rather like a gusset (Fig. 14.4) (Bramble 1982). This procedure requires a full bowel preparation; therefore the patient must be admitted 3 days prior to surgery for this to be carried out. Postoperatively they will require 24–48 hours of nasogastric aspiration and intravenous fluids, and 8–10 days of suprapubic catheter drainage. On the 8th postoperative day the catheter may be clamped and voiding commenced. Initially the catheter should only be clamped for short periods 1–2 hours, and after voiding the clamp should be released to drain off any residual urine. If spontaneous voiding is impossible, a self-catheterisation regime must be instituted.

The addition of the intestinal patch to the bladder will increase the capacity so that the interval between voiding is increased. The presence of the patch disrupts detrusor continuity, interrupting the transmission of hyperreflexic contractions and reducing the detrusor pressure—hopefully to a level below that of the outflow obstruction. In this way the augmentation cystoplasty may also improve urinary continence.

The increase in bladder capacity may not be immediately evident and initially there may be little if any improvement, but over the next 6–12 weeks the capacity will increase and the patient may learn to recognise the new sensation of bladder fullness. It is, however, to be recommended that

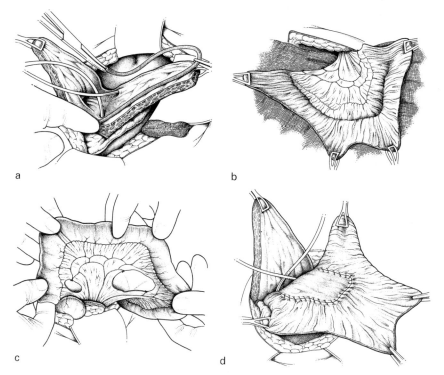

a

b

c

d

Fig. 14.4a. The right side of the bladder has been incised such that the bladder is now completely bisected apart from a bridge of about 1 cm on either side of the bladder neck. The circumference of the bisected bladder is being measured with a length of tubing. **b.** A section of terminal ileum equal in length to the measured circumference of the edge of the bisected bladder is isolated on its vascular pedicle. **c.** After restoring continuity of the ileum, the isolated segment is opened to produce a patch. **d.** The posterior suture line is complete.

regular voiding is instituted as overdistension of the augmented bladder may lead to problems.

Substitution cystoplasty

When the bladder is contracted and thick-walled, augmentation may not be technically possible and the replacement of the bladder with an alternative urinary reservoir is necessary. In these circumstances subtotal cystectomy is carried out, leaving the trigone and bladder neck intact. The substitute bladder is fashioned from intestine, preferably the right colon, which is mobilised and isolated on its own vascular pedicle. In neuropathic patients it has been found necessary to detubularise the intestine to ensure an adequate reduction in contraction pressures in the reservoir (Nurse et al 1988). The intestinal pouch is sutured onto the bladder neck and trigone, and the ureters are implanted into the pouch.

This procedure requires full bowel preparation; the child must be admitted 3 days prior to the operation for this to be carried out. Following a substitution cystoplasty the child will require 3–5 days nasogastric aspiration and intravenous fluids. He will have ureteric stents (drainage tubes) and a suprapubic catheter draining urine for the first 8–10 days. On the 10th day the stents should be ready to come out; if there was any difficulty with the procedure a cystogram may be requested prior to the clamping of the catheter and the institution of a voiding regime as described above.

Problems with cystoplasties

In the early postoperative phase the complications associated with abdominal surgery involving enteric anastomoses may occur. There may also be leakage from the cystoplasty suture lines; this rarely persists if adequate catheter drainage is achieved. Mucus is continuously produced by the intestinal segment used in the reconstruction, and may present problems with catheter blockage; this is usually cleared by gentle bladder lavage.

Late complications include:

1. *Poor cystoplasty emptying*, as a result of the lower pressures and uncoordinated contractile activity of the bowel as compared with the detrusor muscle. This is easily dealt with by instituting a regime of intermittent self-catheterisation.

2. *Mucus obstruction of urinary flow*. The incidence of problems can be reduced by the use of acetylcysteine bladder lavage as often as is necessary.

3. *Incontinence due to high pressure cystoplasty contractions* is rarely a problem since the need for detubularisation of the intestinal segment in neuropathic patients was recognised. If it occurs, a reduction in activity

may be achieved with pharmacological agents, or surgical intervention to patch the cystoplasty may be required.

47% of those patients with ileal augmentation, and 85% of those with substitution cystoplasties will have asymptomatic bacteriuria on random MSU culture (Nurse & Mundy 1989). This may have significance in relation to aetiology of malignant change in the cystoplasty, but this is not proven.

Patients who have undergone uretero-sigmoid urinary diversion are recognised as being at risk of developing a carcinoma at or adjacent to the uretero-sigmoid anastomosis. Patients who have undergone cystoplasty procedures may be at similar risk and these patients should be followed up for life.

Following either of the described cystoplasty procedures, patients may experience a variable period of disturbance of bowel function. This is the result of the bowel preparation and possibly the peri- and postoperative antibiotics. In the vast majority of patients, bowel control returns to normal, i.e. to the preoperative state. There have been a small number of patients who report persisting difficulty in re-establishing a controlled pattern of bowel activity, and they are prone to occasional problems with uncontrolled diarrhoea.

INSERTION OF AN ARTIFICIAL URINARY SPHINCTER (AUS)

The Brantley Scott AUS (Fig. 14.5) is currently the best available method of achieving near normal continence in these patients. The device consists of three components: an inflatable cuff, which is placed around the

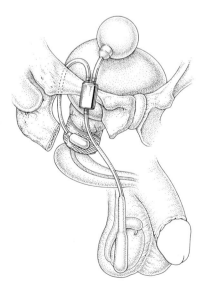

Fig. 14.5 The Brantley Scott Artificial Urinary Sphincter—anatomical position in the male. (Reproduced with permission, from Mundy A R (1987) Cystoplasty. In: Mundy A R (ed) Current operative surgery: Urology. Baillière Tindall, Eastbourne.)

urethra; a reservoir balloon, placed extraperitoneally in the iliac fossa; and a control pump placed in the scrotum in the male and in the labium majorus in the female. These components are connected by kink-resistant tubing and the whole system is filled with a water and contrast medium mix so that the device will be easily seen on plain abdominal X-ray. When the sphincter is activated, the inflated cuff compresses the urethra and stops urinary leakage. The pressure in the cuff is controlled by the reservoir balloon, which exerts a pressure predetermined at the time of manufacture. When the bladder is full and the patient wishes to void, he squeezes the pump; this moves the fluid from the cuff to the reservoir balloon, allowing the urethra to open and urine to pass. The cuff refills over the following few minutes and if, at the time, voiding is incomplete the device can be used again immediately. If the patient is undergoing a bladder reconstruction the sphincter will be implanted at the same time. In those patients undergoing augmentation cystoplasty who have a lesser degree of sphincter weakness incontinence, a sphincter cuff may be placed around the membranous urethra at the time of the cystoplasty; in many, this will provide continence without needing to be inflated.

The implantation of the AUS is a major operation. For an AUS alone the child may be admitted the day before surgery and will require Savlon baths as the only special preparation. An indwelling catheter should be removed 3 days preoperatively and the procedure is covered with 5 days of intravenous antibiotics commencing at induction of anaesthetic. Once the antibiotic course is completed and the wounds are satisfactory the child may be discharged home. At this time the sphincter will be deactivated and the child will still be incontinent. This incontinence should be managed with pads or external appliances. Indwelling catheters should be avoided as their presence in the urethra in the early postoperative period may precipitate urethral erosion over the cuff. Intermittent self-catheterisation to remove large residual volumes is permissible.

The complications seen in relation to AUS implantation are few. Mechanical failure is rare, occurring in 1%. Infection of the device, with erosion of the cuff or pump through the overlying epithelium, occurs in 5–10% of cases. In these circumstances the device will eventually need to be removed; replacement is usually possible but cannot be carried out immediately—it is necessary to wait at least 3 months.

The commonest 'complication' is in fact a feature of the design of the AUS. Stress incontinence may occur with some activities. This is because the system is pressurised at a level controlled by the reservoir balloon. If the pressure in the bladder rises above the pressure in the cuff, urine will leak through the cuff. This affords some protection to the kidneys in the event of high intravesical pressures. If the stress incontinence is a major problem involving the loss of large urine volumes during mild activity, it is sometimes possible to change the pressure-regulating balloon for one with a higher pressure range. A small amount of stress incontinence, requiring a small pad or no special precautions, must be regarded as acceptable.

Some patients with low pressure bladders and an adequate outflow obstruction will be left with voiding difficulties and problems with urinary infection secondary to incomplete emptying. For these patients the solution is intermittent self-catheterisation through the sphincter.

URINARY DIVERSION AND UNDIVERSION

Urinary diversion still has a place in the treatment of the neuropathic patient with vesico-urethral dysfunction. In some severely handicapped children, intermittent self-catheterisation may not be possible. In others, although the technique can be mastered, the effort and time involved in performing the task 3-hourly makes it unacceptable. In a third group, lack of motivation to perform catheterisation or to comply with correct use of the AUS makes ileal conduit diversion the treatment of choice. There are some patients with severe physical deformities that make surgery difficult and occasionally impossible. In this group, urinary diversion may be an option if there is a suitable abdominal site for a stoma. If not they will be best managed with an indwelling catheter or sphincterotomy, and an external appliance.

Undiversion is the term used to describe a variety of procedures that are used to convert the patient from conduit drainage to a continent 'bladder'. This is possible in any patient and may involve utilising the patient's own bladder (if it is still present), the conduit and other intestinal segments to construct a urinary reservoir and outflow. The latter may be a neo-urethra opening in the usual place or it could be a small catheterisable conduit opening onto the abdominal wall (Mitrofanoff procedure). In both cases the conduit is implanted into the urinary reservoir in such a way that the reservoir is continent and no external appliances are required. Voiding is achieved by self-catheterisation.

Careful consideration should be given to undertaking prolonged and complex surgery in patients who are otherwise well and not experiencing any problems. It is important to give a full explanation of the extent of the undertaking, pointing out that several operations may be required, and it is not possible to create a normal bladder. This last point, although stating the obvious, is extremely important. If, at the end of this, they are still motivated to proceed, then we will perform the operation for them.

REFERENCES

Bates C P, Whiteside C G, Turner-Warwick R 1970 Synchronous cine/pressure/flow cystourethrography with special references to stress and urge incontinence. British Journal of Urology 42: 714–23

Borzyskowski M, Mundy A R, Neville B G R et al 1982 Neuropathic vesicourethral dysfunction in children. British Journal of Urology 54: 641–644

Bramble F J 1982 The treatment of adult enuresis and urge incontinence by enterocystoplasty. British Journal of Urology 54: 693–696

Crooks K K, Enrile B G 1983 Comparison of the ideal conduit and clean intermittent catheterisation for myelomeningocoele. Paediatrics 72: 203–206

Diokno A C, Sunda LP, Hollander J B, Lapides J 1983 Fate of patients started on clean intermittent catheterisation therapy 10 years ago. Journal of Urology 129: 1120–1122

Finkbeiner A E 1985 Is bethanechol chloride clinically effective? A literature review. Journal of Urology 134: 443–449

Lapides J, Diokno A C, Silber S J, Love B S 1972 Clean intermittent self-catheterisation in the treatment of urinary tract disease. Journal of Urology 107: 458–461

Lapides J, Diokno A C, Love B S, Kalish M D C 1974 Follow up on unsterile intermittent catheterisation. Journal of Urology 111: 184–186

Lapides J, Diokno A C, Gould F R, Love B S 1976 Further observations on self-catheterisation. Journal of Urology 116: 169–171

Lyon R P, Scott M P, Marshall S 1975 Intermittent catheterisation rather than urinary diversion in children with myelomeningocele. Journal of Urology 113: 409–417

Minns R A, Dag J C, Dujsy S W, Brown J K, Stark G, McClement E 1980 Indwelling urinary catheters in childhood spinal paralysis. Zeitschsrift für Kinderchirurgie 31: 387–347

Mundy A R, Borzyskowski M, Saxton H M 1982 Videoureodynamic evaluation of neuropathic vesicourethral dysfunction in children. British Journal of Urology 54: 645–649

Mundy A R, Shah P J R, Borzyskowski M, Saxton H M 1982 Sphincter behaviour in myelomeningocele. British Journal of Urology 57: 647–651

Nurse D E, McCrae P, Stephenson T P, Mundy A R 1988 The problems of substitution cystoplasty. British Journal of Urology 61: 423–426

Nurse D E, Mundy A R 1989 Assessment of the malignant potential of cystoplasty. British Journal of Urology 64: 489–492

Raezer D M, Benson G S, Weir A J, Dukett J W 1977 The functional approach to the management of the paediatric neuropathic bladder: a clinical study. Journal of Urology 117: 649–653

Rickwood A M K, Thomas D G, Philip N M, Spicer R D 1982 Assessment of congenital neuropathic bladder by combined urodynamic and radiological studies. British Journal of Urology 54: 512–518

Robinson R O, Cockran M, Strode M 1985 Severe handicap in spina bifida: no bar to intermittent self-catheterisation. Archives of Disease in Childhood 60: 760–762

Whiteside C G 1972 Videocystographic studies with simultaneous pressure and flow recordings. British Medical Bulletin 28: 214–219

15. The neuropathic bowel

U. Agnarsson

INTRODUCTION

Over 90% of children with meningomyelocoele, and a substantial proportion of those with cerebral palsy, suffer from faecal incontinence. It is clear that the neural damage, with its effect on the anorectum and other parts of the gastrointestinal tract, is of primary importance in its development. Constipation is also common in both conditions, and here diet, poor fluid intake, skeletal deformity, decreased mobility and intelligence play important roles.

THE PATHOLOGICAL BOWEL

Much of what we know about anorectal function in handicapped children

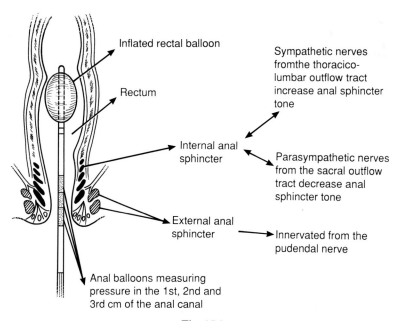

Inflated rectal balloon

Rectum

Internal anal sphincter

External anal sphincter

Anal balloons measuring pressure in the 1st, 2nd and 3rd cm of the anal canal

Sympathetic nerves fromthe thoracico-lumbar outflow tract increase anal sphincter tone

Parasympathetic nerves from the sacral outflow tract decrease anal sphincter tone

Innervated from the pudendal nerve

Fig. 15.1

has been gained by investigations using anorectal manometry. This involves passing a flexible anal probe approximately 15 cm long into the rectum and anal canal (Fig. 15.1). On its distal end is a large balloon, which is used to inflate the rectum, and on its stalk are smaller balloons used for measuring the anal pressure. The following measures are used:

1. The mean, maximal and minimal resting anal pressure
2. Maximal squeeze pressure
3. Rectal sensation
4. Observation of rectal and anal muscle activity and its changes during rectal distension.

From these observations valuable information is gained about anal sphincter and rectal function.

In meningomyelocoele and cerebral palsy a lower than normal pressure in the outermost part of the anal canal is found, which is the zone where the external anal sphincter and/or the levator ani (striated muscles) exert their greatest influence (Agnarsson et al 1989a, b). Only about 10% of all children with meningomyelocoele are able to contract these muscles (Fig. 15.2) and these children are primarily those with low spinal lesions (third lumbar segment and below).

The pressure generated by the internal anal sphincter, a smooth muscle responsible for maintaining the resting tone of the anal canal, may be low, normal or high in meningomyelocoele. Unlike its striated counterpart this sphincter functions independently of high cerebral centres and has a close relationship with the rectum.

This relationship is highlighted by the anorectal inhibitory reflex mediated when the rectal wall distension exceeds a certain threshold. The reflex is transmitted by the intramural nervous pathways to the sphincter, which relaxes and allows stool to enter the anal canal in order for it to be expelled.

In meningomyelocoele and other cord lesions the reflex is more

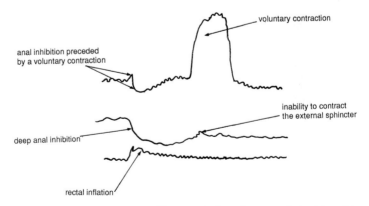

Fig. 15.2 Anorectal manometry trace. Top trace is from the anus of a healthy subject. Middle trace is from a patient with meningomyelocoele. At the bottom a rectal trace is shown.

profound and longer-lasting than in normal children (Scobie et al 1970), and is most clearly found in the lowermost part of the anal canal, where the striated muscles exert their greatest effect. The behaviour of the internal sphincter in children with paralysis of the pelvic floor muscles is a further explanation of the faecal soiling.

Apart from the sphincter impairment, many children—particularly those with meningomyelocoele—suffer loss of rectal sensation, which further exacerbates faecal incontinence. The children are not aware of the rectum gradually filling with stool and that a bowel action is imminent. In meningo-myelocoele the rectum is small and hyperactive with inappropriate small contractions occurring at random. These patients suffer from severe incontinence of small pellets of stool, which can be very difficult to manage.

In meningomyelocoele, defecation is often relatively easy, probably due to the laxity of the anal sphincter. During straining the increased intra-abdominal pressure expels the rectal contents through the low pressure zone of the anal canal. However, many subjects have weak abdominal muscles together with severe structural deformity, and complete emptying of the rectum is therefore rare.

A small number of subjects with meningomyelocoele seem to have a very sensitive bowel, and some of these children suffer from constant soiling of loose and diarrhoea-like stools. It is common for all those with neuropathic incontinence to tolerate gastrointestinal upsets badly, with an unavoidable increase in soiling.

Occasionally, during manometry in children with severe spinal deformity, it is difficult to pass the probe up into its proper position. This gives information about abnormal convolutions in the most distal part of the bowel, which may explain the often explosive soiling seen in some patients.

In cerebral palsy the bowel problem is mainly characterised by constipation, and faecal incontinence is less often seen than in children with spinal cord lesions. Some children with cerebral palsy experience considerable distress with defecation. Presumably this is due to spasticity of the pelvic floor and lack of synchrony as the muscles contract and relax during expulsion of stool. The effect of paralysis and spasticity respectively on the pelvic floor muscles is reflected by the puborectalis muscle sling, which is a part of the levator ani muscle and forms the anorectal angle. The action of this muscle is of great importance during defecation and is thought to play a role in maintaining anal continence.

THE SPINAL LESION

In meningomyelocoele the relationship between the level of spinal lesion and the nature of the bowel problem is unclear. Patients with high spinal lesions (second lumbar segment and above) have incontinence of bulky stools, whilst those with low lesions use laxatives less often but have great problems with incontinence of small pellets of stool. The distribution of the spinal lesion is sometimes asymmetrical, and the extent of the spinal involvement may vary greatly and may indeed be patchy, which further confuses matters.

It is useful to bear in mind the differential innervation of the internal sphincter when this is considered. The parasympathetic and tone-reducing nerve supply to the sphincter occurs through the sacral outflow tract low in the spine. The sympathetic and tone-increasing nerve supply is relayed via the thoracolumbar outflow higher up in the spinal cord (Frenckner 1975, 1976, Lubowski et al 1987).

Anorectal manometry confirms that anal pressure varies enormously in meningomyelocoele, and a clear link with the spinal lesion is not obvious. It is true, however, that most cases of severely reduced anal pressure are seen in low lesions, and this may be related more to the extent of spinal involvement than to the level of the lesion itself. The subjects with the highest anal pressures are also those with low lesions, so it is clearly difficult to generalise about the relationship between manometry and the spinal damage.

The anocutaneous reflex, which has been used in planning bowel management, and which is produced by gently stroking the perianal skin with an orange stick, is seen in 40% of children regardless of whether they have high or low lesions.

MANAGEMENT

Children with meningomyelocoele and cerebral palsy have numerous medical, orthopaedic and surgical problems. It is understandable that these problems are the focus of attention in the first few years of life, so bowel management is often overlooked. This may result in severe problems with constipation and overflow incontinence, which can be a nightmare for parents and child. In a recent survey only 30% of mothers of children with meningomyelocoele had received guidance and advice on bowel care from their doctors (Stellman et al 1983). It is clear, therefore, that there is a strong need for a health professional, such as a community based nurse or health visitor with special experience and training in problems of the neuropathic bowel, whom the parents and children can turn to for advice.

Bowel management usually rests with the mother, especially while the patients are young. The frequent accidents of soiling give an unpleasant smell to the home, are time-consuming to deal with, and may damage furniture, linen, carpets and clothing, and become a financial burden. The incontinence affects the family as a whole, e.g. when on outings and on holidays; in adolescence, emotional problems, depression and social maladjustments are well recognised phenomena. It is clear therefore that bowel management must be started early in life, as the sooner a regular pattern of bowel care is established, the more likely it is to be accepted by the child and its carers.

Before embarking on bowel management, the child's anorectal function is assessed. This includes:

- History and nature of the bowel control and the dietary assessment. This gives an idea about the success of the current bowel management. It is useful to have a bowel diary of the last 3–4 weeks to evaluate the severity of the problems.
- With sensorimotor nerve testing, the level of the spinal lesion is established and the anocutaneous reflex is checked
- The degree of deformity of the spine is noted. The abdomen is palpated for faecal masses and a rectal examination carried out
- The locomotor system is examined and the child's mobility noted
- Psychological assessment and evaluation of intelligence will clearly aid in planning management
- Finally, anorectal manometry may be carried out to give information about anal pressures and anorectal function. If not readily available, referral for this is indicated in children with low lesions who are having problems with faecal incontinence and for whom biofeedback might be beneficial.

When bowel management is planned, there are two points of great importance:

1. The regime has to fit in with the family pattern.
2. The patient should ideally know how to strain effectively.

In a young child the latter can be taught. The intra-abdominal pressure can be increased by asking the child to blow into a balloon, or in the case of an older child to take a deep breath and hold it while bearing down.

Bowel management can be divided into regular toileting, diet and physical assistance.

Regular toileting

This should be started in infancy before the rapid gastrocolic reflex diminishes (Shurtleff 1980). The child is positioned on the toilet or potty, shortly (5–15 minutes) after a meal to take advantage of the gastrocolic reflex. It is important to give plenty of encouragement in order to make these sessions as pleasant as possible. In very young individuals it may be appropriate to have the child lie on a couch or a bed initially while straining is being taught. He/she should sit on the toilet or lie on the bed and strain well for 10–15 minutes. After this time some, but not all, of the stools in the distal colon may have been expelled. Therefore in very cooperative children it may be advisable to place the patient on the toilet again 15–30 minutes later to see if the rest of the stool, now having presumably been pushed further distally by the previous straining, is evacuated. This may have to be repeated 2–3 times every day, i.e. after all main meals.

Regular toileting is important for all patients who have severe faecal incontinence, but in particular those who have severely reduced anal pressures on manometry and low lesions. At the end of the session a finger can be passed into the back passage to check for remaining stool. If emptying is incomplete a suppository may be given or a small manual evacuation may have to be carried out. Initially this may be required often, but gradually, with time, one may anticipate that it will be needed less frequently.

Proper positioning on the toilet is often difficult due to deformity or spasticity. One should try to keep thighs apart and flex the head forward to facilitate the transit of bolus through the anus. Avoid extension and arching back, which is sometimes seen in cerebral palsy.

Diet

Generally it is advised that patients should eat food with a reasonable amount of fibre. This helps with constipation, and generally softens stools and makes them bulkier and easier to pass. However, in children with low spinal lesions and a small empty rectum with low pressures on manometry, a diet rich in fibre may exacerbate faecal incontinence. Here a low residue diet may be advisable.

Physical assistance

This includes manual evacuations, laxatives and other oral medicines, suppositories, enemas and biofeedback.

Manual evacuations

Manual evacuations may have to be carried out in severely deformed subjects with high spinal lesions who are unable to sit on the toilet or cannot strain properly due to weak abdominal musculature. Later, perianal pressure synchronised with the child's own efforts may become effective, and with increasing age and maturity satisfactory bowel evacuation may be obtained by voluntary effort alone.

Laxatives

Laxatives commonly used include the following:

1. *Bulk-forming agents* (methylcellulose, ispaghula husk and sterculia), which increase the faecal mass.
2. *Faecal softeners* (lactulose, danthron, dioctyl sodium sulphosuccinate), which lubricate and soften the faeces, but if given in too large dosages may make voluntary defecation more difficult.
3. *Stimulant laxatives* (senna, bisacodyl), which increase colonic motility and are useful to initiate defecation, but stools can easily be made too loose if the dose is too high.

With stimulant laxatives the exact timing of maximal activity in individual patients is hard to predict. It can be anything between 2 and 18 hours, and to fit it in with the toileting routine is a matter of trial and error to begin with. The rule with laxatives in general is that the dosage is increased gradually until the desired effect is obtained. Too big a dose may result in worsening of the incontinence.

Other oral medications

These include antimotility drugs such as codeine phosphate, which has been used in severely faecally incontinent patients with low spinal lesions and very severely reduced anal pressures on manometry. It should be remembered that giving these drugs can lead to constipation.

Suppositories

Suppositories (glycerine, bisacodyl) are useful in regulating bowel action and in acting as an adjuvant to regular toileting when the latter fails to clear the rectum of faeces. However, in patients with very lax anal sphincters suppositories tend to slide out again and can be very difficult to keep in place.

Biofeedback

Biofeedback has been used in treating faecal incontinence in meningo-myelocoele. Earlier reports were encouraging (Wald 1983), but doubt has been cast recently over the effectiveness of this therapy (Loening-Baucke et al 1988, Whitehead et al 1986), and its success seems similar to that of a well regulated behavioural modification programme. As with anorectal manometry, biofeedback involves placing a balloon into the rectum, which is then inflated with increasing amounts of air to establish the degree of rectal sensation. At the same time pressure is recorded in the anus. The patient is able to see the manometry traces on a computer screen and so is aware visually, if not otherwise, of the rectum being distended and of the responses of the anal sphincters. This is the visual feedback.

He is instructed to attempt squeezing (contracting) with his anus when the rectum is distended, and positive verbal encouragement and praise are given for each correct response. The verbal and visual feedback is intended to make the patient aware of his anorectal sensations and of his capacity to use his striated pelvic floor muscles to contract and control immediate incontinence. Gradually all visual—and later verbal—feedback is withdrawn, and the patient has to rely on his own sensations to squeeze correctly.

Many patients confuse squeezing with pushing, and rectal contractions are produced resulting in a bowel evacuation. If the patient understands what to do and is able to perform correctly, this is repeated on a weekly basis for 6 weeks. The strength of the external sphincter squeeze is measured on each occasion. If there is no improvement in its strength, biofeedback is usually abandoned after three sessions.

An objective assessment of faecal soiling is made during the initial training period and on follow-up of 6–12 months improvements in faecal incontinence of up to 90% have been reported in some children. This therapy relies on the patient having some rectal sensation. Biofeedback would seem to be ideal for those patients with *low lesions* and *rectal sensation* and some *capacity to squeeze* the external anal sphincter. *Motivation* and *intelligence* are also important for patient selection.

REFERENCES

Agnarsson U, Gordon C, McCarthy G et all 1989a Anorectal function in children and adolescents with spina bifida. Gut 30(5): A715

Agnarsson U. Gordon C, McCarthy G et al 1989b Anorectal function in children with severe cerebral palsy. Gut 30(9): A1474

Frenckner B 1975 Function of the anal sphincters in spinal man. Gut 16: 638–644

Frenckner B 1976 Influence of autonomic nerves on the internal anal sphincter in man. Gut 17: 306–312

Loening-Baucke V, Desch L, Wolraich M 1988 Biofeedback training for patients with myelomeningocele and faecal incontinence. Developmental Medicine and Child Neurology 30: 781–790

Lubowski D Z, Nicholls R J, Swash M 1987 Neural control of internal anal sphincter function. British Journal of Surgery 74: 668–670

Scobie W G, Eckstein H B, Long W J 1970 Bowel function in meningomyelocoele. Developmental Medicine and Child Neurology 12 (22):150–156

Shurtleff D B 1980 Myelodysplasia: management and treatment. Current problems in pediatrics. Year Book Medical Publishers, Chicago. January: 41–53

Stellman G R, Gilmore M, Bannister C M 1983 A survey of bowel management experienced by families of spina bifida children. Zeitschrift für Kinderchirurgie 38(11): 96–97

Wald A 1983 Biofeedback for neurogenic faecal incontinence: rectal sensation is a determinant of outcome. Journal of Pediatric Gastroenterology and Nutrition 2(2): 302–306

Whitehead W E, Parker L, Bosmajian L et al 1986 Treatment of faecal incontinence in children with spina bifida: comparison of biofeedback and behaviour modification. Archives of Physical and Medical Rehabilitation 67: 218–224

16 Rehabilitation after acute neurological trauma

J. Middleton   M. Jones   V. Moffat   L. Wintle
P. Russell

INTRODUCTION

In this chapter we will look at acute trauma to the brain and the complexity of problems that can arise, whether temporarily or permanently. We will also look at the levels of expected recovery and will discuss how and to what extent rehabilitation can enhance recovery, not only in terms of physical functioning, but also in terms of communication, daily living and cognitive functioning. Finally we will consider rehabilitation from a wider perspective, the psychological implications of acute neurological injury on the child's sense of self, his personality, how the trauma to the child affects his family, and what a rehabilitation team can offer to help and support.

CEREBRAL INJURY

Traumatic damage to the brain caused by a head injury accounts for over 40 000 children and adolescents under the age of 14 being admitted to hospital each year (Department of Health and Social Security 1987). Under the age of 2 years the majority of injuries are caused through accidents in the home, with falls from stairs and playground equipment being the major cause in middle childhood. Most severe injuries in late childhood and adolescence arise from accidents on the road (Rutter et al 1984). A small proportion (approximately 4%) are caused through physical abuse (Craft et al 1972).

Apart from dynamic injury to the brain, other injury can arise from a variety of causes: (a) infection (meningitis or encephalitis); (b) hypoxia caused by severe status epilepticus, drowning, cardiac arrest or postoperative shock; (c) cerebro-vascular accidents (malformations or blood clotting defects); and (d) cerebral oedema caused by severe diabetic coma etc. Although not so acute in onset, space-occupying lesions (whether benign or malignant) and malnutrition may also cause permanent and severe cerebral insult.

RECOVERY

Indices of recovery

When a child is severely injured, the primary question for parents is whether he will survive. Once they can be reassured, the extent of expected recovery will be foremost in their minds. The answer, however, is not simple. Both the length and depth of coma measured on the Glasgow Coma Scale (Teasdale & Jennett 1974) or the less well standardized Children's Coma Scale (Raimondi & Hirschauer 1984) can provide some index in helping to predict eventual outcome (Jennett 1976). Level and depth of coma, but not level of acute intracranial pressure, have been found to relate to neuropsychological deficits (Winogron et al 1984). Duration of post-traumatic amnesia (PTA) is also a useful measure (Medical Disability Society 1988).

Shapiro (1985) argues for a multi-axial approach that includes both depth and duration of coma, premorbid functioning, the use of aggressive or conservative immediate surgical intervention, site and type of haematomas, and the extent of diffuse axonal injury and cerebral swelling. Closed head injury tends to result in more generalised disruption of brain functioning in children than in adults (Rutter 1981). The presence of severe multiple trauma is also another factor which will affect outcome (Mayer et al 1981).

Fallacies

Physical improvements as an index of recovery

Some of the early optimism for children's recovery following head injury was based on studies that looked generally at improvements in physical independence and daily living skills (for instance, Bruce et al 1979, Brink et al 1980). More recently clinicians in the field (Johnson & Roethig-Johnson 1988a, Goodman 1989, Middleton 1989a, Furlonger & Johnson 1989) are increasingly aware that the child who makes a good physical recovery can continue to have gross and often complex cognitive problems, which superficially may not be obvious. For parents this is particularly difficult, as they may still be given inappropriately hopeful predictions for their child's final recovery, or may themselves judge levels of recovery from watching their child run around the ward, despite professional caution.

Age, plasticity and experience

The belief that the immaturity of the brain at time of injury confers advantage to children over adults is now questioned. Early optimism was based on work such as that of Kennard (1938) with regard to animal studies and Smith & Sugar (1975) with regard to the recovery of speech and language. However, injury to a child's brain will affect new learning, thus decreasing the ability to add new information to past experience. Secondly this knowledge base itself will be less than that of adults. Thirdly greater plasticity in the young brain need not necessarily mean that new neural connections will be beneficial (Black et al 1971, Goodman 1989). Children are not at an advantage over adults and may indeed recover *less* well.

Recovery time

Clinical experience suggests the search for early rehabilitation is partly fired by a belief that recovery continues only up to about 2 years post-injury. The point is that there is little research on recovery stretching beyond 2–2½ years after injury, and consequently little documented evidence that recovery continues for longer. There are exceptions: Klonoff et al (1977) reports that children in his study were continuing to make progress over a 5-year period. Working with children in a clinical setting indicates that they continue to improve for many years, albeit at an increasingly slow rate, and rehabilitation after 2 years can be beneficial.

Conversely some younger children may appear to have relatively mild problems shortly after injury. However, as their brains continue to develop into their teens, those injured parts of the brain that become increasingly more important in their cognitive functioning may create latent problems. For instance, the frontal lobes, often damaged in head injuries, are not fully myelinated until adolescence. After a period of good recovery, disinhibited behaviour may later emerge, which can cause concern to parents and teachers.

Moderate to mild injuries

It has been long accepted that severe head injury (duration of coma beyond 6 hours or PTA of more than 2 weeks), but not milder injuries, cause lasting effects (Chadwick et al 1984, Fletcher et al 1990). This is being increasingly questioned (Boll 1983, Gulbrandsen 1984, Middleton 1989a) and children with less severe injuries may well display problems, if only temporarily (see below).

REHABILITATION: THE INTERDISCIPLINARY THERAPY APPROACH

An interdisciplinary approach to the patient with a head injury is vital from an early stage. This practice is evolving at both Tadworth Court Children's Hospital and Chailey Heritage. Following assessment, a programme consisting of aspects of speech therapy, physiotherapy, psychology, occupational therapy, recreational therapy, education and nursing is devised. It is carried out daily by members of the team, who may be supported by voluntary helpers and the child's family. Programmes evolve as recovery occurs and each discipline continually reviews their particular input to the programme. Regular reviews are held.

The benefits of this approach are that disciplines observe recovery in all areas and the developing programme provides a written record of progress. Family and carers appreciate the structured framework that everyone can take part in, and benefit from being involved in the programme.

A cognitive rehabilitation therapy programme described by Szekeres et al (1984) consists of three stages of recovery. The focus during the early stages is on sensory and sensorimotor stimulation. During the middle stages, reduction of confusion and retention of cognitive components are helped by highly structured programmes; and in the late stage, the aim is to integrate the functional components and compensating strategies so that there is generalisation of skills.

COMA AROUSAL

Referral may occur at any stage following injury, from coma through to the post-rehabilitation stage when further recovery can still be made at a slower pace.

An active rehabilitation programme should be started as soon as possible after head injury to ensure that patients receive intense and varied stimulation. Johnson & Roethig-Johnson (1988b) stated that 'The coma arousal programme stimulates all five sensory modalities with simple but intense stimuli. Some success has been claimed in arousing severely head injury patients from a coma and improving their chances of recovery'. They described a daily intensive stimulation programme incorporating all senses, using both pleasant and noxious stimuli and demanding as much participation as possible from the patient, and involving relatives as co-therapists to increase the total period of stimulation for the patients.

NURSING MANAGEMENT

In the acute phase, post-injury nursing management will include life-saving care in conjunction with the work of an intensive-care team, including maintenance of airways and breathing, appropriate posture, monitoring of vital recordings, general physical care of the child, and support for the family. Working alongside physiotherapists in order to achieve good positioning and to prevent later contractures is crucial. At this stage care will also include nasogastric feeding, catheterisation, etc., ensuring that children are adequately nourished and hydrated. In addition the care of tracheostomies etc. may be necessary. Depending on the specific area of the brain that has been damaged, problems may occur later. For instance damage to the brain stem may give rise to disturbed sleeping patterns. Other problems may include irregular bodily functions, dysfunctional swallowing and breathing, and poor temperature control.

Nursing management will change as the child recovers. Later in the rehabilitation phase when children are no longer ill, they will not necessarily need traditional nursing care (Roffe 1989). As an equal member of multidisciplinary team, the nurse's role in the management of the child will include carrying out the programmes devised by therapists, creating the link between nursing staff, therapists and parents to ensure that there is a consistent approach to rehabilitation, and encouraging the child's independence as far as possible. Nursing management will no longer involve doing things for children, but often sitting back and allowing them to do it themselves, even if this takes twice as long (see Roffe 1989 for a fuller description).

POST-TRAUMATIC SYNDROME (PTS)

On emerging from a coma, a patient will spend some time in the Post-Traumatic Syndrome. This is often referred to as Post-Traumatic Amnesia (PTA) but it is important to realise that it is not only a memory problem but is characterised as confusion, vagueness, fatigue, poor attention and often agitation. Careful assessment is needed as this state may mask other problems which come to light as the PTS resolves. The duration of PTS is often hard to assess as many patients continue to have long or short memory deficits after they emerge from PTS. These may be modality-specific or general and may affect input, storage or retrieval. (From *Introductory guidelines to the management of head injury.*)

At the point where the child's condition is stable and he is showing signs of waking up, an intensive therapy programme should be started. Initial videoing is very useful in order to establish an accurate baseline, and in the future will help the family and staff to be aware of progress made. Intensive therapy may need to commence in short, frequent sessions, e.g. 15 minutes several times a day, to allow for fatigue and problems in concentration span. This can also enable therapy to fit in with nursing routines. The presence of tracheostomies, catheters and nasogastric tubes should not preclude intensive therapy.

Full multidisciplinary assessment should be carried out at this stage and reviewed frequently with all concerned, including the family, to ensure consistency of aims and handling. The age, abilities, interests and personality of the child prior to the trauma should be taken into consideration. The pattern observed will not necessarily be typical of the developmentally delayed child, as isolated skills may have been retained, depending on location and level of brain damage. Assessment needs to be ongoing as the level of functioning may change from day to day and may be erratic. There may be apparent loss of skills while other areas are being focused upon.

FACTORS INFLUENCING REHABILITATION

Fatigue is a very real factor hindering early rehabilitation. Treatment sessions therefore must be kept short but frequent, allowing time for rest.

Changes in personality and behaviour can occur, which affect progress; for example: aggression tending to increase drive or, conversely, reduce tolerance to therapy; euphoria tending to reduce drive, motivation and insight; disinhibition causing behaviour to be inappropriate, which may, in the long term, override good recovery in other areas and make reintegration into the community difficult.

Sensory function may be impaired, for example visual disturbance, sensory neglect or hypersensitivity. Gross motor skills such as mobility and posture (especially head control) will affect all areas of recovery. Fine motor skills may be impaired by the presence of spasticity, ataxia, tremor or perceptual difficulties. A lack of eye–hand coordination will be apparent during activities such as feeding or writing, and causes a great deal of frustration.

PHYSICAL REHABILITATION

Constant assessment of the child's joint range must be carried out, bearing in mind that the asymmetry may lead to formation of scoliosis, which may need splinting with a thoraco-lumbar-sacral orthosis and possible surgical intervention. Children who present with contractures such as equinus deformities of the feet, or elbow or wrist contractures, may also require surgical release. Unfortunately surgical release is often performed just at the time when the child is recovering most rapidly and causes needless delay. (See also Ch. 25.)

A problem that can arise following head injury is the laying down of bone around the joints (ossification). This is not caused by overenthusiastic physiotherapy in the early stages! The removal of this bone cannot take place until it is fully mature—about 2 years post-injury. Rehabilitation has to take place around the limitation until this time. Intensive physiotherapy will be required post-operatively, working from passive movements and capitalising on any return of ability to maximise active participation.

A good sitting position is necessary as soon as possible after the acute stage to facilitate head control, awareness and normal perception of the environment. Additionally this will permit early mobility and orientation for the child. The seating system selected should be adjustable to allow for a fully upright position as soon as this can be tolerated. It should be easily adaptable to allow each new postural skill or progress in hand function to be maximised, e.g. early removal of headrests or side supports as soon as the child is ready. Routinely locate interesting stimuli to encourage head-turning to the non-favoured side to counteract sensory neglect of the affected side.

To enable maximum stimulation to be given to the child, the chair should ideally be suitable as a car seat, an insert for a wheelchair, *and* an armchair allowing the feet to be on the floor. Constant liaison with the family is needed to allow acceptance of specialised equipment being introduced at this early stage in order for it not to be seen as 'handicapping' the child or as being used instead of therapy.

To reinforce body awareness, a variety of sensory input such as hot and cold, textures, familiar smells, sounds and voices can all be used in the early stage. Reliable discrimination of sound can be encouraged by simple presentation of sounds away from extraneous noise, combined with a meaningful visual stimulus such as the gaining of eye contact while speaking to the patient. Oral stimulation to reduce sensitivity should be applied early, and gradual tolerance to touch, taste, texture and temperature can be developed. Vestibular stimulation, spinning or swinging prone on a large swing, movement over a therapy ball or large roll can be introduced. Taking part in tactile activities such as cuddling, massage and aromatherapy can enable the family to enjoy an intimate experience with the child during intensive care and afterwards. Explanations to family and friends about the benefits of these activities will help motivation where the response is minimal.

REHABILITATION OF COMMUNICATION

The communication deficit is just one of a number of perceptual, organisational, emotional and behavioural aspects of head injury; the language disorder differs from dysphasia in that it may reflect an underlying cognitive disorder rather than being language-specific.

Establishment of a consistent way of indicating yes or no is a priority for reliable assessment of language and cognition. Initially this could include using eye movement or blinking, facial expressions or gesture, until a more sophisticated method is established.

Language may improve spontaneously if training is given in other areas such as orientation, memory and independence. The introduction of an augmentative communication system or aid may be beneficial as an interim measure. This may be a sign, symbol, word or alphabet system.

Voice initiation may present problems, particularly following tracheostomy. Frequent changes of position, weightbearing through limbs and breathing exercises will encourage voice production. Speech will often emerge from mouthing words to whispering before breathing and phonation are coordinated. (See Chs 3 and 26.)

REHABILITATION IN DAILY LIVING

Activities of daily living can be presented initially in a very structured form, gradually reducing the level of structure and raising the initiative expected as/if the child's performance improves. Practice at a theoretical task, e.g. describing an imaginary activity such as getting ready for school or taking a bath, can be presented in stages prior to attempting the practical task. Clear 'recipes' for tasks may need to be available for the child to refer back to while working on the practical task (for example, a shopping expedition or making a cup of tea). Items of equipment may be needed to assist carer and child in bathing, toileting, transferring and mobility. These items should gradually be withdrawn if function improves. The child is likely to be catheterised or in nappies in the early stages and a decision must be reached regarding when and how to try use of the toilet. A supportive toilet seat may be required (see Ch. 33). A toileting programme involving regular visits may be necessary initially. Urinary continence can usually be established (even after long periods of incontinence) through consistent management, provided there is no spinal injury. However, this may take up to a year or even much longer.

Dressing activities can incorporate many aspects of cognitive function. Selection of appropriate clothes, matching and contrasting colour and style can be utilised.

At mealtimes, even in the early stages, the child should be fed sitting in a chair in an upright position. Feeding patterns and head control will not improve while the child is reclined. Nasogastric feeding should be phased out as soon as possible and guidance on nutrition sought to avoid weight loss. Desensitisation and facial and oral stimulation should commence in the first stage of recovery and become a routine procedure—otherwise hypersensitivity builds up, hindering good feeding patterns. The oral stimulation programme will consist of stroking lips, gums, tongue, the use of ice and facilitation of swallowing, but advice needs to be sought from a speech therapist before commencing on this.

A phased introduction to technology at all stages of rehabilitation will allow the child earlier access to means of communication, powered mobility, education, 'Possum' and environmental control. As recovery takes place, the use of switches can be refined from, for example, chin switches to a joystick to normal hand function (if possible). Similarly, powered mobility may be used in the early stages in conjunction with work on walking (See Ch. 26).

COGNITIVE REHABILITATION

Problems

The previous sections have shown how physical and communication problems occur following a head injury. As we have already pointed out, it is often these kinds of difficulties that are initially taken as the most serious impairments following injury by parents, with recovery of motor function and simple daily living skills leading to an overestimation of the extent of learning and cognitive recovery. It is not uncommon that children make superficially good recoveries following head injuries, such that in a controlled and structured environment their very real deficits are more easily ignored or overlooked. It is only when the environmental structures disappear, and the choices before them become complex and multiple, that problems can become apparent. Indeed it is often the cognitive and personality problems which finally create greater dependency and burden on the family than impaired motor function (Livingston & Brooks 1988).

Global intelligence

Global intelligence is invariably affected in the most severely injured, but is not necessarily apparent in moderately injured children. Chadwick et al (1981) have found a relationship between cognitive problems and recovery, and severity of brain injury. Performance IQ on the WISC–R was affected more than Verbal IQ, although it was not clear whether the lower Performance scores were due to the slower speed of information processing (as tests in this scale are timed) or to actual visuo-perceptual problems. Eiben et al (1984) also report that children who have been in coma for over 21 days have a poor long-term outcome in terms of being either totally dependent or at least needing assistance. Winogron et al (1984) also found Performance IQ of the WISC–R related to the severity of the injury, but not Verbal IQ or the Full Scale. However, there was a tendency for those with the most severe injuries also to have lower Full Scale scores.

These learning difficulties do not necessarily disappear with time. Klonoff et al (1977) found that one-fifth of his sample of head-injured children still had poor cognitive functioning 5 years post-injury. Intellectual recovery was slower than the rate of recovery measured on EEG recordings.

Talking in terms of global intelligence quotients is not very helpful, however, when considering children with head injuries. Global measures can easily mask very real specific deficits, so that an apparently normal IQ can mislead professionals and parents to assume that a child has no problems when this is not so. Between each stimulus or intention to act and the execution of a response or purposeful action are a number of processes that can interfere with learning and behaviour.

Speed of information processing

Although there may be a lack of clarity in precisely what is meant by the term, a child's speed of information processing will affect his behaviour. If the rate at which information is presented is too fast for a child's processing ability, then clearly learning can be disrupted. This is, therefore, a vital area to assess.

The findings of both Winogron et al (1984) and Chadwick et al (1981) suggest that low scores in the Performance Scale of the WISC-R may be due to reduced speed of information processing, and that this deficit can persist for over 2 years. Looking specifically at this issue, Bawden et al (1985) tested 51 children with mild, moderate and severe head injuries (approximately 1 year post-injury). They found speeded performance was impaired in the severely injured children compared to the mild and moderate groups, although they did not exhibit a generalised deficit in motor or visual–spatial abilities.

Attention and memory

Other evidence of post-injury deficits is found when looking at levels of attention and memory, whether at the content (verbal, visual, tactile, etc.) or the process. Ben-Yishay et al (1987) identify deficits in the process of attention–concentration as: (a) insufficient alertness and the consequent inability to be aware and focus on stimuli; (b) fluctuations in attention leading to failure to attend selectively to specific stimuli; (c) disturbances in concentration and failure to sustain attention; and (d) response deficiencies. Nissen (1986) adds capacity to hold information in working memory. Fatigue is also a factor.

Another axis is whether attention is automatic or controlled. The former relies on long-term memory, the latter needs conscious, controlled and sustained effort. The problems of capacity and overload occur when skills that were once automatic pre-injury need conscious attention post-injury (Johnson & Roethig-Johnson 1989). The need to attend to these previously automatic skills leads to reduced efficiency and capacity in learning new material.

Evidence of attention and memory deficits in children and adolescents has been found by Levin & Eisenberg (1979) and Levin et al (1982). Using Buscke's (1974) selective reminding test, which assesses verbal learning and memory, and a continuous visual recognition task, they found that, up to 11 months post-injury, adolescents (over 12 years) and children (under 12 years) with severe head injury had persistent memory deficits, although there had been improvements since the initial baseline measures. Not only did children store fewer words long-term—they also had less efficient retrieval. While a learning curve was observed, the slope of the curve was flattened. At follow-up, children, but not adolescents, with severe head injuries also had deficits in visual recognition. Clinical experience indicates that retrieval is often random and disorganised.

Sensory and perceptual skills

A child cannot attend to and remember a stimulus if he is unable to sense it. Consequently, a full range of investigations needs to take place, particularly of hearing (Raglan 1989) and vision. Even if vision and hearing are unaffected by injury, perception of visual and auditory stimuli may be impaired. In terms of visuo-perceptual problems neglect, hemi-inattention, field defects and visual agnosia can also occur although a child may be unable to articulate that there is a problem, or be unaware that they have a problem at all.

Communication skills

Children may show a variety of problems in communication, including dysarthria, dyspraxia and both receptive and expressive dysphasia (see

Moore & Middleton 1990 for a recent review). Word-finding and confrontation naming are the most commonly found expressive disorders in acquired childhood aphasia (ACA) (Alajounaine & Lhermitte, 1965). There is also growing evidence that auditory comprehension deficits are more common than originally thought (Lees, 1989). It is important to realise that ACA in children generally shows a different pattern of symptoms and recovery characteristics than is seen in adults.

Planning and execution

Problem-solving, self-evaluation, planning and other executive skills are also likely to be impaired (Goldstein & Levin 1985). As children become older and these skills become more crucial in their academic work, so their school performance may deteriorate or at least their earlier progress may begin to flatten out.

ASSESSMENT

With the complexity of problems described above it is important that children are carefully assessed, not only for their impairments but also for their assets. Assessment is necessary for estimating baseline levels of functioning, monitoring change, planning programmes and evaluating treatment procedures. Irrespective of the limitations of the child, it is always possible to assess his level of functioning to some degree even if he is unable to communicate verbally and has no use of his hands. Observations of his behaviour, both actual and reported from a variety of sources, can be made using criterion-based assessments, or more formally structured interview procedures (for instance, the Vineland Adaptive Behaviour Scales Revised).

Formalised assessments can be made as recovery continues (see Baxter et al 1984 and Hynd 1988 for detailed discussions). Despite the doubted use of global intelligence scores, perceptive and judicious use of standardised measures such as the WISC-R can give many insights into individual deficits as well as intact areas of functioning. It is often not what the child achieves, but how he achieves it, that can give greater information.

In addition to present functioning it is crucial to gain as much information as possible about premorbid functioning. Pre-injury assessment should cover a number of variables (Middleton 1989b) to include age at injury, time since injury, documented brain damage and premorbid cognitive and emotional status. It is unlikely that most children will have been formally assessed prior to their traumatic injury, but school reports are useful. It is also important to assess present expectations from parents and professionals. Despite the limitations of retrospective data, the use of a structured interview (such as the Vineland), with parents can give useful insights.

COGNITIVE REMEDIATION

Evaluation of treatment efficacy is complex. Improvements in specific or functional skills deficits have to take three factors into account: a) natural recovery, b) development, and c) treatment effects. In addition, important questions arise as to whether treatment focuses on deficits and impairments, or capitalises on intact functioning. It might appear simple to suggest both, but at times there may be a dilemma between independence and social acceptability.

Whatever the level of a child's functioning, it is crucial that rehabilitation is seen as an inter disciplinary process, with parents taking an active part in the team. In order for programmes to be fully effective, isolated therapy input will be neither consistent nor persistent, and consequently will either fail or become half-hearted. A child's cognitive capacity will affect his understanding and cooperation in physiotherapy, while his posture may affect learning and task performance. Traumatic injury will not only result in a loss of classroom experience and learning for a time, but also the disruption in the *processes* of learning (see above).

A child's rehabilitation needs will change as he recovers (Szekeres et al 1984), from early stimulation programmes to highly structured learning tasks in a distraction-free learning environment. Individual work will be necessary at first but needs to be extended into group work in order to prepare him for return to school. External aids such as diaries, timetables and perhaps even electronic organisers may be necessary to prompt and remind children of their daily programmes, as well as help with study skills to structure problem-solving tasks, initially written down but with the aim of children internalising these strategies. Computer-assisted remediation programmes may be helpful. However, all this needs to be generalised to functional everyday living skills.

The following give in more detail some ideas with regard to strategies.

Orientation

Early orientation must be encouraged by all who come in contact with the patient. Talking about news of family and current affairs, weather, time, place is essential even when there is little or no response, as the child may be hearing but unable to respond. Planning and anticipating events in the immediate future is useful. Practice at recalling the day's events and at performing simple sequences of activity may need to be carried out frequently.

Attention

Initially it is necessary to exclude all stimuli other than the activity being practiced. The level of external stimuli can be gradually increased as the child's attention span progresses. It can be helpful to present one idea at a time (avoiding complex language), ensuring that maximum attention can be focused on the activity. Activity periods need to be kept short. Attention deficits are always present in severe head injury and may persist in patients with only high-level residual difficulties, and can quite easily be confused with comprehension problems.

Memory

Two important findings (Levin et al 1988) which affect rehabilitation are:

1. The presence of impaired memory is directly related to the severity of acute head injury as reflected by the Glasgow Coma Scale score on hospital admission and by the duration of impaired consciousness.

2. Severe closed head injury sustained during childhood may result in the delayed appearance of impaired verbal learning and memory during adolescence when elaborate mnemonic strategies normally develop.

An implication is that an apparently good recovery after severe closed head injury in children may be followed by educational disability associated with problems in verbal learning and memory. Consequently introductions may be forgotten, new work is not retained and constant reinforcement is necessary. Strategies need to be taught to help in overcoming memory deficits, e.g. cueing, organising words into categories, mnemonics and external aids such as diaries and electronic organisers, particularly if recall rather than storage is impaired. Family photographs and tapes may also prove useful.

Work to assist memory function may need to commence with sequences of simple commands that are not physically too demanding, e.g. blink, look down, look up. There is no evidence that simple repetition increases memory capacity. Memory is not like a muscle which can be made stronger by simply continuing to flex it. However, strategies may be facilitated by activities such as discussion of recent events, study skills, topic work and perhaps memory games.

Perceptual deficits

Problems with these areas can be approached using the media currently available, such as tracing, copying and drawing activities, if motor function permits. Alternatively, where motor function is severely affected, activities such as matching, sorting and figure/ground or form/constancy work can be presented for the child to indicate with hand/eye (see Ch. 3).

Computer programmes, e.g. Captain's Log, Burden Neurological Institute Rehabilitation Program, can contribute to a visual–perceptual programme. Switch use may be necessary and perceptual programmes can be combined with use of a pointer board, scanner or computer programme.

Paper scanning can be promoted using figure/ground media or computer displays ensuring that the child learns to scan from left to right and top to bottom of the page (Savage 1971).

Awareness of body image should be promoted from the earliest stages, with limbs being touched and talked about during handling, e.g. bathing and dressing. This work can develop as the level of skill in dressing and self care generally improves. Much reinforcement of body awareness in conversation and in a conceptual form (i.e. puzzles, drawings, other people's bodies) should accompany the physical aspects of reinforcement of normal body image. Difficulties with laterality, especially right/left confusion and inability to cross the midline, are apparent and may manifest themselves in writing and difficulties in sequencing letters and words. In adolescents these problems may become apparent in asymmetrical grooming. This underlying difficulty with spatial relationships will ultimately affect other functions such as motor planning, problem-solving and expressive language.

Many patients can only differentiate textures and temperature by visual means and premorbid experiences. Vision-occluded sensory awareness tasks such as tactile games, proprioceptive awareness and stereognosis should be included in the programme.

Motivation

To improve motivation the selection of an activity at an age-appropriate level for the child, bearing in mind premorbid interests and talents and the stage of recovery reached, is often necessary. Tasks need to be analysed to allow the child to achieve success in activities. Having defined the required activity, it needs to be broken down into steps—each step to be practised individually until it is achieved.

Continuous review of progress and revision of the activity programme is necessary. Backward chaining—where the final step is completed by the child, gradually increasing the number of final steps completed by the child until the whole task is successfully achieved—is a useful method. This can help ensure that the child is not in a position of failing the task.

Where the level of motivation is thought to be hindering rehabilitation, negotiation of a contract between staff and child may assist, as goals and aims are agreed and commitments made.

Perseveration

The child may have difficulty moving on to the next task or idea presented. Ensure that each stimulus is clearly finished with and set aside before moving on. This will help to avoid loss of self-confidence associated with the child's realisation of failure.

SCHOOL

Preparation for return to mainstream schooling (or introduction to special education) should commence during the middle stages of rehabilitation. Reintroduction to a group situation and to work in new surroundings must be approached gradually and cautiously, ensuring that the changes do not cause disorientation, confusion or panic.

REHABILITATION OF THE CHILD AND FAMILY

Rehabilitation, however, is more than retraining old skills or teaching new ones to compensate for deficits. It involves working towards as full a recovery as possible in terms of the child's physical, cognitive and emotional development within a psychosocial perspective, seeing the child as part of a family, school and community. This means work with the child and his family to help them come to terms with the trauma that has affected them all.

A changed personality and new construct of self

As children gradually emerge from coma, so they may become slowly aware of the enormous changes in themselves, in how they understand their environment and how people view them. Luria's graphic account of a young solider with a penetrating head injury (1972) illustrates par excellence how experience of oneself and the world is shattered. A child may need to reconstruct his world in order to come to terms with what has occurred (McCabe & Green 1987). The changes in his cognitive functioning may make this reconstruction difficult and can relate to changes in his behaviour and personality. Changes may then be due directly to brain injury, a psychological reaction to loss or injury and/or a consequence of functional loss of social and emotional behaviour (Jackson 1988).

At the same time there would appear to be a higher incidence of psychiatric disorder in children who suffer head injuries than would be expected in a normal population (Craft et al 1972). Brown et al (1981) found this to be the case, particularly in those with severe as compared to those with mild injuries. Children with severe injuries run an increased risk of new psychiatric disorders, which, however, may not differ in type from general psychiatric disorders found in a normal population. The one exception is that of social disinhibition (Brown et al 1981). Boll (1983) argues that irritability and fatigue can result from mild injury, which may have long-term consequences on both behaviour and learning.

Changes in behaviour and personality often cause parents, siblings and friends considerable distress. The slightly disinhibited and socially inept child or adolescent who emerges from coma may be very different from the sensitive, quiet child whom they knew before. Greater lability in mood, with occasionally aggressive outbursts, causes family and friends to be confused and bereft. One parent commented that her daughter 'died' on the day of the accident and she has had to get to know a completely new child. Children themselves may be quite unaware of these changes, and find it frustrating that people react differently to them than before.

The children also experience a variety of losses, including at the very least the period of time just preceding and following their accident, which they cannot recall. Those who have lost the ability to walk independently, who have communication difficulties or who have become partially dependent on others in daily living skills have obvious losses, although clinical experience suggests that some children deny these problems. Those with cognitive problems may experience the loss not only of time away from school, but of the ability to keep up with their peers in academic work. In addition they can experience loss of friends after the initial rallying around at the time of the accident, and the loss of social skills to create new friendships. They may temporarily lose contact with siblings if not parents while they are in hospital, and later they may experience changes in their position in the hierarchy of the family and their status in school. All this may lead to confusion and loss of self-esteem, which can be expressed through frustration, anxiety, depression, verbal and physical aggression, or lack of motivation.

An integrated rehabilitation programme needs to address these issues in a variety of ways, ranging from setting strict boundaries and devising apposite behaviour programmes to play therapy for younger children and counselling in both individual and group sessions for older children. Social skills groups, where peers can give feedback on inappropriate behaviour, may also be useful. Where necessary, use of psychiatric medication may need to be prescribed in conjunction with other interventions.

Families

Rehabilitation should also focus on the families of children who experience acute neurological trauma (see Wardle et al (1989) for a parent's perspective). Polinko et al (1984) describe the pattern of parents' reaction over time following the initial shock—anxiety and helplessness, denial, guilt, anger and possibly despair. They may experience rejection of their child, and when the problems are severe they may inwardly question whether the child would have been better off dead, leading to later feelings of guilt and shame at such thoughts.

Throughout this time they will need support and help. Initially this may mean clear information in appropriate amounts, often repeated and perhaps written down. In the acute phase the presence of a third party, such as a nurse or social worker, to interpret medical information and allow the opportunity for discussion can be helpful. Later help may involve facilitating grief for the loss of their past hopes and expectations for their child, advice in coping with the present problems, and help in planning for the future. Many parents can be intimidated by the intensive care unit and neurosurgical ward, feeling helpless when they see their child cared for by strangers. Incorporating them into the team, teaching them new skills to help their child and listening to their priorities are important. Later still, supporting the family when the child returns home is essential if the process is not to be traumatic. The first visit home can cause as much distress as joy if preparations have been inadequate. In addition, parents may need more formal help in dealing with post-traumatic shock syndrome, often when they are over the initial phase in the child's recovery or at specific anniversaries. Grieving may occur at different rates, with one spouse supporting another at any one time. Issues related to guilt and blame by one parent of another may need to be addressed.

In addition, the original trauma is most likely to occur during adolescence, which may be a time of turmoil and adjustment for many young people. Secondly the final outcome of rehabilitation may not be clear for many months or even years. Thirdly physical and behaviourial difficulties may make the special dependency needs particularly hard to cope with as parents of adolescents may themselves have been planning major life changes—a return to work or change of jobs, moving house, accepting responsibility for the care of an elderly relative. The sudden trauma of having a highly dependent child against this background can cause widespread difficulties and disappointments. Help from a psychologist and social worker will be crucial in dealing with them.

The families will have different experiences from those with children born with a disability, who will have acquired a network of professional support services over the years. They will also have seen their children make progress (albeit slow) and have had time to begin to plan for the future. They understand the system and, even it if it does not work well, can usually find their way round it. A late-onset disability presents entirely different problems. Firstly parents are unlikely to know other families with a disabled child. Secondly the family house and life style will have developed to meet the needs of an able-bodied family. Helping a 16-year-old with his toilet and personal care needs is very different to coping with a 4-year-old. Even if the local authority can immediately fund an adaptation to the bathroom and other facilities, there may be a time-lag within which the family have to live with a young adult who needs caring for as if he were a child. Social services support will be essential in bridging these gaps, as will advice from the community occupational therapist about the best types of aids and equipment and the desirability of any major adaptations. Home helps, peripatetic care workers, transport (perhaps to an accessible leisure activity) and respite care may all be crucial to keep the family going.

There is growing interest in providing self-advocacy for children and adolescents in such situations, perhaps encouraging them to join an organisation like Headway or the Spinal Injuries Association. The new

Children's Head Injury Trust can link up families with similar problems. Contact-a-Family may be another source of help. Most importantly voluntary organisations and social services can plan together for the return home, and provide a 'bridge' during the transitional period and beyond if difficulties persist.

Finally it is crucial to consider the other children in the family. During the initial phases they may temporarily experience the loss of their parents who are always by their sibling's bed, while they are cared for by the extended family or friends. Later they too may grieve over their sibling's change. Their position in the family hierarchy may alter and they may receive less attention. Psychological care of siblings is an important part of rehabilitation, exploring their fears and anxieties, and perhaps sense of guilt for being culpable in some way.

SUMMARY AND CONCLUSIONS

Some children may improve substantially, others only minimally, no matter how intensive the programme, but it must be borne in mind that constant repetition of therapy will be necessary to their long-term care.

It has often been observed that families 'freeze' the child at the age when the accident happened, and may need help in adjusting to the fact that the child is getting older and his needs and interests are changing whilst not necessarily making a full recovery. This can become especially acute at puberty and when the child is approaching school leaving age.

The rehabilitation of children with acute neurological trauma is a complex and interdisciplinary process. Rehabilitation bridges the care of children from the acute phase, when medical and surgical interventions are foremost, through to the child's return to his home, school and community.

REFERENCES

Adamovich B B, Henderson J A, Averbach S 1985 Cognitive rehabilitation of closed head injury patients. Taylor and Francis
Alajounaine T, Lhermitte F 1965 Acquired aphasia in children. Brain 88: 653-662
Bawden H N, Knights R M, Winogron W H 1985 Speeded performance following head injury in children. Journal of Clinical and Experimental Neuropsychology 7(1): 39-54
Baxter R, Cohen S B, Ylvisaker M 1984 Comprehensive cognitive assessment. In: Ylvisaker M (ed) Head injury rehabilitation: children and adolescents. Taylor and Francis, London
Ben-Yishay Y, Piasetsky E B, Rattok J 1987 A systematic method for ameliorating disorders in basic attention. In: Meier M J, Benton A L, Diller L (eds) Neuro-psychological rehabilitation. Churchill Livingstone, Edinburgh
Black P, Blumer D, Wellner A E 1971 The head-injured child: time-course of recovery with implication for rehabilitation. In: Head-injury: proceedings of an international symposium. Churchill Livingstone, Edinburgh, pp 131-137
Boll TJ 1983 Minor head injury in children—out of sight but not out of mind. Clinical Child Psychiatry 12(1): 74-80
Brink J D, Imbus C, Woo-Sam J 1980 Journal of Paediatrics 97(5): 721-727

Brown G, Chadwick O, Shaffer D, Rutter M, Traub M 1981 A prospective study of children with head injuries: III. Psychiatric sequelae. Psychological Medicine 11: 63–78

Bruce D A. Raphaely R C, Goldberg A I, Zimmerman R A, Bilaniuk L T, Schut L, Kuhl D E 1979 Pathophysiology, treatment and outcome following severe head injury in children. Child's Brain 5: 191–197

Buscke H 1974 Components of verbal learning in children: analysis by selective reminding. Journal of Experimental Child Psychology 18: 488–498

Chadwick O, Rutter M, Brown G, Shaffer D, Traub M 1981 A prospective study of children with head injuries: II. Cognitive sequelae. Psychological Medicine 11: 49–61

Craft A W, Shaw D, Cartlidge N E 1972 Head injuries in children. British Medical Journal 4: 200–203

Department of Health and Social Secuirty 1987 Hospital inpatient enquiry. HMSO, London

Eiben C D, Anderson T P, Lockman L et al 1984 Functional outcome of closed head injury in children and young adults. Archives of Physical Medicine and Rehabilitation 65: 168–170

Fletcher J M, Ewing-Cobbs L, Miner M E, Levin H S, Eisenberg H M 1990 Behavioural changes after closed head injury in children. Journal of Consulting and Clinical psychology 58(1): 93–98

Furlonger R, Johnson D A 1989 Return to School. In: Johnson D A, Uttley D, Wyke M (eds) Children's head injury: Who cares? Falmer Press, Brighton

Goldstein F C, Levin H S 1985 Intellectual and academic outcome following closed head injury in children and adolescents: research strategies and empirical findings. Developmental Neuropsychology 1(3): 195–214

Goodman R 1989 Limits to cerebral plasticity. In: Johnson D A, Uttley D, Wyke M (eds) Children's head injury: Who cares? Falmer Press, Brighton

Gulbrandsen G B 1984 Neuropsychological sequelae of light head injuries in older children 6 months after trauma. Journal of Clinical Neuropsychology 6(3): 257–268

Hynd G 1988 Neuropsychological assessment in clinical child psychology. Sage Publications, London

Introductory guidelines to the management of head injury. Head Injury Specific Interest Group, CST Bulletin.

Jackson H F 1988 Brain cognition and grief. Cognitive rehabilitation. Aphasology 2

Jennett B 1976 Assessment of severity of head injury. Journal of Neurology, Neurosurgey and Psychiatry 39: 647–655

Johnson D A, Roethig-Johnson K 1988a Stopping the slide of head-injured children. Special Children 15: 18–20

Johnson D A, Roethig-Johnson K 1988b Coma stimulation: a challenge to occupational therapy. British Journal of Occupational Therapy 51(3): 87–90

Johnson D A, Roethig-Johnson K 1989 Life in the slow lane: attentional factors after head injury. In: Johnson D A, Uttley D, Wyke M (eds) Children's head injury: Who cares? Falmer Press, Brighton

Kennard MA 1938 Reorganisation of motor function in the cerebral cortex of monkeys deprived of motor and premotor areas in infancy. Journal of Neurophysiology 1: 477–496

Klonoff H, Low M D, Clark C 1977 Head injuries in children: a prospective five year follow-up. Journal of Neurology, Neurosurgery and Psychiatry 40: 1211–1219

Lees J 1989 Recovery of speech and language deficits after head injury in chidren. In: Johnson D A, Uttley D, Wyke M (eds) Children's head injury: who cares? Falmer Press, London

Levin H S, Eisenberg H M 1979 Neuropsychological impairment after closed head injury in children and adolescents. Journal of Paediatric Psychology 4: 389–402

Levin H S, Eisenberg H M, Wigg N R, Kobayashi K 1982 Memory and intellectual ability after head injury in children and adolescents. Neurosurgery 11: 668–673

Livingston M G, Brooks D N 1988 The burden on families of the brain injured: a review. Journal of Head Trauma Rehabilitation 3(4): 6–15

Lones J 1985 Some educational consequences of spinal and head injuries in the teenage years (Lord Mayor Treloar College). Educare No. 23

Luria A R 1972 The man with a shattered world. Penguin, Harmondsworth

McCabe R J R, Green D 1987 Rehabilitation of severely head-injured adolescents: three case reports. Journal of Child Psychology and Psychiatry 28(1): 111–126

Mayer T, Walker M L, Shasha I, Matlak M, Johnson D G 1981 Effect of multiple trauma on outcome of paediatric patients with neurologic injuries. Child's Brain 8: 189–198

Medical Disability Society 1988 The management of traumatic brain injury—A working party report of the medical disability society. Development Trust of the Young Disabled

Middleton J A 1989a Thinking about head injuries in children. Journal of Child Psychology and Psychiatry 30(5): 663–670

Middleton J A 1989b Learning and behaviour change. In: Johnson D A, Uttley D, Wyke M (eds) Children's head injury: Who cares? Falmer Press, Brighton

Moore D, Middleton J A 1990 Language difficulties following head injury in children. Speech Therapy in Practice (In press)

Nissen M J 1986 Neuropsychology of attention and memory. Journal of Head Trauma Rehabilitation 1(3): 13–21

Poe P M 1988 A model for evaluation of input in relation to outcome in severely brain damaged patients. Physiotherapy (December 1988)

Raglan E 1989 Disorders of hearing and balance. In: Johnson D A, Uttley D, Wyke M (eds) Children's head injury: Who cares? Falmer Press, Brighton

Raimondi A J, Hirschauer 1984 Head injury in the infant and toddler. Child's Brain 11: 12–355

Roffe J 1989 The role of the nurse in paediatric rehabilitation. Paediatric Nursing (December): 11–13

Rutter M 1981 Psychological sequelae of brain damage in children. American Journal of Psychiatry 138: 1533–1544

Rutter M, Chadwick O, Shaffer D 1984 Head Injury. In: Rutter M (ed) Developmental neuropsychiatry. Churcill Livingstone, London

Savage A 1971 Perception and perceptual training activities.

Serial casting to prevent equinus in acute traumatic head injury. Physiotherapy Canada (Nov/Dec 1988) vol 40(6)

Shapiro K 1985 Head injury in children. In: Becker D P, Povlishock J T (eds) Central Nervous System Trauma Status Report. NIH, Maryland

Smith A, Sugar O 1975 Development of above normal language and intelligence 21 years after left hemispherectomy. Neurology 25: 813–818

Szekeres S F, Ylvisaker M, Holland A L 1984 Cognitive rehabilitation therapy: a framework for intervention. In: Ylvisaker M (ed) Head injury rehabilitation: children and adolescents. Taylor and Francis, London

Teasdale G, Jennett B 1974 Assessment of coma and impaired consciousness: a practical scale. Lancet 2: 81–84

Wardle J, Clarke D, Glenconner A 1989 The parent's perspective: through the glass darkly. In: Johnson D A, Uttley D, Wyke M (eds) Children's head injury: Who cares? Falmer Press, Brighton

Winogron HW, Knights RM, Bawden HN 1984 Neuropsychological deficits following head injury in children. Journal of Clinical Neuropsychology 6(3): 269–286

17. The ventilator dependent child

R.O. Robinson   R. Cartwright   W. Fuller   M. Jones   M. Samuels

INTRODUCTION

Children need ventilatory support for two main reasons: severe lung disease (most frequently secondary to cardiac problems), or severe neuro-muscular conditions. The former group are usually ambulant. The latter normally are not, with the one exception of children who have a central disorder of respiratory control which causes them to stop breathing when they sleep. This is called central nocturnal hypoventilation, or more picturesquely 'Ondine's curse' (Ondine being a vengeful Germanic wood nymph). Generally those neuromuscular disorders involving either spinal cord damage or generalised severe neuromuscular weakness render the child effectively tetraplegic; this group share problems such as neuropathic bladders, seating and postural support systems with other forms of disability dealt with elsewhere. This chapter will confine itself therefore to the features peculiar to the state of ventilator dependency.

INCIDENCE AND PREVALENCE

If ventilator dependency is defined as having been on the ventilator—either at night only or throughout the 24 hours—for at least 6 months and without obvious prospect of dispensing with this support, there are 28 such children in the UK (Robinson 1990). During the last 4 years, 3–10 children per year have become ventilator dependent.

CAUSES

The commonest cause in this group is high cervical cord injury, most commonly secondary to road traffic accidents in boys aged 4–7 years, usually as pedestrians. The cord or lower brainstem can also be damaged by infection, vascular accidents or surgical endeavours for resection of tumours. Children can also be started on long-term ventilation if they have congenital myopathies or spinal muscular atrophy, particularly if the diagnosis or the extent of the weakness is not initially apparent. Polio-myelitis is a potential cause in developing countries. Bronchopulmonary dysplasia following prolonged ventilation in the neonatal period for lung immaturity may evolve into long-term ventilator dependency.

VENTILATOR SUPPORT

Ventilator support can be achieved by one of three methods: positive airway pressure, negative extrathoracic pressure, and electrophrenic stimulation. Although positive pressure ventilation is the most commonly used method in children in the UK, there are situations where children may be particularly suited to one of the alternatives. All techniques may prolong life, may improve the child's wellbeing, and when used at home may reduce the need for expensive inpatient care.

To identify whether a child needs ventilatory assistance it is first necessary to establish that there is chronic respiratory acidaemia with or without hypoxaemia (arterial oxygen saturation <95%). In children, this frequently follows an acute incident, involving trauma or infection, where endotracheal intubation and positive airway pressure ventilation has been needed. If weaning from the ventilator is not readily achieved, then a decision to provide long-term respiratory support must be made, taking into consideration the child's prognosis and the potential for support in an appropriate environment.

Recognition of chronic respiratory failure in the child with a neuromuscular problem, and in whom an acute incident has not occurred, is more difficult. Symptoms of respiratory failure may be nonspecific or mild until a crisis develops. It is only with the creation of noninvasive multichannel tape recordings of oxygenation, carbon dioxide levels and respiratory patterns that the presence of major breathing problems in this and other groups of children is being recognised. In children with neuromuscular causes of respiratory failure, the measurement of maximal transdiaphragmatic inspiratory pressure is considered by some to be of value in assessing the course of the underlying disease. It is an invasive technique unlike the simpler peak inspiratory flow. Other respiratory measurements such as lung volumes, airway resistance and lung compliance have a limited role in the long-term management of the ventilator dependent child. Their interpretation is difficult in the presence of a tracheostomy, scoliosis and muscle weakness, and abnormalities may represent either the cause or effect of inadequate ventilation. For too many children, appropriate ventilatory support is still only provided when right heart failure, recurrent pneumonia or lung parenchymal abnormality has already supervened and made treatment more difficult.

To decide which method of respiratory support should be used requires an understanding of the underlying respiratory pathophysiology. Where there is total or substantial dependence on artificial ventilation, positive airway pressure ventilation through a tracheostomy is most suitable. The presence of a tracheostomy tube, however, is associated with problems:

apart from the operative risk, there is an increased risk of chest infection, impairment of vocalisation and the development of speech, problems of humidification and cosmetic disadvantages. It is also potentially more difficult to withdraw treatment, resulting in the inordinate prolongation of life. In spite of this, positive pressure ventilation is the most practised technique for children in the UK.

When ventilatory support is intermittent, the most suitable tracheostomy tube will provide some form of expiratory resistance when off the ventilator. The silver tube (Alder Hey, Down's Surgical) has an appropriate design with a flanged outer tube and two types of inner tube. One has a hinged flap valve that will allow speech, and the other is a plain tube that can be adapted to connect to the ventilator. For continual ventilatory assistance, other less expensive tubes exist (Portex, Shiley, GOS).

Negative pressure ventilation or nasal intermittent positive pressure ventilation may be used where breathing needs assistance, primarily during sleep and where the child is able to breathe independently for substantial parts of the day. Negative pressure tanks are not mobile, unlike domiciliary positive pressure ventilators and electrophrenic stimulators. In addition, negative pressure ventilation is not suitable in patients with quadriplegia who need regular physiotherapy and changes in posture, and where upper airway obstruction is a problem from bulbar palsy. There is less experience with negative pressure ventilation, and least with electrophrenic stimulation in the UK.

There are many positive pressure ventilators currently available for use at home: East Radcliffe RP4 (East, Oxford), PLV 100 (Medicaid, West Sussex), Monnal-D (Deva Medical, Runcorn), Puritan–Bennett 2800 (Puritan–Bennett, Hounslow) and Brompton Pac (Pneupac, Luton). The ideal should be one that is reliable, quiet, portable, mains or battery powered and simple to operate. Unfortunately they were all designed primarily for adults; they are volume cycled, time limited. In infants, when body size is changing rapidly, a pressure cycled ventilator as used on neonatal units may be preferable. In addition, many domiciliary ventilators do not provide an end-expiratory pressure. This is particularly important when a tracheostomy has bypassed the natural mechanism (the larynx) for providing expiratory resistance, which helps maintain adequate lung volume and airway oxygenation. Most ventilators, however, do allow the facility for addition of oxygen to the inspired air.

In children with normal lungs, ventilator settings should result in the use of low airway pressures (<25 cm H_2O) and rates (<25/min). If there has been chronic hypoventilation or parenchymal disease prior to instituting ventilation, then greater minute ventilation and pressures may be required. Adequacy of ventilation best relies on noninvasive monitoring with a pulse oximeter and transcutaneous pCO_2. Intermittent arterial punctures upset the child and this interferes with gas exchange; they are thus of limited value. If respiratory support is adequate, any spontaneous ventilation will usually be synchronised with the ventilator.

Although the ventilators have alarms in the case of mains failure or patient disconnection, the patient should ideally also be supplied with some form of monitor. When the patient is immobile and has no spontaneous respiratory or body activity then an apnoea monitor may be suitable. However, in most cases an oxygen monitor (e.g. Kontron transcutaneous pO_2 monitor) would be the most valuable. The symptoms and signs of slowly progressive hypoxaemia and/or hypercapnia are too subtle and nonspecific to assume that ventilation is always adequate. Even minor infections may have major effects on gas exchange, which result in sudden and rapid deterioration.

AIRWAY MANAGEMENT

Details of airway management will vary from unit to unit. Offered here is the pattern which we have found has suited our patients.

Overnight humidity is added to the ventilator to maintain secretions fluid. As changing position in the morning will usually prompt a request for suction, this is usually a good opportunity for chest physiotherapy. Percussion and vibration are used with ventilation timed using an Ambu-bag, and suction given as required. Soft rubber-tipped tracheal suction catheters with a side hole, moistened with sterile water, are least traumatic. Tracheal suctioning is kept to a minimum — if possible not more than three times during this session. If this is done effectively, suctioning during the day can be quite infrequent unless the respiratory tract becomes infected. After use, suction catheters are soaked and syringed through in bicarbonate solution, sterilized in antiseptic and then allowed to dry. The procedure is therefore clean rather than sterile. During infections we advise humidity during the day also, increasing the frequency of physiotherapy sessions as necessary.

Mucus plugs may escape suction. They cause distress (and frequent requests for suction) and changes in ventilator pressures and effectiveness. Physiotherapy as above can solve the problem, failing which slow removal of the tracheostomy tube may displace the adherent plug also. Suction via the stoma at this point is frequently useful to dislodge any additional secretions before the new tracheostomy tube is inserted. Usually the whole procedure takes less than 15 seconds. It should cause minimal distress to the child, particularly if preceded by careful explanation. In addition, the tube is changed weekly on a routine basis to remove occult crusted secretions.

A non-cuffed plastic tracheostomy tube facilitates speech. The child allows air to pass up the trachea to the larynx during the inspiratory phase of the ventilator. A metal insert provides secure attachment of the ventilator tubing. The whole is secured using tracheostomy tape padded to prevent neck sores.

SAFETY

No alarm systems are infallible. Constant observation throughout life is impractical. In children who cannot operate a buzzer, an alternative is to teach them to produce a 'click' between the back of the tongue and palate. This manoeuvre, relying on intra-oral pressures, does not require ventilation to produce a noise. It follows that there must be someone within earshot to deal with any acute situation. Since an emergency tracheostomy tube change generally requires two people, there should ideally be two people on hand at any time. They should be able to change the tracheostomy tube in any situation whether sitting or lying. Always with the child therefore is the necessary equipment: tracheal dilators (rarely necessary), scissors, replacement tracheostomy tube, disposable gloves, tracheostomy dressing, suction catheters and portable suction apparatus. Another common problem is disconnection of the ventilator tubing from the tracheostomy. This may be effectively prevented by threading the tracheostomy tube, thus creating a screw fitting between the two.

Equipment failure still occurs with trustworthy alarm systems and vigilant staff. We suggest there should be a duplicate on hand of all main pieces of equipment (see list below and Fig. 17.1). This, combined with a regular servicing programme, is the best basis for confidence in the equipment by the child and staff.

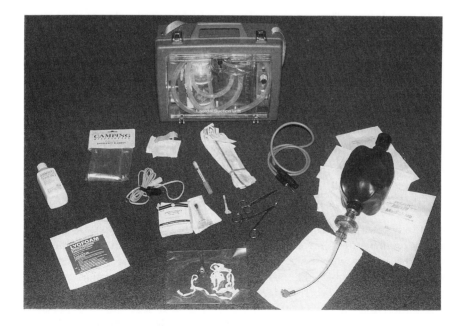

Fig. 17.1 Portable equipment required for suction and tracheostomy tube change.

- 2 ventilators (mains supply)
- 2 humidifiers
- 2 alarm systems
- 1 self-drive powered chair } both with interchangeable
- 1 attendant drive powered chair } portable ventilator
- 1 battery charger for portable ventilator
- 2 suction machines (mains supply)
- 2 portable suction devices
- 2 Ambu-bags with tube attachments
- 3 tracheostomy tube attachments for plastic disposable tracheostomy tubes.

ASSOCIATED PROBLEMS OF VENTILATOR SUPPORT

SCOLIOSIS AND CONTRACTURES

If paraspinal tone is asymmetrical, an active scoliosis can develop rapidly. Absence of paraspinal muscle tone usually means a passive scoliosis appears eventually and may collapse quickly once the Cobb angle is greater than 20°. Either may be prevented by a polypropylene thoraco-lumbo-sacral orthosis (TLSO) worn whenever the child is sitting. Lateral supports to such a jacket with, if necessary, a chin block to prevent neck flexion from occluding the tracheostomy tube, provide adequate stability in a powered chair.

Hip and knee flexion contractures, which can develop during pro-longed sitting, should be prevented, if only to ease recumbency at night. Polypropylene knee–ankle–foot orthoses (KAFOs) at night and ankle–foot orthoses (AFOs) by day are usually sufficient, but should be supplemented by a full range of passive movements morning and night.

Wasting of the lower limbs increases susceptibility to pressure sores. A cotton stockinette, careful moulding of the orthoses over bony points and lambs' wool padding should be adequate to prevent this. Routine checking for early evidence of pressure is crucial. We recommend changing the lying position 2-hourly throughout the night.

AUTONOMIC INSTABILITY

Children with the highest lesions are relatively poikilothermic (body tem-perature dependent on environmental temperature). This may improve to some extent with time, but they remain vulnerable to extremes of temperature. Bradycardia at night may signal hypothermia, which is preventable with thermal underwear and aluminium foil 'space blankets'. An underlying sheepskin not only prevents heat loss but also pressure sores. The temperature of the ventilator humidifier can be a useful addi-tional source of heat.

Children with cervical lesions at any level may also be vulnerable to postural hypotension. Again this usually improves with time (or may reappear after a period of recumbency enforced by illness) but, until it does so, sitting from lying must be taken gradually.

INCONTINENCE

Urinary incontinence is best managed with intermittent catheterisation. The frequent tendency to constipation is usually preventable using a high fibre diet and regular bowel stimulants. It may be possible to predict bowel evacuation after meals, in which case a moulded toilet seat with appropriate trunk support is less messy than nappies. However, as the child gets heavier this may become an increasingly formidable procedure. A colostomy at this point is a reasonable alternative: it promotes maturity and prevents pressure sores.

SEATING AND MOBILITY

Mobility in a powered chair with battery-driven ventilator attached, using head or chin switches, is a reasonable goal (Fig. 17.2). Cushions carefully checked for pressure measurements will allow sitting for several hours without danger of pressure sores.

PSYCHOSOCIAL NEEDS

The fullest form of integration in the community is, of course, achieved by those children who are cared for at home. Almost half the children in the UK are home based, either part or all of the time. As outlined above this is a major undertaking. As such it is perhaps best initiated by the family themselves. However, it must be clear that all those within the family who will be responsible for the child are of one mind, for if they are not, enormous tensions within the family will be generated. Assuming this is the case, the pace at which this proceeds is best dictated by the family themselves. Details of the logistical issues that must be addressed need not be detailed here but include an emergency power supply at home, a telephone, guaranteed availability of instant advice on ventilator malfunction or medical difficulties, regular maintenance and same-day ventilator repair contracts.

However, given the confidence engendered by experience, reliable equipment and safety procedures, many things become possible. Mainstream schooling is one example. Mouthpieces attached to felt-tipped pens and paintbrushes can be used with paper on a board adjustable for height, distance and angle. Mouthpieces can also be used to hold a spoon, knife or other play items. Spring-loaded scissors can be operated with the chin. Mouthsticks have a variety of uses—as a pointer, a page turner, for a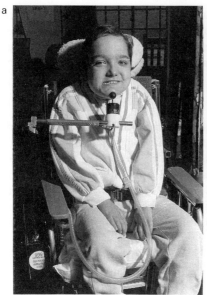

b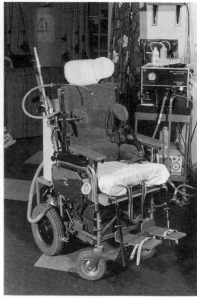

c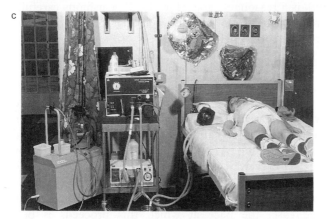

Fig. 17.2   a. Driving powered chair using a chin switch. **b.** Powered chair with Adapta Seat and supportive headrest. The ventilator is on the back of the chair. On the right, behind the chair, is the ventilator used at night. **c.** Child being prepared for school. He is wearing his LSO and AFOs, and is still attached to his night time ventilator; the Ambu-bag and tube attachments are lying beside him on his right side.

changing the television channel with a remote controller, etc. Other examples include the full range of social opportunities accessible to wheelchair users, holidays abroad and even swimming.

Maturation is perhaps only possible when life is seen as not necessarily sheltered. Decisions as to life's shape and direction can then be taken increasingly, as normal, by the growing young person. Attendance, initially all-pervasive and directing, should then assume a more subordinate role and, like the equipment, be used courteously and with discretion.

Self-image and maturation

It should not be assumed that children who have been ventilator depend-ent from birth or infancy regard themselves initially as different, let alone handicapped. We have seen this as a realisation that slowly develops. It is probably dependent upon the definition of self as separate from others. When others are necessary, at first for meeting every need, it is understand-able that the baby's normal egocentricity is prolonged. Since continuing physical dependency precludes the normal learning process of recognising priority for the needs of others at times, this may be a lesson to be formally taught. It may be a painful process. Standards applied from the independ-ent and adult perspective may define the child as 'selfish'. From the child's point of view, the inability adequately to articulate anger is doubly frus-trating. Spitting (which can become very accurate) and food refusal may be the only methods available.

The adjustment that must follow the realization of handicap is neces-sarily more acute when the disability is acquired; anger and depression are more in evidence the older the child, relating as they do to more long-term issues such as fulfilment throughout life in employment and marriage. In this respect the responses differ little in kind to those of children with physical handicap acquired following head injury.

REFERENCE

Robinson R O 1990 Ventilatory dependency in the United Kingdom. Archives of Disease in Childhood 65(II): 1235–1237

18. Neuromuscular disorders

R.O. Robinson   R. Cartwright   M. Jones   P. Russell

This chapter discusses neuromuscular conditions characterised by chronic, usually generalised, weakness, which, apart from the muscular dystrophies, is stable. The static forms include the spinal muscular atrophies and the congenital myopathies. All are inherited, although the mode of inheritance differs. Exact diagnosis is important for accurate genetic counselling. The basic principles of management are broadly similar between the different conditions. It is worth emphasizing to parents at the outset that the conditions are basically painless (although associated contractures may cause pain) and do not affect continence.

MUSCULAR DYSTROPHIES

There are several varieties of muscular dystrophy differentiated according to their age of onset, patterns of muscles affected, speed of deterioration and association with related conditions. All but one—congenital muscular dystrophy—are characterized by an initial period of apparently normal power and motor development.

DUCHENNE MUSCULAR DYSTROPHY

The commonest form of muscular dystrophy is Duchenne muscular dystrophy. It has recently been shown that these boys lack a newly discovered protein normally found in muscle, now called dystrophin. Its exact function is as yet unknown, but it seems important for the maintenance of the structural integrity of the muscle fibre. Lack therefore leads to gradual muscle fibre damage. This fundamental knowledge will almost certainly be the basis for future forms of therapy, which as yet remain to be developed and tested. Being an X-linked disorder, it is for practical purposes only seen in boys.

Early clinical features

The child appears normal initially. Walking may be achieved at the usual time, but is frequently delayed. By this time weakness can be detected. The gait, even in the early stages, is abnormal. There is no spring from the weightbearing foot, and the first signs of the characteristic rolling movements of the hips can be detected. The child jumps and hops inadequately. Running is not properly acquired. It is at this stage that the child is usually referred.

Diagnosis

The diagnosis can be made with a fair degree of confidence from the characteristic pattern of weakness on careful clinical examination. The calves, though weak, may appear bulky. The 'pseudohypertrophy' is due in part to replacement of functioning muscle by fat and fibrous tissue. Rising from the floor is difficult from the supine position. The child rolls to prone, pushes up to a bear-walking position and then extends his trunk on his pelvis by 'walking his hands up his legs' (Gowers' sign).

An enzyme called creatine phosphokinase (CPK), normally concentrated in muscle, leaks from dystrophic muscle into the bloodstream. In Duchenne muscular dystrophy the CPK blood level is very high. This is not only of value in helping to establish the diagnosis, but it is also of value in screening families (see below).

Further evidence of muscle disturbance can be obtained by recording the electrical activity directly from the muscle—an electromyograph (EMG).

Ultrasound of the muscles may demonstrate increased echogenicity. Given a typical clinical picture, elevated CPK and a characteristic EMG, the diagnosis is essentially secure. Some clinicians, in view of the gravity of the diagnosis and its implications, prefer to have the additional certainty of muscle biopsy. In this procedure, which is only transiently uncomfortable, a small piece of muscle is removed either at operation or by using a wide-bore needle, and then examined histologically. Where the clinical picture is atypical the diagnosis can be confirmed on biopsy by demonstration of the absence of dystrophin.

Genetic aspects

Duchenne muscular dystrophy is an X-linked recessive condition. This means that it is carried by asymptomatic females whose sons have a 50% chance of inheriting the condition and whose daughters have a 50% chance of themselves being carriers. In addition, if the mother is a carrier, the mother's sisters also have a 50% chance of being carriers and clearly need to know the risks for any future children they may plan to have. Not all mothers are carriers; the condition may arise de novo in the son. Such women do not have an increased risk of further affected sons.

The recent advances in genetics, and in particular the analysis of the genetic code carried on the chromosomes of the boy and his family have enabled identification in a high proportion of cases—not only who and who is not a carrier, but also whether or not a male fetus carries the gene and is therefore affected. For this work to be carried out it is important that blood samples from all boys with Duchenne muscular dystrophy should be taken, and if necessary stored for further analysis so that appropriate advice can be given, sometimes in years to come, to their female relatives.

Equally important is early diagnosis of the first affected male. A CPK estimation is good practice in the investigation of a 2-year-old boy who is not yet walking, particularly if he also seems generally somewhat delayed. In this way the disaster of the birth of a second affected brother may be prevented.

Progress of the condition

Once the diagnosis has been established the family can be told that the child will become progressively weaker. He will stop walking at 7 to 13 years (Dubowitz 1978) and can be expected to die in the late teens or early twenties. Grim though this picture is, much can be done to alleviate the condition and improve the child's quality of life.

Walking

As weakness advances, walking becomes more difficult and unstable. Continuation of walking is important for some boys and their families. It usually depends upon a reasonably plantigrade foot. Toe-walking tends to counterbalance the destabilising effects of progressive muscular weakness accompanying a hyperlordotic posture. Progressive talipes equinovarus frequently develops towards the end of the walking period. It may be retarded, but rarely prevented altogether, by daily passive dorsiflexion of the feet combined with either polypropylene ankle–foot orthoses as night splints or even occasionally inside the shoes. Similarly, as more time is spent in sitting, hip and knee flexion contractures begin to occur. If prolongation of walking is going to be attempted, the contractures must be relieved. This can easily be achieved by percutaneous tenotomy. Discussions between the child, his family and all the professionals involved are essential before surgery takes place. The decision to proceed depends upon the child's motivation, his parents' capacity to support this, and a suitable home and school environment to provide continuing opportunities. It is rarely possible to mobilise a child effectively if walking has been abandoned for more than 3 months.

Percutaneous releases are followed by walking training in ischial bearing plasters and then, in the shortest time possible (usually within 1 week) lightweight polypropylene knee–ankle–foot orthoses with intensive physiotherapy walking training (Fig. 18.1). Walking continues with treatment

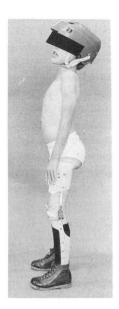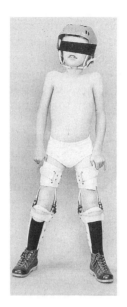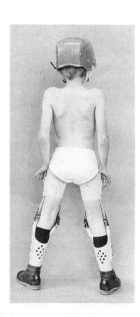

Fig. 18.1   Boy wearing ischial-bearing KAFOs to enable ambulation. Note his lordotic posture and the cantilever knee locks, which can easily be released.

for an average period of a further 2 years. Occasionally walking may continue as late as 17 or 18 years old. When walking is abandoned, contractures are almost inevitable. Bedrest for whatever reason, even for a few days, frequently causes a decline in power, which may prove impossible to reverse.

During walking, however achieved, preparations should be set in hand for the inevitable transition to a wheelchair. It is advisable to consult the local community occupational therapist at this early stage for advice on adaptations and available funding. Ramps for access to the home should be laid, doors should be widened, and toilet and bathroom facilities should, if possible, be provided downstairs. A stairlift is an alternative option. At school, decisions must be made about the most appropriate setting architecturally, be it mainstream school with a classroom helper or a special school. To smooth the transition into a wheelchair, early introduction to sports wheelchairs and adapted tricycles for use in games and in the playground can help to make their use a positive experience. Pre-empting problems in this way smooths the transition to a wheelchair; the change does not then assume to proportions of a crisis.

Sitting

The wheelchair should be self-propelled for as long as possible, although a powered chair is eventually inevitable. The wheelchair should be fitted with a lapstrap to prevent the child being tipped out. Around the time of abandoning walking, transfers from wheelchair to bed, car, lavatory and so on should be taught to maintain independence for as long as possible. Transferring to a bed depends on the correct bed height; it is made easier by a firm mattress with a board underneath. Advice on techniques and appropriate equipment should be sought from a local physiotherapist or occupational therapist.

Sitting on the toilet can be stabilised using various special toilet seats with straps (see Ch. 33). Cleansing can take place from the front while sufficient sitting balance and hand strength are maintained. For micturition a wide-based urinal with a U-shaped cut-out cushion can be used to allow the child to remain in the chair.

Scoliosis

As the condition progresses, breathing exercises, postural drainage and percussion of the chest need to be taught to parents so that they may carry them out when necessary. Walking is associated with an exaggerated lumbar lordosis. When seated the majority of boys tend to slump forward and lose this lordotic curve. It is thought that in this position the back is more susceptible to forces from the side; the posterior articular facets become unlocked. A small percentage retain their lordosis spontaneously, which may become increasingly rigid, protecting them from scoliosis.

A progressive scoliotic curve (Fig. 18.2a and b) adds greatly to the difficulties. It is often associated in time with a pubertal growth spurt. Asymmetrical ischial pressure makes comfortable seating progressively difficult. One arm becomes dedicated to propping, with loss of two-hand function. With increasing instability the back becomes less comfortable; the problems of accommodative seating become overwhelming, whereupon a bedbound existence may begin. Thoracic involvement in the curve causes a pulmonary ventilation: perfusion mismatch with additional vulnerability to hypostatic pneumonia. By this time hip and knee flexion contractures have frequently been acquired, which prevent self-turning in bed. Since it may be necessary for the boy to be turned every 2 hours, this is an additional strain and affects the family's ability to cope. A suitable mattress (e.g. polystyrene bead, ripple, Spenco, or Roho) may alleviate the problem (see Ch. 33).

Institutional life may begin therefore at a time when the boy needs the comfort and support of his home and family. This catalogue of deterioration may not be inevitable if scoliosis can be prevented. One way of attempting this is to fit a light polypropylene jacket (TLSO), which accentuates the lumbar lordotic curve (Fig. 18.2c and d) (see Ch. 17). Such a jacket can be worn under ordinary clothes. It is hoped that this method may retard or even prevent altogether the development of scoliosis.

If, despite these measures, scoliosis progresses, surgical spinal fusion should be considered (see p. 363). Much less traumatic than previously, the Luqué and similar procedures allow rapid mobilisation so that even

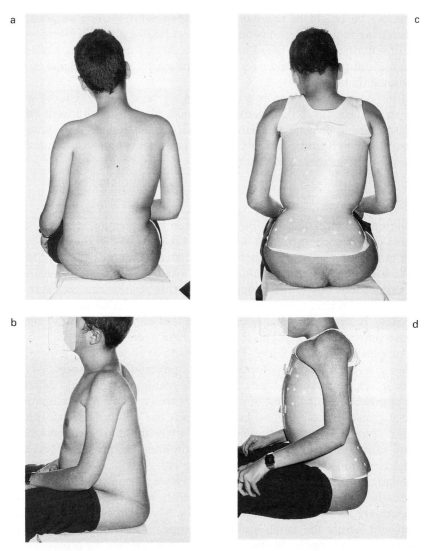

Fig. 18.2 a and b. Scoliosis developing with loss of lordosis. **c and d.** TLSO gives support and accentuates the lordotic curve.

within a day or two the boy can be sitting out of bed without his jacket (Fig. 18.3). If the decision for surgery is too long delayed, ventilatory reserves will be diminished sufficiently to preclude operation. Respiratory function should therefore be carefully assessed preoperatively in order to gauge the anaesthetic risk. As the heart muscle and its blood supply can also be affected, cardiac assessment should be carried out preoperatively as well. During surgery, and in the immediate postoperative period, the ECG should be continuously monitored to allow the rapid detection and reversal

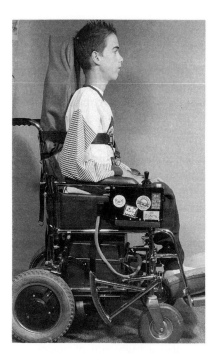

Fig. 18.3 Boy after spinal surgery sitting without a spinal orthosis. The powered chair has an extended backrest to give support when driving.

of cardiac arrhythmias. Grave though these considerations are, with this sort of approach the risks can be minimised. Successful surgery undertaken before it is too late can transform the last years of a boy's life.

Continuing weakness

Hand and arm function can be assisted, even in the face of profound weakness, by correctly positioned arm supports if the child is willing to accept them. These may allow the continuing use of electric typewriters or microwriters at a time when the use of a pen is no longer possible. Similarly, lightweight cutlery with padded handles to assist grip, and beakers or straws, allow independent feeding and drinking to a late stage (see Ch. 33).

Once the child can no longer transfer for himself, the height of the bed may need to be raised so that the parents may turn him more easily at night and dress or undress him on the bed. Parents' backs are always at risk. They should be taught how to lift taking the strain off their backs at an early stage. Hoists may need to be provided by the bed and bath. Bath seats and rails are useful initially, but later a shower or 'shallowbath' insert may be invaluable (see Ch. 33). Further discussion with the community occupational therapist is advised.

With increasing immobility, obesity is a not infrequent problem with these boys. It need hardly be said that not only does this compound the effects of muscle weakness, but also places an additional burden on those caring for him. It occurs for four reasons:

1. Many do not reduce their intake with decreased activity
2. Over-eating may assuage depression and anxiety
3. Over-feeding may be a mother's response to her child's condition
4. Perhaps most commonly, over-eating may be a response to boredom, particularly in those boys with limited intellect.

Appropriate hobbies to encourage include CB radio, computer activities, chess, fishing and photography. Swimming may continue for a period after walking becomes impossible. Eventually the weight of the water induces dyspnoea, at which point it should of course be abandoned.

Intelligence

An accompanying feature of Duchenne muscular dystrophy is mental handicap. The normal distribution of intelligence is shifted 15–20 points 'to the left'. The average IQ therefore is around 80–85. The mental handicap is nonprogressive and is present before the weakness. It has been shown that the performance level is better than the verbal level; reading may be retarded. Not surprisingly there is also a high rate of emotional disturbance (Leibowitz & Dubowitz 1981).

Social and psychiatric aspects

Duchenne muscular dystrophy is different from most other conditions treated in this book in that it involves gradual progression and relatively early death. These families are entitled to informed discussion and well coordinated help. Much appreciated advice on practical aspects can be found in *With a little help* published by the Muscular Dystrophy Group of Great Britain. Many families find sharing problems with others in a similar situation a great source of strength. It is sometimes said that these boys and their families face three crises: diagnosis, stopping walking and dying. The shock of diagnosis is a little different from breaking the news of most forms of handicap. First of all the child may be little affected at the time of diagnosis, and incredulity may predominate. Secondly the repercussions of only one partner transmitting the condition can lead to guilt on the one hand and recriminations on the other. These feelings need to be brought into the open, together with the usual bereavement for the loss of the normal child, before the parents can be expected to cope realistically.

Stopping walking is a crisis in the sense that this is the most inescapable evidence of continuing deterioration and all that is implied by that. Its effect may be ameliorated for the child by suitable forward planning as outlined above.

The realisation of the reduced life expectancy usually comes slowly to the child. Death itself is rarely feared, although the mode of dying may be. This needs careful exploration with the child, usually at a time he chooses with the person he chooses. He needs to know that death is neither painful nor uncomfortable, taking place in the setting usually of increasing drowsiness. This not infrequently relieves unspoken fears.

OTHER CHRONIC NEUROMUSCULAR DISORDERS

There are a great many of these. Most are rare, but the group of spinal muscular atrophies is the commonest. This presents a spectrum of severity. The most profoundly affected (those with Werdnig–Hoffmann disease) present at, or shortly after, birth with severe hypotonia and weakness. Such children do not have enough strength to overcome gravity with their proximal muscles, and consequently they do not achieve independent sitting and may not be able to reach out. Rehabilitation as such is not a realistic goal for this group. Swallowing and ventilatory weakness combined make death from hypostatic pneumonia inevitable within the first 2 years.

At the other end of the spectrum is the Kugelberg–Welander type. Here weakness does not become apparent until, at the earliest, the second year. Initially this may be confined to the lower limbs and pelvis, with subsequent involvement of the arms. The course is relatively static, with a continued waddling gait and lumbar lordosis identical to that seen in the milder dystrophies and myopathies. Respiratory insufficiency is not a problem.

Between these two extremes fall a number of children who achieve sitting unaided at the normal time, but who do not acquire standing or walking alone. As in the other varieties, the arms are not as involved as the legs. Reaching is possible but may be obviously weak. As with the most severe forms, fasciculation of the tongue, a hallmark of the disease, is unmistakable when present. A number of children have been seen who initially resemble the Kugelberg–Welander type and acquire walking, but subsequently deteriorate more rapidly, and become unable to walk and have greater arm weakness within a few years. It is in these two latter groups that rehabilitation has most to offer.

The diagnosis is supported by EMG findings of denervation, characteristic of anterior horn cell disease, and the muscle biopsy typically shows large group atrophy, interspersed with fascicles containing markedly hypertrophied fibres.

In another important group of disorders, the congenital myopathies, the problem lies within the muscle structure. For an exact diagnosis in this group a muscle biopsy is essential.

In neither the spinal muscular atrophies nor the congenital myopathies is intelligence affected.

REHABILITATION

Prevention of scoliosis

This happens relatively soon after loss of independent sitting and can occur very rapidly. Anything less rigid than a polypropylene jacket seems ineffective. This should be applied at the earliest sign of a postural curve, irrespective of whether it corrects fully on suspension. It would seem logical to incorporate a full lumbar lordosis as for the children with muscular dystrophy. For surgical management, see Chapter 22.

Promotion of walking

If the child can bear some weight on his feet he may acquire walking using lightweight polypropylene orthoses. He will almost certainly need a pelvic band, and possibly higher support, depending on trunk strength and the presence or otherwise of scoliosis. In either case confident balancing is only likely with the aid of some kind of support sticks. There must therefore be enough residual arm strength for these. If the child is too weak even with this support, an Orlau swivel walker may be considered (Stallard et al 1978). This depends on the ability to shift weight from one leg to the other (see p. 208). With this movement the apparatus swivels around an eccentric hinge, bringing the non-weightbearing leg with it. It can be fitted if necessary to a child wearing a spinal jacket. While it may produce a kind of 'walking' and be of benefit for that reason alone, the child with spinal muscular atrophy who cannot walk in long calipers with support sticks is unlikely to be able to get into or out of the swivel walker independently. In addition, the swivel walker is useful only indoors on very flat surfaces, and cannot at this time mount door sills or other minor hurdles.

An alternative to walking is a powered chair. This can be fitted with adapted hand controls with microswitches as necessary. Adequate support must be given, particularly to the neck, to prevent any whiplash effect from rapid acceleration or deceleration forces (see p. 285).

In the event of limited arm strength, an overhead gantry with slings on elastic or springs above a tray can permit independent feeding, play and writing.

RESPIRATORY SUPPORT

With increasing weakness, breathlessness may become the predominant symptom. Whilst the long-term ventilatory support of young people with chronic neuromuscular disease is a complex and controversial area, it needs to be clearly separated from the relief of dyspnoea, which is always justified. This problem may also present as disturbed sleep or actual sleep apnoea with consequent daytime drowsiness. Ventilatory support can be effected by a variety of methods including nasal oxygen, face-mask continuous positive airways pressure, a trunk cuirass or actual body box providing intermittent negative pressure (Heckmatt et al 1989).

SOCIAL WORK INVOLVEMENT WITH NEUROMUSCULAR DISORDERS AND MUSCULAR DYSTROPHY

Living with a degenerative condition poses heavy and changing problems for a family's ability to cope; many families with a child with muscular dystrophy will have more than one affected child. Their primary needs, therefore, will be for practical help and advice in managing their day to day lives. The 1989 surveys on disability in Great Britain carried out by OPCS (Office of Population and Census Surveys) give some clear pointers to the nature of the help parents need and frequently do not receive.

Report 6 (Disabled children: services, transport and education) of the OPCS shows that families pay on average £6.54 extra each week on caring for a disabled child. This sum is exclusive of major purchases like furniture or wheelchairs or other mobility aids. As the same Report shows that families with disabled children have lower equivalent incomes than their counterparts in the general population, any increase in cost is significant. Many parents in the survey spent money on transport to hospital, incontinence and other practical aids, extra heating and food. Some of these costs could have been covered from other sources. But only 12% of parents of disabled children living at home routinely saw a social worker! Hence their sources of information on available help were severely limited.

The OPCS surveys give us a clear picture of what families want from social services departments. Although most parents would have welcomed respite care as a means of giving themselves a break (and offering a change of environment and activity to their children), only 4% of the parents interviewed actually got such help. Furthermore 63% did not know that respite care schemes existed in their locality. Additionally 38% did not know of any voluntary organisations they might join. Social services are often primary sources of information on local self-help groups, but only if they see the transfer of information on other sources of help as a priority. The importance of belonging to a voluntary organisation is clearly demonstrated by the Contact-a-Family evaluation of their project in Wandsworth (Hatch & Hinton 1987). This study showed that parent members were more likely to use existing services like respite care, were more articulate about their needs, and were much more confident because of the local friendships and networks which they were able to develop.

One characteristic of the neuromuscular disorders in children is that the access and mobility problems increase as the child (and parents) get older. The OPCS studies show that 56% of parents with children with significant mobility problems had paid for all the adaptations to their homes themselves. Another 35% of parents felt that their home needed some kind of adaptation such as shower, bathroom or toilet in order to make their care role easier. In addition to major adaptations, many families would have welcomed help with smaller aids and gadgets to help children with reaching or stretching or dexterity problems. A major role for social services, therefore, should be *assessment* of need (with an occupational therapist) together with advice about sources of funding. Since many applications for adaptations take several years to process, parents may need counselling and sensitive support in planning for the future and acknowledging that the 7-year-old who can struggle up the stairs to the bathroom with a good deal of help may be quite unmanageable when he is 14 and unable to walk at all. In addition to supportive parents, appropriate aids and adaptations permit the disabled teenager to be as independent as possible in his own personal care, avoiding the unnecessary indignity of being washed and helped to the toilet simply because a door needs widening or a hoist fitted in the bathroom.

The OPCS reports have been published at an appropriate time, since the Government's response to the Griffiths Report on Community Care clearly endorses the role of social services departments as *case managers* of services for people with disabilities. However, the success of that role will also depend upon the willingness of the district handicap and community mental handicap teams, child development centres and hospital services to work with social services and to achieve a 'seamless service' for children and their families. The 1981 Education Act, with the statement of Special Education Needs, offers a framework for wider assessment and coordinated planning. This Act links in turn with the 1986 Disabled Persons Act and assessment for adult life. The Children Act 1989 similarly interrelates to educational and other legislation with the intention of avoiding the fragmentation of services of the past and providing a preventive service to support families and avoid breakdown.

Families with children with degenerative conditions do not, however, only require practical help. Lansdown (1982, 1987) has outlined a range of personal and social needs for both child and family, in terms of feeling able to discuss the disability, the possibility of death and the support services that may be needed. The death of a child is, for many people, an unimaginable and terrible event. Professional carers, friends and the local community may also feel a sense of loss and uncertainty about how to cope. For children with terminal illnesses, coping with death will mean coping with dying and the pain and exhaustion which comes with it. Many families will experience feelings of bereavement following the diagnosis of a life-threatening condition. At this point preexisting family stress and practical needs must be recognised and support offered. Families may be desperate for sources of advice and counselling.

As a child's condition temporarily stabilises (or if, as in the case of diagnosis of muscular dystrophy, there is no immediate deterioration) families may appear to develop coping strategies. However, there may be denial, or a cover for seeking alternative 'miracle' treatments. As the child begins to deteriorate, the old fears reawaken. Anticipatory mourning may mean that parents are preoccupied with fears of dying and may have great difficulty in talking to their children. They may also see contemporaries of their son or daughter dying—and the fear of death becomes a reality. At this stage the child may need special counselling and support. Denial by parents will not convince a teenager, who in any event will have seen television programmes on the subject, as well as observing the condition of school-friends. Sometimes at this point respite care is necessary to give the child a break from family stress. Many social services departments have access to respite care programmes, often in ordinary families' homes. The use of specialist provision such as children's hospices is an option but should be linked to the child's need for specific medical care.

Siblings are often forgotten (Russell 1989, Lansdown 1987) but they may suffer not only from fears of loss of a brother or sister but also because parents have less time—and they themselves may feel guilty about being alive and well. If a sibling is also affected by a similar disease, losing a brother or sister will also mark the inevitability of their own death. Many parents feel they cannot talk about death in the family with their children. Others may feel able to do so with support. Social services departments should be able to provide the personal support necessary and to access parents to relevant voluntary organisations like the Muscular Dystrophy Group of Great Britain or the League of Compassionate Friends. Meeting other parents is likely to be one of the most positive experiences in an otherwise bleak future, and can provide the kind of ongoing support that is difficult for any statutory service to offer. Many voluntary organisations have trained counsellors. All are likely to know their way around the maze of local services; but perhaps their greatest strength is that they can offer hope of survival even when life seems at its most difficult. However, many families will not become part of local networks of support if social services do not adopt the role of 'honest broker' envisaged in the Griffiths Report (1988) and make sure that the families know all available sources of help and are encouraged to use them.

REFERENCES

Dubowitz V 1978 Muscle disorders in childhood. W B Saunders, Philadelphia
Griffiths R 1988 Community care: agenda for action. A Report to the Secretary of State for Social Services, HMSO
Hatch S, Hinton T 1987 Self help in practice: a study of Contact a Family. Social Science Monographs/Community Care
Heckmatt J, Loch H L, Dubowitz V 1989 Nocturnal hypoventilation in children with non-progressive neuromuscular disease. Paediatrics 83(2): 250-255
Landsdown R 1982 More than sympathy. The everyday needs of sick and handicapped children and their families. Tavistock Press, London
Landsdown R 1987 Brief lives: living with the death of a child. Tavistock Press, London
Leibowitz D, Dubowitz V 1981 Intellect and behaviour in Duchenne muscular dystrophy. Developmental Medicine and Child Neurology 23: 577–590

Office of Population Census and Surveys 1989. Report 6. Disabled Children: Services, Transport and Education. HMSO, London.

Russell P 1989 The wheelchair child, 3rd edn. Souvenir Press, London

Stallard J, Rose G K, Farmer I R, 1978 The Orlau swivel walker. Prosthetics and Orthotics International 2(1): 35–42

19. Arthrogryposis

R.O. Robinson   R. Cartwright   J.A. Fixsen   M. Jones

Arthrogryposis is a word derived from the Greek meaning 'curved joint'. It refers to the clinical condition of babies born with stiff contractures of the joints. These contractures arise from prolonged fetal immobility. This may occur if a normal fetus is cramped in the uterus, either because the uterus itself is abnormal or because the amount of liquor is insufficient. Alternatively the problem may be with the fetus itself. Over 100 conditions have now been described associated with arthrogryposis (Hall 1985). Some of these conditions are genetically inherited; others carry their own additional complications. It is important therefore that these children are assessed by someone, usually a paediatric neurologist or clinical geneticist, who is aware of these conditions. Examination should be directed towards the integrity of the central nervous system and the exclusion of other congenital abnormalities. Investigations should include nerve conduction velocities, EMG and muscle biopsy (which is often most conveniently performed during other surgery). When all the evidence is in, the majority are found to be sporadic, belong to the neuropathic group and have in common selective depletion of anterior horn cells in a greater or lesser number of spinal cord segments, (Wynne-Davies & Lloyd-Roberts 1976). The cause of the anterior horn cell depletion is unknown. An analogous condition, with a similar pathology occurring in a variety of domestic animals, is caused by the Akbana virus (Whittem 1957). While a viral aetiology would furnish an explanation for the apparently worldwide epidemic of arthrogryposis that occurred during the 1960s, symmetrical involvement of affected joints is harder to understand on this basis.

CLINICAL FEATURES

In approximately equal numbers either all four limbs are involved or the legs only are involved, with a minority having affection of the arms only. The pattern of deformity depends ultimately on the length of affected spinal cord segments. A muscle with a long length of innervation, for example pectoralis major (C5–T1) is likely to escape total paralysis, whereas a muscle with a restricted segmental innervation such as the quadriceps (L3–4) or pronator (C7) is more likely to be selectively involved. If not all muscles across a joint are affected, the joint will tend to become locked in a position dictated by the residual muscle power in a manner similar to the lower limb deformities occurring in spina bifida. If, however, all the muscles across the joint are affected so that the joint is flail, it will become stiffened in the position dictated by fetal folding.

This provides some justification for the suggestion that myopathic cases of arthrogryposis (generalised muscle weakness) are characterised by flexion contractures (fetal folding), whereas neuropathic cases more frequently have fixed extension, particularly in the arms. Similarly, clinical clues afford a basis for speculation about timing of the presumed insult. Many joint spaces exist 7 weeks after conception, and by 8 weeks the limbs are seen to move. At 11–12 weeks skin creases form across the plane of joint movements. It may be inferred therefore that in cases where the skin creases are abnormal the fetus became affected between the eighth and twelfth weeks. A characteristic feature of arthrogryposis is the dimples seen near joints. These imply close fetal contact between skin and bone secondary to an early fetal failure to develop subcutaneous tissue. The muscles of the head and neck are usually spared. However, the temporomandibular joint may be ankylosed, leading to early feeding and speaking difficulties. This may be accompanied by micrognathia and, sometimes, a small larynx — a point sometimes of considerable anaesthetic significance. While scoliosis can happen, and be progressive, this is unusual. Longitudinal growth is frequently reduced.

MANAGEMENT

Management depends on a delicate balance between therapists, orthotists and orthopaedic surgeons. The right balance is most likely to be struck by drawing upon the experience gained from following a number of individuals throughout childhood and adolescence. It follows therefore that the best results are obtained by involvement of referral centres with this experience. This may take the form of an initial assessment, major intervention in the form of surgical correction, fitting of orthoses and intensive physiotherapy, or minor interventions in the form of advice about dressing or feeding aids. Rare though the condition is, sufficient experience has been acquired about certain aspects of management.

With the exception of lower limb flexion contractures (see below) less emphasis should be placed on straightening limbs than on maximising the functions of residual movement, for the fact is that an independent existence is possible with trunk and head mobility alone.

In the newborn the joint surfaces themselves are remarkably little affected. However, they become distorted with time and lack of movement. Initially the deformities are caused by periarticular soft tissue contractures, which are often amenable to considerable stretching, particularly in the young. Thus at birth the limbs often appear very stiff, but daily passive stretching by the parents with supervision by a physiotherapist usually gains a considerable increase in joint mobility (but not strength). This may be continued for the first year, at the end of which time a decision is necessary about how to tackle lower limb deformities prior to walking.

Lower limb

After the maximum effect has been gained by passive stretching and postural management, further correction can be obtained by serial plasters. Hip abduction and flexion and knee flexion can be corrected simultaneously. Feet can be corrected separately. The plaster is applied with the limb in the 'best' position obtainable and then removed 2 weeks later, to be followed by intensive physiotherapy. It will then be found that further correction can now be gained. However, serial plasters rarely correct deformities sufficiently to allow conventional equipment to be worn to aid walking. One of two possible approaches, each with its own merits, can be made at this point.

Surgical correction aimed at achieving a plantigrade foot and extended but reasonably flexible knees and hips

If this approach is followed it is best to start with the foot, which is usually either in severe talipes equinovarus or is of the rocker-bottom variety (vertical talus).

For the former, a posterior or posteromedial release may be sufficient. If adequate correction is obtained, rigorous splintage is essential to hold the correction, at least until the child is ready to stand. This can be achieved by well-fitting Denis Browne hobble boots incorporating a heel-retaining strap, or, alternatively, by specially moulded splints. However, frequently the foot deformity is so severe that adequate correction can only be achieved by talectomy. The position of the foot on the tibia is maintained postoperatively for 8 weeks by a Kirschner wire and plaster, following which long-term splintage is applied as above. This may correct the hindfoot very well, but further surgery to the forefoot may be necessary later.

A rocker-bottom foot (vertical talus) does not of itself preclude walking. However, it is likely to give rise to severe problems later and can only be corrected surgically. Once the child is established in walking, surgical correction may be considered. The heel equinus is corrected by soft tissue release. The navicular, which is dislocated dorsally on the talus, is returned to its correct alignment. Sometimes this makes the medial border of the foot too long, and the navicular may have to be removed altogether. If the lateral border of the foot is very contracted, a lateral release of the foot may also be necessary.

Surgical correction of knee flexion is difficult as the anatomy behind the knee is frequently very abnormal. For this reason a tourniquet is best not used, so that vascular structures remain identifiable. It is usually necessary to divide everything but the nerves and blood vessels behind the knee, including the posterior capsule of the knee joint. Even after this, further serial plasters to get full extension may be necessary. This must be followed by rigorous long-term splintage to try and prevent recurrence. It is always tempting to perform a supracondylar osteotomy of the lower femur in a resistant case. This temptation must be resisted if at all possible until near maturity, otherwise subsequent growth produces a disabling and unsightly anterior angulation of the femur.

A hyperextended knee that does not respond to serial plastering will probably require a quadricepsplasty to release the tight quadriceps and achieve a functional position with some joint mobility.

At the hip, resistant flexion and abduction may require, as in the knee, extensive soft tissue release down to and sometimes including the joint capsule. Deformity is frequently accompanied by disclocation. Since this is already of long standing at birth, it is irreducible. If it is unilateral it should be reduced surgically to avoid the problems of leg length inequality. If the dislocation is bilateral it should probably be left alone since the required extensive surgical programme frequently leaves stiff, poorly functional hips and risks the complications of myositis ossificans or femoral fracture secondary to immobilisation osteoporosis.

The development of lightweight extension prostheses enabling walking in the presence of considerable residual deformity (Fig. 19.1)

Provided extension of the hips and knees can be obtained to within 30°, no further surgery is necessary. The position of the foot is accepted, and weightbearing is shared between a number of sites on the orthosis. The use of the limb in the prosthesis is then encouraged by physiotherapists, either with or without underarm crutches depending on the extent of arm involvement (see below). These prostheses have the added advantage to the child that he thereby achieves the same head height as his peers, and can wear normal shoes.

Summary. Which of these two approaches is adopted must depend on the availability of orthopaedic and orthotic expertise. The merits of the extension prostheses have been outlined. The surgical approach has the merit of getting the child into conventional calipers, and is of particular benefit for selected problems where residual functional muscle is available.

Upper limb

These children rarely have a single problem in the upper limb. It is most

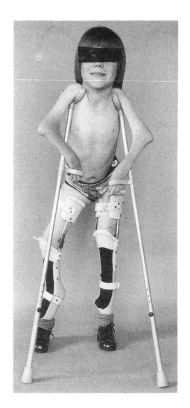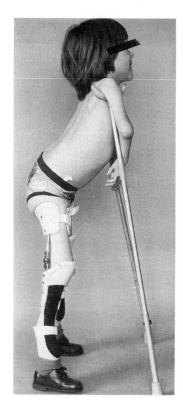

Fig. 19.1 Boy with four limbs affected wearing lightweight extension prostheses and using lightweight underarm crutches with custom-made hand pieces.

important to observe them very carefully before considering surgery. Often a child will use his deformity to function well, in which case 'correction' of the deformity may be unhelpful. Therefore surgery in the upper limb is rarely undertaken for very small children.

Where upper limbs have a very limited range of movement, it can be helpful to obtain active extension of one elbow for toileting and menstruation hygiene, and active flexion of the other for feeding. Whether or not this can be achieved obviously depends on the extent of muscle involvement. Thus if both elbows are stiff in extension, a posterior soft tissue release on one side may be followed by either a Steindler flexor plasty (which may leave an increased flexion deformity at the wrist), or anterior transfer of the triceps tendon to the radius. Alternatively the pectoralis muscle can be transferred to the biceps (which, however, creates a very extensive chest wall scar). Since the humerus is frequently internally rotated at the shoulder, elbow surgery can usefully be combined with external rotation osteotomy at the humerus to get the arm into a more functional position. It must be borne in mind that where there is arm flexion on one side and extension on the other, mobility using crutches will be less symmetrical.

Sometimes, in the more severely involved child, none of this is possible due to lack of functioning and accessible muscle.

Flexion deformities of the wrist are common, but may be a positive advantage with limited elbow flexion for feeding. Stiff hypoplastic fingers are rarely amenable to surgery, but severe adduction deformity of the thumb in the palm may be worth correcting in order to obtain a palmar grasp. Arthrodesis of the wrist may be requested by the older patient for cosmetic reasons and may be of some functional benefit; it can be considered at the age of about 12–14 years when the wrist nears skeletal maturity.

Occupational therapy for the upper limb is directed towards solving a range of functional difficulties, usually by a combination of trick movements and individualised items of equipment. Since much depends on the distribution of residual power and mobility, solutions will tend to be individual to each child. Work proceeds jointly between the child therapist and family, experimenting to establish which are the best options. Many children with arthrogryposis possess considerable ingenuity, motivation and insight, and discover solutions before the therapists!

Mobility

Initially, one of the commonly available prams, and then a pushchair or baby buggy will nearly always be found suitable without further adaptation. If there is a tendency towards scoliosis, correct seating must be introduced very early and continued throughout the child's growth. Meanwhile the parents are taught how to encourage the baby to roll, sit and then progress by whatever method seems most likely to succeed. Many children learn to transfer using their head and feet as pivots. It is important that flexion of the spine is encouraged early as it is vital for daily living activities. Even at this stage the emphasis is less on the mode of movement than on the motivation for movement. The reward afforded by play for acquisition of movement cannot be overemphasised. Orthotic support may be required for mobility but it should not be forgotten that orthoses are frequently relatively task-specific, and in the young they should be discarded for periods in the day for play on the floor when other forms of learning may take place. Underarm lightweight crutches with custom-made handle pieces may be required if the arms are straight and weak (Fig. 19.2). Stairs may be negotiated with these by (1) getting the back against the wall; (2) wedging the uppermost crutch; (3) moving the uppermost leg onto the next step; and, after adjusting the second crutch for maximum support (4) lifting the second leg onto the step followed by the second crutch. Orthoses for the child with mild involvement of the lower limbs may consist of simple lightweight polypropylene support.

For longer distances, wheelchairs such as the Turbo (Fig. 19.3) have proved invaluable although many children will manage a self-propelled chair. Ease of transfer must be a consideration when selecting any wheel-

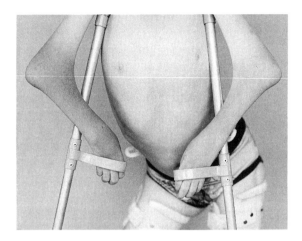

Fig. 19.2 Custom-made hand pieces. Note webbing of the elbows.

chair. Certain children will tend to have a preference for sitting or standing but it is important that periods of the day are spent in both positions to maintain spine and hip mobility.

Feeding

Feeding problems from birth are not uncommon in arthrogryposis. They are most frequently associated with involvement of the jaw and/or tongue. Adequate nutrition may initially only be secured by tube feeding. Thereafter calorie supplements may be required. Problems appear to diminish

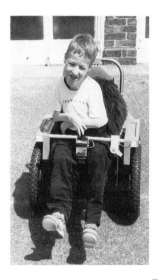
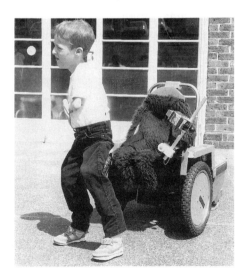

Fig. 19.3 Turbo wheelchair.

with jaw and tongue growth, but during this period support from a speech therapist interested in training early oral skills is very important.

Many children with severe upper limb involvement learn to eat directly from the plate in a most clean and acceptable way; they may also drink from a light cup or mug gripped between the teeth. These methods may not continue to be acceptable to either the child or companions as they grow older, however, and adapted spoons may become necessary. A rocker spoon (Fig. 19.4) or a pivoting block with a specially adapted spoon (see p. 303), used in conjunction with a non-slip mat, may enable children to feed themselves in a more socially acceptable way, as can the use of flexible drinking straws.

A child with a degree of elbow flexion plus some lateral movements of an arm may cope with a light spoon with an extended handle if the grip is contoured to fit within or around the hands, with the possible addition of a strap.

Care must be taken to ensure that the child is learning to eat in the most functional position. Seat height (or whether to stand to eat) plus precise table height can be critical when range of movement is small. Assessment using adjustable height chairs and tables is strongly recommended.

Toileting

Potty training can generally be carried out on supportive potty chairs such as the Mothercare type (see p. 555). Older children generally use a standard lavatory and may require some adaptations to enable independent use. For instance:

1. A small backrest can help, both with transfer onto the lavatory and balance while sitting
2. A drop-down grab bar can often help the child maintain balance

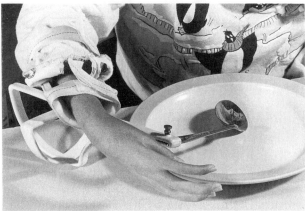

Fig. 19.4 Rocker spoon.

3. Non-slip matting under the feet can prevent sliding while transferring and can aid stability

4. A raised toilet seat can be useful when calipers are worn.

Problems may also be encountered if the child has to transfer sideways onto the lavatory. Often a gap between chair and lavatory is inevitable and a sliding board is not always of use. The lavatory height needs to be similar to that of the wheelchair seat.

For boys, where reach is too short for directing the flow of urine while standing, an aid may be required to help the child's accuracy and avoid splashing.

Acquisition of independence involves a sequence of skills, which will not all be acquired at one stage of development.

Management of clothes for toileting can be a problem and is exacerbated by the need to stand while adjusting clothes over the lumps and bumps of calipers.

Cleansing is ideally carried out in the sitting position. Children with extended arms frequently require no equipment and learn to cleanse themselves by flexing the trunk to increase their reach. Toilet-paper aids can be obtained (see Ch. 33) where the child's reach is insufficient.

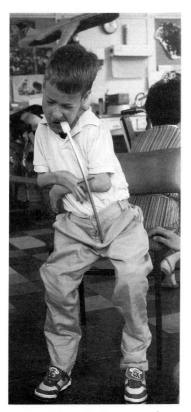

Fig. 19.5 Dressing stick used for a zip.

Dressing

Choice of clothes is most important when considering independent dressing skills. Loose-fitting clothes with easy fastenings, e.g. velcro, large buttons, zips with loops, are ideal.

Dressing sticks with two-way hooks or pimpled rubber ends can be helpful (Fig. 19.5), often in conjunction with tape loops sewn inside the waistband of pants and trousers. Crosspieces on dressing sticks can also be helpful, as can the use of a dressing stand or wall-mounted bars and hooks.

Bathing

For small children a foam support or soft bathmat may be sufficient to allow comfort and stability in the bath. Most children will need very few aids but, if the child is unable to transfer, use of the head and shoulders as a pivot in conjunction with a shallow bath may allow independence. Transfer will be from a bench or chair (Fig. 19.6). Lever taps can be helpful where the wrists are immobile (see Ch. 33)

Schoolwork

The relative positions of seat and work surface need to be checked. The desk-top and/or the chair should be adjustable.

For mouth-writing, an orthodontic mouthpiece may be required, but a

a

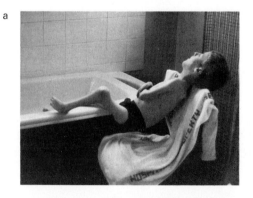

b

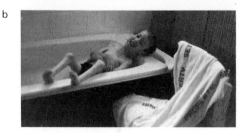

Fig. 19.6 a and b. Transferring from a chair to a shallow bath.

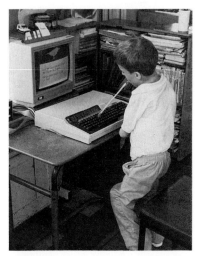

Fig. 19.7 Using a computer keyboard with a mouth stick.

a

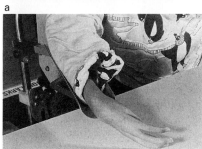

b

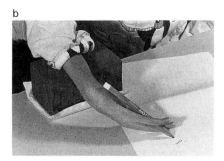

Fig. 19.8 a. Arm support attached to wheelchair. **b.** Using a foam block as an arm support.

piece of polythene tubing over the pencil may suffice. Hand splints incorporating the pencil may be necessary, and metal boards and magnets for stabilising the paper can be useful. Early introduction to a keyboard (computer or electronic typewriter) is advisable (Fig. 19.7). Arm supports (Fig. 19.8) or pointers (mouth or hand held) for use on the keyboard may be required. Spring-loaded scissors may be needed for cutting (see Ch. 33).

REFERENCES

Hall J G 1985 Genetic aspects of arthrogryposis. Clinical Orthopaedics 184: 44–53
Whittem J H 1957 Congenital abnormalities in calves: arthrogryposis and hydranencephaly. Journal of Pathology and Bacteriology 73: 357–387
Wynne-Davies R, Lloyd-Roberts G C 1976 Arthrogryposis multiplex congenita: search for prenatal factors in 66 cases. Archives of Disease in Childhood 51: 618–623
Wynne-Davies R, Williams P F, O'Connor J C B 1981 The 1960 epidemic of arthrogryposis multiplex congenita. Journal of Bone and Joint Surgery 63B: 76–82

20. Limb deficiency

I. Fletcher   R. Cartwright   M. Jones

A child may be born with one or more limbs either partially or completely absent. The person responsible for breaking the news to the parents must do so with considerable care and compassion, for whatever is said to them on that day will be permanently ingrained upon their minds.

Experience has revealed that it is essential for the mother to see *and hold* her baby as soon as possible after the birth. Failure to do so adds to the maternal torment and may even lead to rejection. The majority of limb deficient children are quite normal in all other respects and compensate well for their handicap, often excelling in a wide variety of activities.

NOMENCLATURE

In recent years a new nomenclature for the classification of skeletal limb deficiencies has been introduced. This replaces that devised by Frantz & O'Rahilly (1961), which had a Greek derivation. Unfortunately confusion arose and frequently terms were used incorrectly.

Formerly, the limb deficiencies were divided into three main states: transverse, longitudinal, and intercalary. The latter has now been included in the longitudinal category. We now state 'right' or 'left' followed by either 'transverse'—with the level of absence, implying that all bones distal are missing—or 'longitudinal', with the names of all bones affected.

STATISTICAL ANALYSIS

Of 830 limb deficient patients dealt with by the author (I.F.), the ratio of males to females was 3:2. Those with defects of one or both upper limbs accounted for 70%; lower limb anomalies *alone* 14% whilst the remaining 16% had a combination of upper *and* lower limbs affected.

Of all new patients attending the various limb fitting centres, about 27% of those with upper limb loss are of congenital origin. In the lower limb category, less than 2% are congenital.

AETIOLOGY AND FAMILY HISTORY

The majority of limb deficiencies are idiopathic; only about 1% are hereditary, e.g. split (or 'lobster-claw') hands and feet. Most mothers have uneventful pregnancies and a family history of the same, or a similar, condition is extremely unlikely. The affected child may be the oldest or the youngest of a large family and may even be one of twins, the sibling being normal.

Thalidomide and its derivatives (withdrawn in 1961) accounted for approximately 11% of all the limb deficient patients dealt with by the author.

DISABLEMENT SERVICES CENTRES

There are 28 Disablement Services Centres (formerly Artificial Limb and Appliance Centres) in Britain, each with full-time doctors capable of dealing with limb deficient children. In England the Service came under the aegis of the Department of Health and Social Security but joined the National Health Service in 1991. In Scotland and Wales the Service was already regionalised within the NHS.

A neonate with a malformed limb should be referred to the nearest Centre as soon as possible after birth. *Both* parents should be encouraged to attend for the first consultation so that family histories can be obtained and the baby examined. The doctor is then able to outline a programme, which will include the wearing of prostheses (if indicated), the type of schooling recommended, sporting activities and other leisure pursuits. It may also be possible to allay any fears regarding hereditary factors being responsible and subsequent parenthood of the child. All these matters are of vital importance to the distressed family. Later a meeting with an older and similarly affected child and his parents can often prove beneficial.

In 1978 a group of parents, each with an arm deficient child, formed an association called 'REACH' and it would be well worthwhile for parents of a newly born, arm deficient baby to join this organisation. Information may be obtained at any limb fitting centre.

UPPER LIMB ANOMALIES

TRANSVERSE TYPES

Forearm deficiency

The commonest major limb deficiency is absence of one hand and approximately two-thirds of the forearm. The ratio of left to right is 2:1. The stump is rounded at the end but, despite its appearance, it is *not* a congenital amputation. Close inspection will reveal the presence of rudimentary digital buds (Fig. 20.1). Elbow flexion is normal, but an excessive degree of hyperextension is usual (although no cause for concern). Pectoral muscles should be carefully examined, as very occasionally they are deficient on the affected side. The end of the stump is often considerably cooler than the skin on the normal forearm and cyanosis is frequently

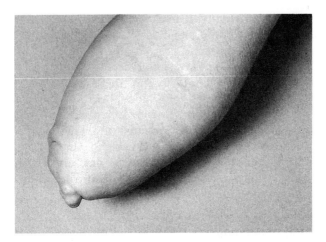

Fig. 20.1 Right below-elbow deficiency showing ridge of rudimentary digital buds. Note the invaginated fold of skin near the tip.

present. Despite this, problems rarely occur. There is an exquisite sense of touch terminally and two-point discrimination is similar to that of a normal finger pulp (2–3 mm); this is the essential difference between congenital absence of a forearm and an amputation.

The ulna is always longer than the radius, the head of which appears on X-ray to be dislocated, yet flexion of the elbow is unrestricted. This is an important fact to be recognised should an injury occur in later life. Fortunately open reduction has been prevented at the last minute, in more than one instance, after the surgeons concerned had been acquainted with this congenital anomaly.

Prostheses

A soft lightweight one-piece prosthesis with a little cosmetic foam hand should be supplied at about the sixth month. This accustoms the infant to limb wearing. The socket, which encloses the stump, is similar to that used on the functional prosthesis, which should be supplied during the second year. This has a rigid forearm and wrist mechanism which allows rotation, both of the hand and of an interchangeable gripping device. The latter is activated by a cord, which is attached to a simple ribbon-like harness appendage used for suspension of the prosthesis. Opening of the gripping device is achieved by the child extending the elbow, coupled with a few degrees of shoulder flexion—an action quickly learnt.

At about 3½–4 years of age a myoelectric hand prosthesis may be supplied. Although substantially heavier than the foregoing these are well tolerated unless the child has a very short stump (less than 5 cm). Two electrodes are incorporated in the proximal part of the socket. They are sited to make contact with the flexor and extensor muscles respectively, just below the epicondyles. The mechanical hand opens and closes when the child contracts the appropriate muscles. The index and middle fingers are pivoted, to operate as a single unit, to 'open' and 'close' against a fully opposed thumb, which also moves simultaneously.

Connected by a trailing flex to the prosthesis is a 6-volt rechargeable battery. This may be carried in a convenient pocket or small pouch suitably positioned on the child's clothing. Provided the stump is not too long, the older child can have the battery incorporated within the socket. This makes the unit neat and self-contained, also less liable to damage.

It should be appreciated, however, that the mechanism controlling the prosthetic hand is contained within the wrist and palm, thus limiting the space available for the battery should the stump be long.

Unilateral hand deficiency

The second commonest limb deficiency is either complete or partial absence of a hand, and again the ratio of left to right is 2:1. Often there is a strong, fully mobile wrist although a radiograph may show a reduction in the number of carpal bones. The forearm is minimally shorter than its fellow in infancy, and in full maturity may be 1–2 cm shorter. Pronation and supination are usually normal, but very rarely these movements are lacking due to proximal radio-ulnar synostosis. Digital buds can always be identified but in different individuals they vary in maturity from small nodules to pedunculated rudimentary fingers bearing tiny nails.

Other hand anomalies include absence of the distal portion of the palm and one or more digits. The latter, however, may exist as proximal stumps looking very much like amputations or rudimentary fingers (see Fig. 20.2).

Treatment

Because of the excellent sense of touch at the end of the stump, a prosthesis should *not* be fitted, certainly during the early years. The lack of grip, which seems to cause great concern both to surgeons and others dealing with the child, is of *no consequence*. Surgical intervention (to fashion a cleft) should definitely not be performed. It is mutilating and ugly, and can seriously interfere with the highly developed sense of touch. Experience in dealing with a large number of children and adults born without a hand has revealed that they have negligible difficulties. A few who have had the misfortune to undergo surgery have requested a cosmetic prosthesis to hide the mutilation, thus rendering them one-handed!

Appliances

In rare instances an opposition device is indicated, particularly for use in carpentry—when it is necessary to hold a chisel, for instance.

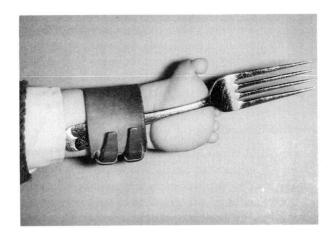

Fig. 20.2 Leather wrist band used to hold a fork when there is either partial or complete absence of the left hand. Note the rudimentary thumb and finger buds.

One social problem is the inability to hold two eating utensils at the same time. To overcome this the author (I.F.) has devised two simple types of wrist band: (1) a plain one with two strap-and-buckle fastenings (Fig. 20.2) so that the handle of a fork may be held firmly to the wrist. This is for use when the left hand is missing; and (2) a similar band with a slot above a pocket to take the handle of a knife, which is ideal for use on the right side. These wrist bands are extremely well accepted by a large number of people, many of whom were originally issued with the appropriate one at about 3½ years of age.

Alternatively it is possible to have purpose made cutlery that has stainless steel rings/extensions attached. These can be slipped on and off by the child and are easy to wash. They must look as similar to normal cutlery as possible.

For babies, it is often a good idea to make an attachment for a plastic spoon allowing them to 'play' with their food, similar to their pens.

In the early teens, some boys and girls request a cosmetic hand for occasional social use. However, the decision must be theirs and theirs alone.

Bilateral forearm deficiency

Because of the excellent degree of sensation at the end of a forearm stump, prostheses will be rejected if supplied to children born with *bilateral* absence. Left to their own devices these individuals become very adept with the bare limbs. Fastening quite small buttons can be accomplished in 2 or 3 seconds. Writing is usually performed with the pen held between the two stump ends and is as speedy as normal. A fork or spoon, held in a similar manner, can be dextrously swivelled so that eating presents no difficulty.

Bilateral hand deficiency

Children born with absence of *both* hands also prefer to use the bare limbs. However, when eating they may choose to wear either one or two wrist bands as described above. Some youngsters are also well able to tie shoe-laces, using their teeth and both stumps.

Above-elbow and through-elbow deficiency

A transverse terminal deficiency above the elbow is very rare, particularly as a single entity. When it does occur it is usual for the condition to be either bilateral or for one or both lower limbs to be affected. As growth proceeds the end of the arm stump becomes very pointed. Despite this, surgical trimming of the humerus should be resisted as ulceration (so common following an above-elbow *amputation* in childhood) is very un-likely to occur. If, however, the bone is sectioned, repeated surgery will be necessary until growth has ceased.

Slightly more common is the complete absence of the forearm with a full-length, although slightly shorter, humerus with poorly developed epicondyles. The stump end is well rounded with the possible presence of a dimple. This is invagination of the flesh that was probably destined to have been the forearm and hand.

Prostheses

The age of 1 year has proved to be the best time to supply a prosthesis for either the through-elbow or above-elbow deficiency. Initially it is advisable to prescribe a one-piece 'limb' (without either an elbow or wrist joint). A light plastic socket extends from the shoulder to the stump end and is blended, with a gentle curve at the elbow, to become continuous with the forearm to which is attached a little cosmetic hand. The prosthesis is secured to the infant by a ribbon-type harness, which passes across the nape of the neck to encircle the opposite shoulder and axilla. At about the age of 2½ years the child should be ready for a 'limb' with an elbow joint incorporating a locking mechanism. A wrist unit is also fitted to allow the hand to be removed and a gripping device substituted when necessary. This is activated by means of a Perlon cord attached to the back of the harness appendage.

Complete absence of one or both arms

This condition, formerly known as *amelia* (meaning 'no limb'), is rare but the absence of both upper limbs occurs more frequently than unilateral absence. The scapulae are small and the acromion processes are upward-pointing but very mobile. A firm grip can be achieved between the jaw and shoulder (a method frequently used for carrying objects). A small dimple is nearly always present in the approximate position of the glenoid and, at puberty, hair grows in this area. While some individuals have complete absence, others have a single flail digit at shoulder level, almost invariably on the right side only. This should *not* be removed.

Children with either the bilateral or unilateral condition will almost certainly reject prostheses. Not because they have little to offer but because they are, inevitably, cumbersome and limit activity, particularly during playtime. It is extremely difficult to convince parents (and others intimately involved) that provided the lower limbs are normal a child with bilateral loss will become very adept with his feet. Prehension develops naturally and should never be discouraged. Hip mobility, which allows either foot to reach the mouth and back of the head, must be maintained. During the growing years the child will exhibit dominance for one or other foot, usually the left, and the opposite hip will lose much of its flexibility unless checked. The importance of maintaining the extreme degree of movements of both hips is a safeguard for the child should the dominant limb ever be injured. In the author's experience this has happened to two armless youngsters.

In the early months of life, parents may be worried because the child is late in walking. It is usual for armless infants to have no inclination to stand until 20 months or more. This is because the child is unable to support himself when learning to stand and whilst on his feet he cannot use them for prehension—which is much more interesting than walking!

The baby tends to move about by shuffling on his bottom, but ultimately balance is learnt and both boys and girls engage in a variety of sporting activities. Many enjoy swimming; it is advisable for them to learn a backstroke prior to attempting any face-down methods.

Children with either one or both arms missing can usually manage at ordinary schools. In the early years they prefer to sit on the floor when writing but it is important for them to learn to use a chair, and write and eat comfortably, with the appropriate foot on a table or desk slightly higher than the chair. Leaving this until later in their school life makes it harder to learn and may present a social problem.

When the child is very young, parents have to be more indulgent, but independence is of vital importance and must be encouraged. Short-term admission to a specialist unit for 'aids to daily living' is essential.

LONGITUDINAL/TYPES

Radial deficiency

Partial or complete absence of the radius (a pre-axial defect) is quite a rare anomaly and results in a 'radial club-hand' deformity, the hand being acutely deviated to the radial side of the wrist. The thumb is often rudimentary or absent and there is a reduced number of carpal bones also related to the radial side. Sometimes the elbow lacks the normal mobility, in which case it is in the extended position.

Surgical correction

Because of the ugly appearance of the deformity, consideration should be given to surgical correction if the condition is unilateral. Such a decision must only be taken after very careful assessment of hand function: it is advisable to refer the child, with both parents, to a surgeon specialising in such corrective procedures (Lamb 1977).

Children with the bilateral condition are in a very different category and may fare better without surgery. Function is of prime importance and all aspects of daily living *must* be taken into account. If, eventually, correction is contemplated, only one side should be chosen, but *not* unless the elbow can be *actively* flexed to at least 90°. It should be noted that the digits always lack full mobility and that the ulnar-sided fingers are responsible for prehension.

Ulnar deficiency (Fig. 20.3)

Absence of the ulna, whether partial or complete, is a rare type of skeletal arrest, usually associated with a short radius that is fused to the humerus (radio-humeral synostosis). The hand is never complete and only one or two digits are present. These are rudimentary and syndactyly is an additional feature. There is a wide variation in the types of ulnar deficiency. Some forearms are almost normal in length while others are very short and devoid of a hand. The digits appear to be extensions of the humerus although there is no articulation. When there is severe shortening the condition is likely to be bilateral and reasonably symmetrical. Sometimes both lower limbs are malformed.

Prostheses

When the forearms are only moderately short and one or two fingers exist it is best to allow free use of the limbs. The two used together become very adept at prehension and quite small objects can be handled safely and confidently. The highly developed tactile sensibility well outweighs any functional ability of even the most sophisticated prosthesis.

Sometimes a child with a unilateral malformation will request either a cosmetic or activated prosthesis. Such can be supplied, although after a trial period rejection may occur.

A *single* limb with an extremely short fused radius, minus any digit and resembling an elbow disarticulation, can reasonably be fitted with a conventional activated prosthesis. However, *none* should be supplied when *both* arms are affected.

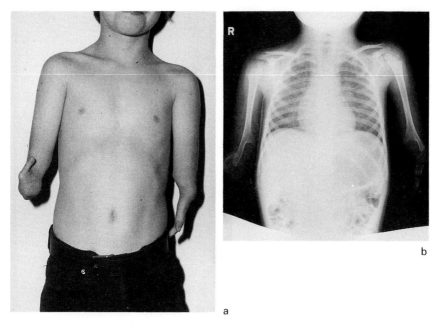

Fig. 20.3 a. Boy with bilateral ulnar deficiency and radio-humeral synostosis. There is a single digit on the right arm and two fused digits on the left. **b.** Radiograph of same child. The medial spur-like projection on each humerus is probably the medial epicondyle.

'Flipper' hand

This is a very rare and complex deficiency, previously described as *phocomelia* (seal-like limb). However, this name is still used to describe a hand (or foot) *without* an intervening long bone, attached directly to the body—an exceptionally rare condition (Fig. 20.4).

The flipper-like limb, which usually has an ulna but lacks a humerus and radius, is a pre-axial defect. Many of the people affected by thalidomide had either bilateral or quadrilateral 'flipper' limbs.

The absence of a humerus and therefore a shoulder joint results in a flail limb that does not have the fulcrum so necessary for elevation of the arm. Sensation appears to be normal, but lack of reach and power are the main physical difficulties. Very rarely is an arm prosthesis accepted because it deprives the wearer of natural hand function. However, some people with only one limb affected may decide to wear a purely cosmetic arm. In the author's (I.F.) experience many children with the bilateral defect discarded prostheses at an early stage and it is clear that they should not be supplied as frustration will be inevitable.

Arm training

Many of the Disablement Services Centres have facilities for arm training

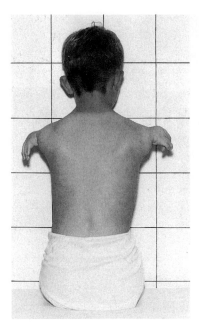

Fig. 20.4   Boy with true phocomelia.

and 'aids to daily living'. Following the supply of his first activated prosthesis, the child should attend the nearest Centre, where the occupational therapist responsible for training will instruct the child *and parents*, and then outline a programme. Further visits are recommended, particularly when a more sophisticated prosthesis such as a myoelectric limb is issued. Care of the prosthesis and stump hygiene should be fully discussed.

Bimanual activities are taught to encourage the use of the prosthesis, and frequent visits during the growing years are strongly recommended so that advice may be given when different skills are needed.

Children with bilateral limb deficiencies, who will not be wearing prostheses, should also be encouraged to attend training sessions, accompanied by one or both parents. Independence is vitally important and must be taught early. However, there is little inclination on the part of a multi-handicapped child to dress, undress and become fully toilet trained at a young age. Gentle persuasion and considerable patience are essential!

Clothing may need to be adapted and velcro substituted for buttons. The less modification the greater the tolerance, and when the child reaches his teens he will wish to be attired the same as his peers, irrespective of the difficulty in dressing! It is of the utmost importance to allow this, as it is a major step nearer 'normality'.

LOWER LIMB ANOMALIES

Malformations of the lower limb are comparatively rare and they differ greatly from those of the upper limb. Whereas a transverse deficiency is common in the latter, it is rare—certainly as a single entity—in the lower limb.

The most frequently occurring condition is a short limb due to a deficiency of one or more of the long bones. Those involved may be aplastic (absent) or hypoplastic (poorly developed and short).

LONGITUDINAL TYPES

- *Femur*—A partial deficiency of this bone is *always* proximal, even when it is represented by a mere nodule. The mild form is referred to as proximal femoral focal deficiency. It may or may not be associated with a malformation of one or both the long leg bones.
- *Fibula*—Usually completely absent but occasionally represented by a very narrow proximal rudiment.
- *Tibia*—Very rarely absent (but a condition seen in many people affected by thalidomide). There is usually complete absence, but if any rudiment does exist it is proximal and sometimes this and the fibula are individually covered with skin (Fig. 20.9).

Fibular deficiency

The most frequently encountered lower limb anomaly is an absent fibula with a short tibia. The latter is curved anteriorly, the apex being situated at the junction of the middle and lower thirds of the bone, referred to as a 'tibial kyphos'. Overlying this is a dimple, which is adherent to the tibia. The foot is small, everted and devoid of the lateral one or two rays and lateral tarsal bones.

The tendo calcaneus is thin and has the appearance of a tight subcutaneous cord, which draws the heel upwards causing a fixed equinus. Because the bony structure of the foot has been distorted in utero, an elongation of the tendo calcaneus fails to improve the deformity.

Treatment

Extension prostheses. An artificial foot, ankle, and possibly a shin may be supplied to fit over the affected limb, to obtain the correct length. Reasonable cosmesis must also be achieved. For the extension prosthesis to be acceptable, both functionally and cosmetically, the malformed limb needs to be shorter than the length of the foot, since this has to be accommodated in maximum equinus. Provided it lies neatly in the long axis of the tibia the effect is very good. So often, the foot is in uncorrectable eversion and, as growth proceeds, the deformity becomes more obvious and very difficult to mask. Amputation (as mentioned later) should therefore be considered.

About 10–12 months is the ideal period for the supply of the first prosthesis, which can be made of plastic. Alternatively, a light leather 'bootee socket' may be fitted. This extends to the knee and encloses the foot comfortably in full equinus. Duralumin side-struts connect the socket to a shaped 'platform', to which is added a flexible foot. An ankle joint is not recommended until the child is about 8 or more years of age.

For the older child an enclosed extension prosthesis is supplied. This has very good cosmesis and consists of either plastic or leather in the form of a bootee. The latter has a front zip or lace fastening and the whole is then encased in a shaped shin-like container contoured to match, as near as possible, the contralateral leg (Fig. 20.5 a–c). Provided there is sufficient room, an ankle joint is incorporated. The fully enclosed type is not recommended for very young children because pressure areas may develop as the leg grows and it is essential for these to be identified immediately so that adjustments can be made to the prosthesis.

If an extension prosthesis is fitted to a leg with the amount of shortening appreciably less than the length of the foot, the latter will protrude and be very unsightly. A raised boot will therefore be necessary unless surgery is performed (see Ch. 23).

Surgery. The options are:

1. *Leg equalisation.* This is not recommended unless *full* length can be guaranteed and the foot is not only plantigrade but the same length as its fellow. (Odd-sized shoes are *not* acceptable.)

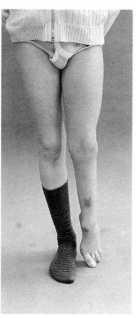 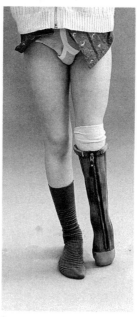 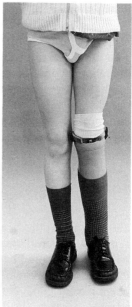

a   b   c

Fig. 20.5   Boy (10 years) with an absent fibula. **a.** His foot is well in line with the long axis of the tibia. Shortening is only just sufficient for a metal enclosed prosthesis. **b.** Wearing a leather bootee socket with zip fastening. **c.** Bootee entirely contained within a metal shin complete with foot. The amount of shortening is insufficient to permit an ankle joint.

2. *Amputation.* If, at birth, the rudimentary foot is markedly everted then disarticulation at the ankle should be performed in order that a cosmetically acceptable prosthesis may be fitted before the first birthday. Disarticulation should also be considered when there is no likelihood of the foot being plantigrade and there is insufficient shortening to allow the fitting of an extension prosthesis. There are, however, intermediate degrees of shortening and deformity, which must be individually assessed—preferably by a medical practitioner working in the field of prosthetics.

Prostheses. If the foot has been removed within the first few months of life (or if the child has been born with a short tibia and an absent foot) then the initial prosthesis should be supplied at about 10–12 months. It consists of a lightweight plastic shin with a detachable soft liner. There is no ankle joint and the foot is flexible.

Children who have the foot amputated and are subsequently supplied with a prosthesis not only walk without a limp, but run and are able to play all the usual games. Rugby, soccer, hockey, cricket and athletics are a few of the activities in which these young amputees engage. Also, of considerable psychological importance, is the fact that ordinary shoes can be worn and the general appearance of the prosthetic limb is excellent.

Tibial deficiency

Absence of the tibia is very rare but when it occurs it is usual for the fibular head to lie alongside the lateral femoral condyle. The foot is reasonably well formed but grossly inverted.

Treatment

Whether the defect is unilateral or bilateral, disarticulation at the knee is the ideal method of treatment *provided* the hips and upper limbs are normal. Following ablation the prosthesis of choice is the same type as that used for a through-knee amputation.

Femoral deficiency

The femur may be entirely absent or exhibit varying degrees of hypoplasia and, as already mentioned, it is the proximal portion of the bone which is deficient. The tibia, fibula and foot are usually normal but deficiencies of these are occasionally encountered. A radiograph is essential to determine the state of the hip joint as this influences the treatment very considerably.

Treatment of femoral deficiency with stable hip joint

Extension prostheses. A platform-type extension prosthesis, extending up to the knee, is usually all that is necessary. This may consist of a leather 'bootee socket' embracing the leg and maintaining the foot in equinus. Alternatively an enclosed prosthesis can be fitted. (Both these types are described above.)

Surgery. Sometimes the hip, although stable, is acutely flexed and it may be considered advisable to disarticulate the leg at the knee joint after surgically reducing the hip flexion as much as possible (full correction is rarely obtained). A conventional above-knee prosthesis is then fitted.

A procedure known as the Van Nes rotationplasty (Van Nes 1950) has occasionally been performed on a limb with a very short femur and the foot level with the contralateral knee. A rotation osteotomy of 180° is performed, thus turning the foot back to front. The heel then acts as a knee joint and the foot as a leg stump. A reasonably conventional below-knee prosthesis is then supplied. There are various methods of achieving this rotation, (Kostuik et al 1975, Kritter 1977) and some of the earlier operations, performed when the children were very young, resulted in derotation after a few months. Apart from this complication an important psychological one remains: a few patients have requested amputation during the teens due to the appearance and feebleness of the foot as an effective stump. Great care and thought should therefore be taken before subjecting a child to this very drastic and major procedure.

Treatment of femoral deficiency with unstable hip joint

An extension prosthesis with a blocked leather socket is fashioned from a cast of the *whole* limb and buttock. Full ischial tuberosity bearing is essential. The socket is attached by means of jointed side steels to an artificial shin and foot. The natural foot should be allowed to hang free but secured to the side members by means of a detachable strap across the dorsum. A pelvic band with a hip joint should also be incorporated to prevent excessive rotation and abduction of the limb when walking. (Fig. 20.6).

TRANSVERSE TYPES

Although a transverse terminal deficiency is the commonest congenital malformation of the upper limb, it rarely affects the lower. However, when it does occur other limbs are almost invariably involved.

Foot deficiency

The whole foot, the forefoot or merely the toes may be absent. It is of interest to note that when the forefoot is missing there is no associated equinus deformity, which so often occurs following an amputation at the same level.

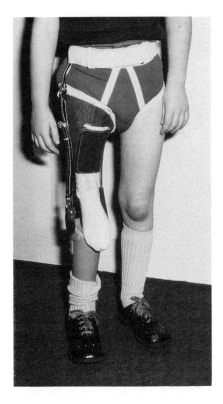

Fig. 20.6 Boy with complete absence of the right femur fitted with an extension prosthesis. Full weight is taken on the ischial tuberosity and the foot is unsupported. A joint, with a lock, is situated level with the left knee and is released when sitting.

Prostheses

For complete absence of the foot, a standard Syme prosthesis is supplied. As the child grows there is a likelihood of slower development of the tibia and two malleoli. Paradoxically the cosmetic effect is therefore enhanced.

There are two types of prosthesis for absence of the forefoot:

1. A plastic dropped-foot type, extending from the calf to the under-surface of the rudimentary foot; here it is curved to a right angle and continued to a blocked toe-piece. This will fit neatly into an ordinary shoe (Fig. 20.7). Some very active youngsters, however, maintain there is insufficient support with this type when they play rugby or football.

2. A Chopart type of appliance is the alternative. This consists of a soft leather bootee with central lacing and a polished hard wood (beech) insole.

Through-knee and above-knee deficiency

When a child is born with absence of one or both legs, whether at or above the knee, it is advisable to have a radiograph of the hips. Quite often there is either congenital dislocation or proximal femoral focal deficiency, causing a hip flexion deformity. If either exists, walking will be extremely slow and difficult to accomplish, particularly if bilateral.

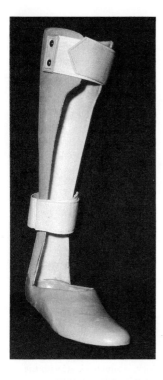

Fig. 20.7 Dropped-foot type of prosthesis for a forefoot deficiency. Made from Ortholen, whch is flexible and allows some movement of the ankle when walking or running.

The stumps are well rounded at the end with a fleshy pedicle, either at the side or posteriorly. The femoral condyles are lacking but children with *normal* hips and bilateral femoral defects have no such problems—they are able to run well on the bare limbs.

Prostheses

During infancy a simple non-articulated prosthesis is supplied. This has a metal socket with an internal end-bearing pad and a light hip joint incorporating a pelvic band. A foot is fitted unless the stump is short, in which case a small 'rocker' is preferable since it is lighter and easier to manage. In due course a larger prosthesis is issued, incorporating a knee joint. The child learns quickly to walk with only the merest trace of a limp. Most youngsters take part in many of the usual games although it is necessary to convince school teachers that the activities are not only possible but beneficial. The prostheses for youngsters with bilateral loss are similar, but when knee joints are introduced it is advisable to incorporate manually operated locking mechanisms on one or both. Provided the hips are normal, balance is soon acquired and the locks can be omitted on subsequent limbs.

For recreational purposes a pair of short leather sockets, with ischial bearing and stout ends (but no shins or knees) can be supplied. These enable the child to run about more easily on grass and asphalt playgrounds.

Absence of the lower limb

There are two types of this rare complete lower limb deficiency, often referred to as lower limb amelia.

Type A. Absence of all the lower limb bones with an intact pelvis, but unformed acetabulum on the affected side.

Type B. A hemi-pelvis in which the whole of the limb and associated half of the pelvis is missing (Fig. 20.8). This is an extremely rare phenomenon. The ipsilateral kidney and testis may also be absent. Whether or not the two kidneys exist, incontinence is a possible but not invariable complication.

In type A it is usual to find a small fleshy nodule on the lateral side of the pelvis, which is probably a rudimentary limb bud.

Although early radiographs show no evidence of any long bone, a palpable mass is occasionally present in the hip region. By the time the child reaches adolescence, a radiological examination may well reveal a segment of bone with an epiphysis. This is most likely to be a *distal* end of femur, as mentioned earlier.

Prostheses

Unilateral absence. At about 10–12 months a lightweight non-articulated prosthesis is fitted with a socket embracing the lower portion of the trunk and both hips. Because mechanical hip and knee joints are heavy it is

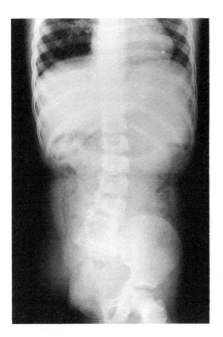

Fig. 20.8 Radiograph of a girl with congenital absence of the right side of the pelvis and lower limb. The right kidney was also absent.

inadvisable to incorporate them until the child is older and walking well. They may be added sometime between the ages of 3 and 5 years, after which it should be possible to walk with a 'free' knee within a short space of time.

Bilateral absence. Because an infant without either lower limb is unable to maintain a sitting posture a special supportive device is necessary at the age of 6 months. This is a 'sitting socket' mounted, like a saddle, on a little wooden dog. This in turn is on a platform to which four castors are fitted. While the child sits comfortably a parent can move it from room to room. This device is based on the original Chailey plaster of Paris 'flower-pot' design, used by many thalidomide affected children in the 1960s.

Swivel walkers

At about 10–12 months of age a new socket is made, beneath which are mounted two non-articulated legs with a spring-loaded swivel action. In order to walk the child sways from side to side.

The age at which separate prostheses are supplied varies considerably with the development of the child, and initially these limbs are also non-articulated. The two sockets (which are connected, back and front, by straps and buckles) fully embrace the respective hip and buttock.

Having been securely fastened into the prostheses the child should be able to achieve a 'swing-through' gait with the aid of crutches. As the height is increased, there may be a need to introduce hip and knee joints, but these will add very considerably to the weight of the limbs. It will be appreciated that the child is in a permanent sitting position despite the appearance of standing. Removal of the prostheses for transfer to a wheelchair or private car is a simple matter; therefore non-articulated limbs can be worn until the teens.

It must be remembered that when the legs are removed the trousers stay with them! It is therefore essential that a pair of shorts (with the leg apertures sewn up) are worn as an undergarment.

OTHER LIMB ANOMALIES

Multiple asymmetrical limb anomalies

Many people are born with multiple limb deficiencies that do not fit into any recognised pattern. There are, however, certain specific features: always three, and often four, limbs are affected, and they tend to be different from one another and asymmetrical—quite unlike the thalidomide types of deformity, which are bilateral (or quadrilateral) and usually symmetrical.

The cause is obscure but a few affected individuals are known to be one of twins, the sibling being normal.

Treatment

Because of the diversity of the conditions it is not possible to outline a specific method of treatment. However, experience has shown that the greater and more numerous the malformations, the less likely it is that multiple prostheses will be accepted.

'Lobster-claw' deformity

The bifid hand or 'lobster-claw' deformity is considered to be hereditary, due possibly to an autosomal dominant trait (Temtamy & McKusick 1969). Functionally the hands are capable of excellent grip but, for psychological reasons, surgical closure may be advisable at an early age.

When the feet are also affected (which is usual) standard shoes can rarely be worn. Corrective surgery should, however, be tempered with caution since discomfort can result. Surgical shoes should be prescribed, certainly during the early years; then, in due course, the patient can have a say in the ultimate treatment.

Apart from the deformed feet the lower limbs may be grossly affected with distal tibial hypoplasia, the proximal rudiment of which presents as a separate entity and is covered completely by skin (Fig. 20.9).

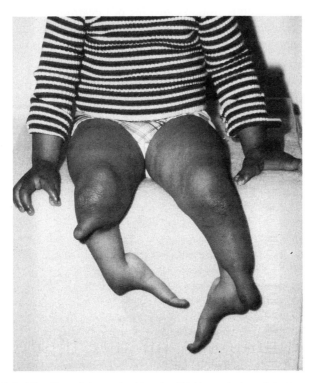

Fig. 20.9 Hereditary 'lobster-claw' hands, tibial hypoplasia and single-ray feet.

Treatment

In this condition the feet are far from normal and the removal of whatever rudiment exists is the treatment of choice. Fusion of the tibia to the fibula is ideal *if* it can be achieved. When there is wide separation between the two bones, considerable difficulty is experienced when surgical approximation is attempted. Reasonably standard below-knee type prostheses can be fitted, but great care has to be taken to prevent pressure sores if the tibial segment starts to migrate, as growth proceeds.

Ring constrictions

A baby may be born with one or more fingers (or toes) only partly formed, giving the appearance of an encircling band. Although a deep sulcus is present there is never any evidence of an actual ligature. The condition is almost invariably multiple and the terminal part of one or more limbs may also be missing or, if present, may be devoid of bone distal to the constriction (Fig. 20.10).

Treatment

When the constriction is around either leg or forearm it may be advisable to remove the pendulous portion of the limb and fit an appropriate prosthesis.

When fingers or toes are affected surgical intervention is *not* advised unless requested by the patient after reaching full maturity.

Absence of the lumbar spine and sacrum

When a baby is born with absence of the lumbar spine and sacrum the

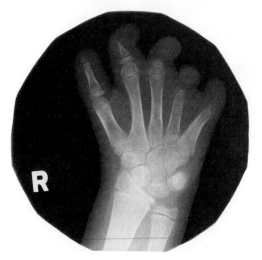

Fig. 20.10 Radiograph of a child's hand showing multiple ring-constrictions. Other limbs were affected. Note absence of bones distal to the lesions.

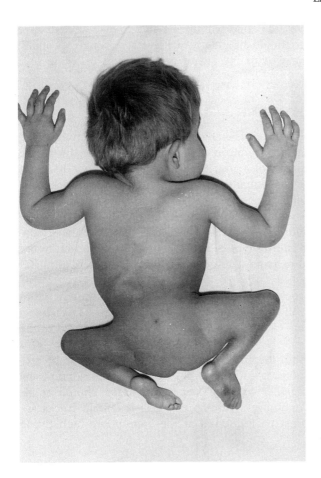

Fig. 20.11 Boy with absence of lumbar spine and sacrum. External rotation, abduction and webbing of both lower limbs produces a frog-like appearance.

lower limbs are usually paralysed, abducted and externally rotated at the hips. The knees are acutely flexed, often with webbing of the skin between the thighs and calves, giving a frog-like appearance (Fig. 20.11). The two iliac bones are joined posteriorly and double incontinence is the rule. In addition there may be rectal atresia and hypoplasia of the pelvic organs.

Treatment

Provided the popliteal webbing is not too severe it should be possible for the infant to have a 'sitting socket' at about 6 months and later a pair of swivel walkers (see p. 322).

Surgery. Major surgery has something to offer for the severely flexed lower limbs. Bilateral disarticulation at the knees may be performed followed by subtrochanteric osteotomies to correct the abduction and rotation. Prostheses may then be fitted, but *thickly* padded, rigid, pelvic bands are essential since the ribcage rests heavily upon them. Because of the paralysis from the waist level, the child will not be able to take any effective stride with either leg but should be able to achieve a reasonable walking speed, over short distances, with the aid of crutches and resorting to a tripod gait.

STUMP CARE AND HYGIENE

Whenever a lower limb prosthesis is worn it is usual to wear a stump sock; these may be of wool, nylon or cotton and are supplied, free, by all the DSCs. Owing to the difficulty of manufacturing the great variety of shapes and sizes of socks for the congenitally malformed lower limb, a stockinette is frequently used, particularly by those with bilateral 'flipper' limbs. The material is fashioned like a pair of short trousers and easily sewn to shape. Many limb deficient children sweat excessively and they find the stockinette most acceptable. Whatever type of sock is worn, it is important to use a clean one each day and to avoid detergents when washing them as rashes can easily result.

The inside of plastic sockets should be wiped with a clean damp cloth each evening and carefully dried, ready for morning use. Detachable leather sockets, and others with a leather lining, should be exposed to the air overnight.

Apart from his daily bath the child should have the affected limb carefully washed night and morning and thoroughly dried prior to donning the prosthesis. The latter, together with the suspension straps, should be inspected periodically to minimize serious breakages. If telltale cracks are seen, an appointment must be requested at the appropriate limb fitting centre for urgent repairs.

OCCUPATIONAL THERAPY AND PHYSIOTHERAPY

GENERAL PRINCIPLES

Full movement in all remaining joints is essential and must be encouraged from the beginning to achieve independence in daily living later. Changes of position and play are vital so that the child can investigate his environment using hand, stump, mouth, body and feet. Teeth take undue strain, so regular dental appointments are essential.

Children with problems balancing when sitting are going to need initial help, perhaps the Chailey 'flower-pot'. When they achieve sitting balance, encouragement may be needed to move onto bottom shuffling. The 'flower-pot' can be made from plaster of Paris or other materials. It totally encloses the lower half of the trunk and pelvis, leaving apertures for the feet. The device can be mounted onto a chair with castors to enable parents to push it from room to room.

Children with severe limb deficiencies have reduced sweating surfaces and feel the heat excessively; therefore they need to be lightly clad in loose cotton clothing. Dehydration also occurs very quickly if the child is unwell, and so fluid intake must be increased at such times.

Bony areas around the feet of phocomelic children may become painful; socks continually wear out due to constant shuffling, and may need protection in the form of polypropylene 'spats'. Leather patches on the seats of trousers help to prevent undue wear.

Children with short or absent arms take time learning to stand and may be nervous of falling without arm protection. Supported standing in a baby walker or using adapted reins will give confidence until they are ready to take the plunge. Falling needs to be taught. Chins and heads are vulnerable and a crash helmet may be worn (local cycle shops now stock these). Another reason for late walking is that the feet are used for prehension and open-toed socks and shoes are necessary with these infants.

Children with abnormalities of all four limbs learn to walk on their own feet, if present, but there are a few who need to have the experience of the upright position in prostheses before they do this. Crutches tend to upset the balance, and the length of the stump of the upper limb will determine whether the child is able to control a prosthesis for the lower limb at an early stage. Those with long arm stumps can use adapted crutches to aid walking. When balance is precarious a standing table can be used.

Gradually, independent standing and walking are encouraged. As these are achieved, mobility is increased to include curbs, steps and stairs. When a child is wearing two rigid artificial legs and has very short or absent arms, the best way to go up and down stairs is sideways using the wall, but this depends on the width of the stairs. It may also be helpful to have a high bannister with stops on it so that the chin or upper limb can help a child going up or down stairs. Mobility should be continually encouraged—for example, sitting to standing, and rising from the floor to standing—so that these lead to functional activities such as being able to get in and out of the bath and on and off the toilet. A potty chair may be necessary to aid balance for toileting. A swimming aid (see Chailey brochure or Ch. 33) is useful for both swimming and bathing.

Some adaptations to eating utensils may be required (see Ch. 33).

PSYCHOLOGICAL EFFECTS

It is understandable that parents will feel very upset when they learn they have produced a malformed baby. There are usually feelings of guilt (although groundless) and one parent may well blame the other. Turmoil of this nature, if it persists, will become apparent to the child even though not fully understood, and he may feel unwanted and insecure. The majority of handicapped children with a good home background and parents who do not *show* anxiety over the limb condition are very well adjusted. To aid this the parents must have sympathetic and often repeated counselling to reassure them during the early years of their child's life.

Comments *will* be made by other children, but if a rational explanation is given to an enquiring child, without anger, it is likely to have a good effect. To hide the affected part and make a mystery of it will only arouse curiosity and invite numerous questions and comments.

Malformations most likely to cause psychological problems are those concerning a hand rather than more proximal deficiencies. A well-rounded stump seems to be accepted by the lay public better than a deformed hand. Many people with a limb deficiency, and others with an amputation, tend to compensate by indulging in a variety of sporting activities at which they usually excel. These should be encouraged and some of the many youth organisations are beneficial in this respect. The psychological trauma experienced by a limb-deficient person varies quite considerably. It is clear, however, that the greater the understanding and acceptance by the parents and others, coupled with a good stable home, the happier the child will be. Those closely involved with limb-deficient children should make light of their handicaps and encourage independence, while steering them towards as 'normal' a life as possible and remembering that overprotection causes frustration. Recognition of any potential, however bizarre it may seem, should be fostered to the full. Life has presented a very real challenge to limb-deficient people and they will meet it and overcome it, often having greater determination than the so-called able-bodied. What handicapped persons want more than anything else is acceptance and recognition of their *ability*, not an emphasis on their so-called disability.

It must be remembered, however, that in the privacy of their homes they know they are different from their peers, and there may be occasional bouts of depression. Perhaps they may take comfort from the words of Shakespeare:

In Nature there's no blemish but the mind;
None can be call'd deform'd but the unkind.

REFERENCES

Frantz C H, O'Rahilly R 1961 Congenital skeletal limb deficiencies. Journal of Bone and Joint Surgery 43A: 1202–1224
Kostuik J P, Gillespie R, Hall J E, Hubbard S 1975 Van Nes rotational osteotomy for treatment of proximal femoral focal deficiency and congenital short femur. Journal of Bone and Joint Surgery 57A: 1039–1046
Kritter A E 1977 Tibial rotation-plasty for proximal femoral focal deficiency. Journal of Bone and Joint Surgery 59A: 927–934
Lamb D W 1977 Radial club hand. Journal of Bone and Joint Surgery 59A: 1–13
Sorbye R 1977 Myoelectric controlled hand prosthesis in children. International Journal of Rehabilitation Research 1: 15–25
Sorbye R 1980 Myoelectric prosthetic fitting in young children. Clinical Orthopedics and Related Research 148: 34–40
Temtamy S, McKusick V A 1969 Synopsis of hand malformations with particular emphasis on genetic factors. In: Bergsma D S, McKusick V A (eds) Clinical Delineation of Birth Defects, vol. 4 Williams and Wilkins, Baltimore

Van Nes C P 1950 Rotationplasty for congenital defects of the femur: making use of the ankle of the shortened limb to control the knee joint of a prosthesis. Journal of Bone and Joint Surgery 32B: 12–16

FURTHER READING

Atkins D J, Meier R H 1989 Comprehensive management of the upper-limb amputee. Springer–Verlag, New York

Burtch R L 1966 Nomenclature for congenital skeletal limb deficiencies: a revision of the Frantz and O'Rahilly Classification. Artificial Limbs 10(1): 24

Department of Health and Social Security 1981 Report on the trial of the Swedish myoelectric hand for young children. DHSS, London.

Fletcher I 1980 Review of the treatment of thalidomide children with limb deficiency in Great Britain. Clinical Orthopedics and Related Research 148: 18–25.

Fletcher I 1982 The management of limb deficient children. Maternal and Child Health 12

Henkel L, Willert H-G 1969 Dysmelia—a classification of congenital defects of limbs. Journal of Bone and Joint Surgery 51B: 399–414

Kuhne D, Lenz W, Petersen D, Schoneberg H 1967 Defekt von Femur und Fibula mit Amelie Peromelie oder ulnaren, Strahldefekten der Arme-Ein Syndrome. Humongenetik 3(3): 244–263

Mallinson V 1980 None can be called deformed. Arno Press, USA (Previously published in 1956 by William Heinemann, London)

Mazoyer D 1975 L'amputé congénital du membre supérieur. Réflexions à propos de 50 cas. Annales de médecine Physique 18: 3

Murdoch G, Donovan R G 1988 Amputation surgery and lower limb prosthetics. Blackwell Scientific Publications, Oxford

Robertson E 1978 Rehabilitation of arm amputees and limb deficient children. Baillière Tindall, London.

21. Osteogenesis imperfecta

A. Wisbeach   G. T. McCarthy   J.A. Fixsen

Osteogenesis imperfecta (OI) is a group of disorders characterised by abnormally fragile bones, hence the common name 'brittle bone disease'. The associated features are thought to be due to the generalised connective tissue defect. It is a genetically determined disorder and in the past decade information on the molecular basis of the condition has been determined (Marini 1988). Many individuals with OI have been found to have defects in type I collagen protein (Pope et al 1985).

The incidence of OI identifiable at birth is between 1 in 20 000 to 30 000. This does not include those people with very mild manifestations who do not come to medical attention.

The severity of OI varies greatly. Some children have multiple fractures before birth, and may have over 100 fractures in childhood. Others have few fractures and live a relatively normal life. A small number of more severely affected children may live for only a short time, but most survive to adulthood and have a good life expectancy. Fractures may occur from apparently minor trauma, such as being lifted, or in extreme cases when lying still. Conversely there may be times when a child falls heavily but does not fracture. The number of fractures a child has does not relate directly to the severity or prognosis of the disorder.

It is helpful for the family to know what type of OI the child has, so that they can be given a more accurate idea of the problems they are facing. It is also important in offering advice concerning further pregnancies.

CLINICAL CLASSIFICATION

The classification most often used is based on that proposed by Sillence in 1979 and later expanded by him and others. This clinical, radiological and genetic classification divides OI into four types (Table 21.1).

Genetic counselling

It can be seen that genetic counselling may be very difficult in OI, particularly as there is variability of expression and clinical types may overlap. It is possible for individuals with the mildest symptoms to be carriers, and for

Table 21.1 Classification of osteogenesis imperfecta

Type	Genetics	Incidence	Skeletal involvement	Blue sclerae	Dentinogenesis imperfecta	Hearing loss
I	Autosomal dominant	1 in 30 000	Mild without deformity	+	+	+
IA			Mild to moderate short stature	-	+	-
IB				-	-	-
II	Autosomal dominant or Autosomal recessive	1 in 62 487*	Perinatal *death* with multiple fractures in utero, growth retardation in utero, large soft head, beaded ribs, short broad thighs, long bones broad and crumpled, "accordion" appearance on radiographs.			
III	Autosomal recessive	Rare — about 20% of total†	Severe fragility, progressive deformity, multiple fractures in utero, large head, triangular face, extreme short stature, kyphoscoliosis. Useful walking not possible for many.	+/-	+	-
IV	Autosomal dominant	Rarest type‡	Fragility more severe than type I. Tend to fracture at birth or in the first year of life. Early radiographs may be normal, leading to suspicion of non-accidental injury. Bowing of long bones, growth retardation, joint hypermobility in some cases.	-	-	-
IVA				-		
IVB				+		

* Sillence et al (1979)
† Lubb & Travers (1981)
‡ Paterson et al (1983)

children with the severest symptoms to be spontaneous mutations. The purpose of genetic counselling is to give parents as accurate a picture as possible of the clinical type, in order to give some idea of prognosis and risk of recurrence in future pregnancies.

There are a number of centres carrying out research into collagen disorders and it may be helpful for families to be referred for skin biopsy and fibroblast culture.

Prenatal diagnosis can be made, using ultrasound detection of long bone deformities or skull abnormalities, as early as 17 to 20 weeks gestation. More recently chorionic villus sampling has been carried out at 8 to 10 weeks gestation allowing examination for the same collagen defect as the affected child. This would allow diagnosis as early as 16 weeks and termination of a severely affected fetus if the parents wished.

CLINICAL FEATURES

Fractures and deformity

The most obvious features of OI are recurrent painful fractures and angulation deformities of the long bones (Fig. 21.1). Marked deformity may be present despite few known fractures. It is thought to be the result of stronger muscle groups pulling the pliable bones into a bowed position. The deformities most typically (but not exclusively) seen are:

- Lateral bowing of the femora
- Anterior bowing of the tibiae and humeri
- Latero-posterior bowing of the radii and ulnae. (This bowing tends to be seen with associated rotation.)

For children who spend much of their early life supine there may be noticeable skull flattening anteroposteriorly. The skull is often described as

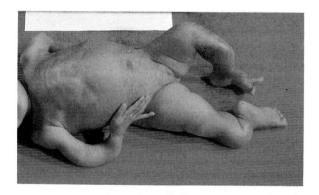

Fig. 21.1 Child with severe OI showing typical deformities of the limbs and 'bee-hived' ribs.

triangular or 'Tam o' Shanter'. The anterior fontanelle may show delayed closure. In more severely affected children, the ribcage may be 'beehived' (see Fig. 22.1), and kyphoscoliosis may develop.

Sclerae

A frequently noted feature of OI is the blue or grey colour of the sclerae. This may be due to the underlying choroid pigment showing through the unusually thin sclera. It has also been suggested that the colour is caused by a decreased scattering coefficient rather than just thinness, (Lanting et al 1985). The majority of more severely affected children have normal scleral colour.

Although no clear evidence exists, many families report that their child's sclerae become a darker blue just prior to or at the time of fracture. Some of these children also seem particularly sensitive to direct sunlight.

Skin

The skin may be thinner than normal in some children and wounds may heal slowly, with marked scarring (see Fig. 21.10b). Bruising may occur more readily as a result of rupturing of the small blood vessels, and there is a greater risk of haemorrhage during operations. Nosebleeds may occur frequently and unexpectedly.

Joint laxity

This may be limited to the extremities but may also be seen in the elbow, shoulder, knee and hip joints. Whilst this may lead to functional difficulties such as dislocations, it might well prove useful in helping children compensate for restriction of movement caused by bone angulation.

Muscle weakness is thought to be a result of the collagen defect.

Fatigue

Children with OI often tire easily, possibly because the generally low muscle tone requires them to exert more energy to fulfil normal motor activity. This is particularly difficult for more mildly affected children, who may be thought of as lazy or clumsy.

Sweating

Some affected children sweat excessively in response to environmental temperature or anxiety. This means that they may be uncomfortable during hot weather or in a centrally heated room. As most parents dress young infants warmly this can leave some children with OI wet with perspiration. It is not unusual for some children to wear summer-weight clothes throughout the year, and to dislike having many bedclothes.

At night-time it is important to get the right balance of room temperature and bed clothing. This will avoid the child becoming chilled from lying on a patch of cold sweat.

Chest infections

A small proportion of children suffer from recurrent chest infections and require careful supervision to prevent chronic respiratory difficulties. Breathing may be rapid and shallow.

Conventional chest physiotherapy is contraindicated as this may result in rib fractures, although postural drainage with the child on his side is possible, accompanied by gentle tapping with a finger or cup, as in neonates.

Some children are prone to recurrent collapse of the lungs and require re-expansion using positive pressure ventilation with a self-triggering ventilator and mouth-piece.

Feeding

Many of the more severely involved children are slow feeders, and take small quantities of food more frequently than their peers. This is in contrast to usually expected infant intake. Attempts to increase the volume of feed may result in vomiting or prolonged feeding times, which cause anxiety to both mother and child.

Increasing food intake does not correlate directly with increased growth in height of the child, and may in fact lead to obesity. This in turn will increase pressure on the skeleton and muscles, and lead to decreased activity. Correct feeding management is essential and parents need support during this difficult time.

An additional problem is colic, which can make mealtimes more fraught and disturb the child's sleep pattern.

Constipation

This is particularly prevalent in more severely affected and less mobile children. It can cause considerable discomfort and distress to the child, and may result in delayed bowel control in some. The situation usually improves with increased independent mobility and upright posture. Dietary management and medication often help to relieve the situation and should be instituted early. Modification of the seat of a potty chair may help with posture.

Routine advice and support is important to maintain regularity and avoid distress. Hernias sometimes develop due to weak abdominal musculature.

Hearing loss

Hearing loss may occur, usually in the second or third decade. This is usually a conductive loss as a result of damage to the stapes. Some in dividuals have been shown to have a sensorineural loss affecting high frequencies.

Hearing aids are helpful and some people have found a stapedectomy beneficial.

Dental problems

Whilst some individuals have normal dentition (with the usual range of dental problems) others have tooth abnormalities, so-called *dentinogenesis imperfecta* (see Table 21.1, p. 332). The primary dentition is generally more severely affected. Discolouration of the teeth, with chipping or even wearing down to the gum margins is seen. It is caused by a collagen defect in the dentin.

Routine dental visits are important, along with dietary advice. Fluoride drops are recommended in non-fluoridated water areas.

Sleeping difficulties

Some children establish disturbed sleep patterns, which can be exhausting for the parents. Possible explanations include: lack of movement; pain or discomfort; fear of pain ; seeking reassurance or attention. Advice and support are important to help the parents establish a more acceptable routine.

Growth

Impaired growth is a common feature in children with more severe types of OI. Virtually all children with type III OI, and as many as 50% of types I and IV are affected (see Table 21.1). Although this may be caused in part by the skeletal deformities, there is evidence to suggest neurosecretory deficiency of growth hormone, or abnormalities of somatomedin production. Further investigations of this aspect are in progress.

Behaviour problems

The fear and anxiety of new parents often make them extremely alert and attentive to the needs of their new 'special baby'. They have to be especially careful to avoid fractures; if there are young siblings playing close by, the parents will need to protect the baby from being accidently knocked or from having toys dropped on him/her. Whilst this becomes an accepted part of daily life, the child gradually learns to take responsibility for himself and becomes more socially and emotionally independent. The severe motor handicap imposed on some children can, however, lead to difficult and demanding behaviour. They may become overdependent on one parent, or scream if their needs are not met.

Parental support and counselling is important in addition to channelling the behaviour into a more constructive form of environmental control and providing increased independence skills.

Development

More mildly affected infants will follow the usual developmental sequences (Fig. 21.2) although there may be some variations caused by immobilisation from fractures, or parental restraint in an attempt to avoid injury.

More severely affected infants tend to follow a supine developmental sequence (Fig. 21.3) with great variability in the age at which skills are achieved and the final level of achievement.

MANAGEMENT

Other than following fracture or surgery, the emphasis is on management and handling, rather than treatment. Given the opportunity, most children will attempt to be as active and independent as their condition will allow. It is important for the children to be confident in their own abilities.
Key issues for independence in more severely affected infants include:

- *Side-lying* — For skull moulding; gradual weightbearing of the long bones; exploration of hands together; development of hand/eye activities
- *Independent sitting* — For development of cognitive/fine motor skills; self-help activities; feeding, toileting, dressing; use of mobility aids
- *Bottom shuffling* — For independent mobility and transfers
- *Half-kneeling* — For climbing on/off chairs; up/down stairs; pull to standing
- *Standing* — For transfers and walking.

Early handling

To avoid the infant becoming overdependent on parents, it is important

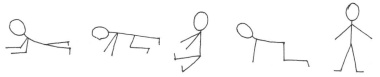

Fig. 21.2 Prone developmental sequence.

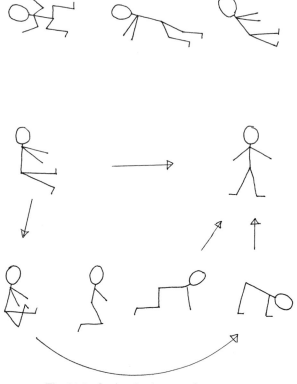

Fig. 21.3 Supine developmental sequence.

to encourage regular handling by family and friends. Parents rapidly become experts at holding their baby, and they can share this skill. Although
this may be initially stressful, it will ultimately increase the child's confidence, and enables the parents to spend time together while the child is
cared for by others. This will expand the child's experience of life.

All young babies are handled carefully and the infant with OI is no exception. However strong the inclination, it is not necessary to carry the
baby in a protective cocoon, or on a pillow. Babies can be safely lifted by
supporting their head with one hand, and their pelvis and back with the
other (Fig. 21.4). Many enjoy the experience of being rocked from side to
side or up and down when held like this.

The baby should always be talked to and told what is going to happen
next, as sudden movement or sounds may startle and upset. By exercising
this practice at the beginning, it will become an automatic process by the
time the baby is able to understand.

Whilst the majority of mildly affected babies are happy to be placed in
prone, most moderately and severely affected babies prefer to be supine.
Provided sufficient alternative positions are introduced, this does not adversely delay motor development.

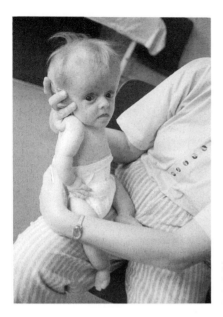

Fig. 21.4 A baby being supported correctly—the head and neck supported with one hand, and the pelvis and back with the other.

Unless the baby moves into prone, this position should be avoided as the cervical vertebrae are flattened resulting in a short neck which is difficult to extend. The head is often disproportionately heavy creating a mechanical disadvantage. Breathing tends to be diaphragmatic and shallow, and is restricted in the prone position. Rib fractures and shoulder dislocation and fractures of the humeri may occur on attempting forearm support.

As an alternative to the prone position, the child may be placed in a semi side-lying position. Place the baby supine on a towel or blanket. Use a lure to encourage visual following and reach. As the baby reaches, raise the opposite side of the blanket so that he gently rolls towards the toy. Make sure that he is not completely on his side initially as the weight on the supporting limbs may cause fractures. As the baby's tolerance and confidence improve, he will reach out further for toys. Remember to lay the baby on alternate sides to discourage skull moulding and promote symmetry. This is also a good sleeping position for the baby.

Alternatively the baby can be propped on a wedge, in a reclined car seat (Fig 21.5) or in a bouncing cradle with a play frame. If there is a tendency to slump to one side, place a foam cushion either side of the trunk to correct.

Many of the more severely affected children prefer straight-leg sitting, but if the baby is unhappy with his legs straight, sit him on another small block of foam which extends as far as his knees.

The baby can be held upright, facing against the adult's shoulder, initially giving maximum support, and reducing gradually as the child's head and trunk control improve (Fig 21.6). Although adults tend to be more

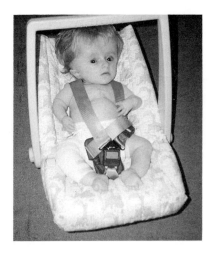

Fig. 21.5 A reclined car seat can be adjusted to different angles.

comfortable carrying on one side or the other, it is important to alternate for symmetry.

Once some head and trunk control has developed, lap sitting can allow the baby to be reclined or more upright. To begin with, it is a good idea to cup the chin lightly between thumb and index finger to prevent sudden falling forwards.

Lifting by the ankles should be avoided when nappy changing. The baby should be placed on a towel or a changing mat. The nappy can then be undone and rolled up. The baby should be cleaned and then gently lifted from the bottom, as when carrying, and the dirty nappy slid out and replaced by the clean one.

Babies with OI enjoy the same kinds of stimulation as others. Although

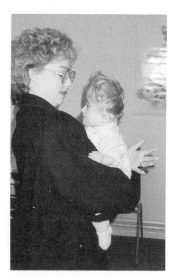

Fig. 21.6 If the baby is held upright against the adult's shoulder, support to the head and back can gradually be reduced to encourage head and trunk control.

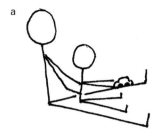
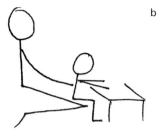

Fig. 21.7 Sitting positions for play. **a.** Between the adults's legs using them for support. **b.** On the adults's knees supported with a low table in front.

sudden noises may cause fright, they do not need special toys. As the babies are small it may be necessary to find small toys which they can grasp. Hard or heavy toys do not have to be avoided, provided they will fit the child's hand. The babies are happy to wave and bang solid toys and this encourages their strength and coordination.

As they become older there are numerous puzzle, construction, car and miniature doll activities to enjoy, as well as craft activities. Independent sitting can be encouraged by allowing the child to sit between your legs (Fig 21.7). The adult can lean back initially but gradually become more upright as the child's ability increases. As a precaution place a pillow in front of the child to protect from falling forwards and suddenly transferring all the weight through the femurs. This will also provide a play surface and

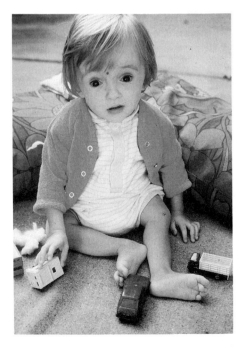

Fig. 21.8 When the child is able to sit independently, cushions can be positioned to protect from falling, and toys placed to encourage rotation to the side.

a
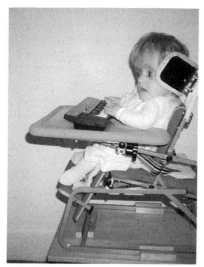

b
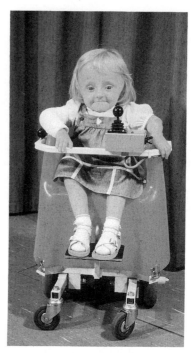

Fig. 21.9 a. A specially made chair with adjustable support and tray; the head rest can be removed. (Chailey Heritage Rehabilitation Engineering Department.) **b.** Children enjoy the freedom of powered mobility from an early stage.

encourage forward propping. Toys can be placed along the adult's legs to encourage side propping and rotation.

As the child's ability increases, the adult can gradually move further back and eventually place cushions around the child for safety. Once the child can floor sit, toys can be positioned to encourage rotation to either side (Fig 21.8).

When the child is able to rotate easily, he will probably bottom shuffle spontaneously. A few children may need encouragement by example. For children who cannot achieve this skill, a self-propelling or powered trolley may be needed. Once the child realises the advantages of mobility it may achieve bottom shuffling later, or at least become adept at manoeuvring a trolley or wheelchair.

Chairs and wheelchairs may need to be modified or specially made to accommodate femoral shortening and allow the child to sit with the hips and knees at right angles (Fig 21.9).

NURSERY PLACEMENT

With the current emphasis on mainstream education, the majority of children with OI attend their local Nursery Group. A few children may initially go to an Opportunity Group or Special Needs Nursery, and later may also go to a local Nursery. Staff are often quite anxious at the thought of having a child with 'brittle bones' in the classroom, and will need guidance and support in coping with the situation. It is helpful to provide basic information on the nature of the disorder and the likelihood of fractures occurring, with a procedure for their management should it be necessary. In addition they will need to know about the child's specific needs and abilities. The majority of children with OI have normal intelligence despite what might be a severe motor impairment. It may be that wheelchair-bound children are in fact easier to deal with in the classroom as they are protected by their chairs, whereas children who are mobile are more in danger of slipping or tripping up. A protocol for fracture management should be agreed with the parents; for example, this might be:

1. Make the child comfortable
2. Telephone the parents
3. Telephone the emergency service.

It is always worthwhile remembering to take a second or third telephone number in case the parents cannot be contacted. The staff need to be aware of special details, such as whether or not the child goes into shock or how they react to fractures. They will also need guidelines on lifting.

In the initial stages of school placement it is advisable to have a care assistant within the classroom specifically for the child with OI, who can take special responsibility for lifting and activities that the child is unable to manage independently. The care assistant should spend time with the child and his family prior to nursery admission, in order to learn the skills of caring for the child. Most children, particularly as they become older, are quite happy and able to instruct assistants on how best to help them.

Furniture may present some problems, and needs to be looked at before children are introduced to nursery to make sure that they can sit in the school chairs, reach the tables, manoeuvre around the classroom, and manage the toilet. Thought may need to be given on the positioning of equipment so that children are able to reach and do as much for themselves as possible.

EDUCATION

The majority of children with OI move from Opportunity Group or nursery placement directly into mainstream school. Staff guidelines, fracture management and care assistants continue to be appropriate. However, a number of other issues arise, particularly as secondary levels of education are reached. Transport should be arranged to enable children to go to school independently, and advice will be required concerning suitable car seats, or transporting children in their wheelchairs in an ambulance or minibus. It may also be necessary to negotiate who is going to move the child in and out of the car or minibus.

It is important for the child with OI to become as independent as possible. This may be facilitated by appropriate furniture or modifications to the environment, particularly to allow the child full access to the national curriculum. Particular areas of difficulty are frequently encountered in the domestic science room, the science lab and the woodwork area. Structural alterations may be needed in order to make these more suitable for the wheelchair-bound child. Space for manoeuvring is also a frequent problem due to the size of some classes.

If the child is in a wheelchair, it is important to look at their manoeuvrability and the various seat heights that are necessary in order to access the desks, toilets and workbenches. More than one wheelchair of different types may be necessary. In addition, the child might need an outdoor chair or a pushchair for school excursions. Some children will transfer from their wheelchair onto a standard school chair, whilst others will sit in their wheelchair in the classroom. Very small children may benefit from a powered chair with a variable height platform.

The entrances of the school will need to be looked at for wheelchair access, as will the toilets. Some toilet areas need modification of increased door widths and space for the wheelchair to be positioned for independent transfers. In some situations, particularly in primary education, a changing bench may also be necessary.

A short-term issue that may arise is that of going to school when in a plaster cast. This does not present a problem to children who are mobile with arm fractures or with a leg in plaster and using crutches, but can cause more difficulty to wheelchair bound children. They may need the temporary loan of a wheelchair or simply an alteration of the position of the control box of their powered chair from one side to the other depending on which arm is broken. Leg rest extensions can also be provided to support a straight leg in plaster. The children should be encouraged to go back to school as soon as possible following fracture, both to encourage them to continue being as active as possible and to relieve boredom.

Some mobile children with OI seem to fatigue more easily than their peer group and may need a pushchair or bicycle for coping with longer distances. Alternatively, a brief rest usually helps them to regain their energy quite quickly.

Some children are thought to be clumsy because of the tendency to trip over, but this is likely to be due to the generalised muscle weakness particularly around the ankles.

As to pen and paper skills, most children with OI cope extremely well, even those with marked deformity of their upper extremities. The increasing amount of written work as they get older may cause fatigue and in some instances word processors are indicated, but this is unusual.

Many children with OI succeed academically and go on to further education.

Physical education (PE) can give rise for concern, and it is generally not advised to engage in contact sports. However, many children with OI enjoy competitive games such as table-tennis, badminton, racing, swimming, etc. It is also a useful time for the children to explore as much of their movement as possible during activities such as movement to music and hydrotherapy. PE provides an excellent opportunity for the child to practise independent transfers getting from floor to wheelchair or wheelchair to chair, and also for dressing skills.

ADOLESCENCE

The self-image of the child with OI is of great importance. Integration into mainstream schools helps the child to identify with the peer group and share the same dreams and expectations for the future. Some individuals have great difficulty in coming to terms with their imagined self and their real self as they become older and realise the restrictions imposed on them by their deformity and fragility. They require sensitive handling to enable them to express their feelings and to learn to appreciate themselves as individuals. In addition to discussing personal relationships with their peers and parents, it is often helpful to have access to a counsellor who has experience of other young people with disability.

Menstruation may be difficult to manage for some girls with severe deformity, but with the wide range of tampons and panty liners currently available, most can be completely independent.

Eventually the school discussions become a reality and adolescents suddenly have to face their sexuality, independence, leaving home, career choices and financial responsibility. Their mobility is limited and thereby their opportunity for establishing social and subsequently sexual relationships is restricted. There is a great need for them to have as much contact as possible with their able-bodied peers to enable them to mature emotionally, intellectually and sexually. They are subject to the same pressures as their able-bodied peers to establish boy–girl relationships, and adequate sex education is especially important due to their limited opportunities for acquiring knowledge by contact with their peers. The difficulties likely to be experienced in sexual activity are those imposed by deformities and the possibility of fractures. These will be different in each case and each couple will have to arrive at their own solution (Sillence 1981).

Career choice, as with all young adults, is very varied but there will be some limitations caused by the physical difficulties. Fortunately because of their good intellectual abilities, many have successful careers in law, teaching, computing and the arts.

Many find difficulty in approaching the issue of leaving home. A major concern is how to tell the parents who have cared for them so lovingly and tirelessly over the years that they no longer want to live in the family home.

The new-found freedom of adolescence is enhanced by the ability to drive, the goal of most youngsters. Unfortunately, the reality is a little more difficult. Although the Mobility Allowance has made a definite improvement to the prospects for outdoor mobility, and option schemes such as Motability have enabled some individuals to exchange their Mobility Allowance for a leased car, there are still many shortfalls. Specialised centres such as Banstead Place now exist for a thorough assessment of the driving needs of the individual. The centre will recommend modifications needed, suggest the type of car that might be suitable, and give advice on financing. However, this still leaves the individual with the need to find at least a deposit for the car, if not the total amount. In addition, before they can take driving lessons, it is necessary for them to have the car adapted.

PARENTHOOD

Whilst the majority of mildly or moderately affected individuals become parents, an increasing number of severely affected individuals are also having children. It is important for women with severe problems to seek advice from a sympathetic obstetrician before embarking on pregnancy.

Whichever partner has OI, the management of a child who might be similarly affected introduces a whole new set of challenges, which can only effectively be dealt with by regular visits. Often, customised equipment must be made and management routines established.

TIMES FOR INCREASED THERAPY

Whilst therapy support (rather than active treatment) is important for developmental and management advice, a more rigorous regime is useful after fractures or surgery.

Following removal of plaster of Paris or traction, the child needs to build up his general strength and confidence. Initially this can be done in hydrotherapy and gradually phased into a graded mobilisation programme during which activities can be built up to achieve the previous level of ability.

If the child has the potential for weightbearing, he may need external support initially such as with a 'spacesuit' or lightweight orthoses. Both tend to be restrictive, so although they may be helpful in encouraging initial weightbearing they are not usually compatible with active mobility and independence.

Walking aids are important and children may graduate from using parallel bars to a rollator, and then to clumpers and finally crutches. Some children may be unable to take sufficient weight through their upper limbs, either because of fracture or dislocation. In such instances, some form of 'lobster-pot' walker with a slung seat may be appropriate. Parents are naturally anxious to protect their child when they begin to weightbear, but there is no failsafe solution, particularly when walking free. Some have found it helpful to sew long pockets along the inside of each trouser leg. Into each of these can be slipped two lengths of large size bubble pack, facing each other, and a layer of small size bubble pack sandwiched in between. These can be simply sellotaped together. If the child falls and a bubble bursts, it can be replaced by sellotaping another in its place. They can be easily removed for washing or once the child has a well-established walking pattern. Important considerations to bear in mind are the child's fear of further fractures or joints 'giving way' if there are unstable knee joints. Often children who present with unstable and hyperextensible knees also present with instability of the pelvis and ankle joints on examination. Recurrent pain and their motivation to walk must also be taken into account.. As children become older those who have only been minimal household walkers may find far more independence from their wheelchair.

ORTHOPAEDIC MANAGEMENT

It is important to be aware of the extreme anxiety of parents and children with OI. Management therefore depends on the development of confidence in handling the child. Parents become expert in diagnosing their child's problems and most soon learn to use light splints or immobilise limbs with elasticated net or bandages, and use analgesia effectively when necessary. In the first year, fractures should be splinted as simply as possible. The aim is to immobilise the child as little as possible and return to early weightbearing. If gallows traction is required, children can often be nursed at home, particularly if there is paediatric nursing back-up in the community.

The family with a child with OI should have open access to their local children's department and a plan of management agreed with their orthopaedic surgeon. It is not always necessary to radiograph a painful limb—parents can usually be relied on to know whether their child has a fracture or the injury is less severe. Adequate analgesia is important, using opioids initially and tailing down to paracetamol as the pain is controlled.

Once a vicious cycle of repeated fractures leading to further immobilisation and osteoporosis is established it is vital to adopt a more radical approach. There are a number of methods of straightening and strengthening bones using internal rods (Fig 21.10). Expanding rods have been developed, but they are more difficult to insert and have an increased incidence of complications.

Another ingenious way of supporting the weak bones is the pneumatic orthosis described by Morel (1971). This is based on the pilot's 'G' suit, and provides all-round support for the legs, allowing weight to be taken partly through the inflated tubes of the suit. Before the suit can be fitted

a 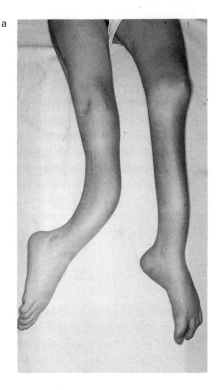 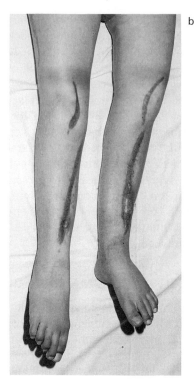 b

Fig. 21.10 a. Severe bowing of the tibiae and fibulae. **b.** Same legs following surgery using intramedullary rodding. Note the marked keloid scarring.

the limbs must be reasonably straight, as the child cannot tolerate areas of high pressure over the bony prominences.

Sofield rodding can be used to correct the bony deformities. Alternatively, Morel uses multiple closed osteotomies followed by traction for 6 weeks and then the immediate fitting of the suit to the straightened limbs.

The pneumatic orthosis can be very successful in getting the child onto his feet for the first time. It can also be used for the child who has become immobilised by repeated fractures, and who needs to regain confidence in walking. However, it is cumbersome and restrictive and many children will want to discard it once their confidence is regained. It takes considerable time and expertise to manage children in these suits.

Although fractures and deformities of the upper limbs are less common than in the lower limbs, they can be a problem. It is possible to use intramedullary rod fixation on the humerus, but it is much more difficult on the small forearm bones. It is important to avoid causing stiffness of the elbow where movement is more important than cosmetic appearance.

Subluxation of the radial head is common in OI.

Hyperplastic callus

This is a rare and remarkable response to fracture in OI. Following a minor fracture, or occasionally intramedullary rodding, (McCall & Bax 1984), or even spontaneously, the limb becomes hot, swollen and tender. The child runs a low-grade pyrexia and the alkaline phosphatase becomes raised. Not surprisingly the condition is frequently thought to be an infection or even a tumour.

Radiographs show exuberant callus which develops rapidly, causing increase in size of the limb. Immobilisation of the limb is important as movement seems to exacerbate the process. This is a selflimiting condition but the limb is left permanently enlarged and thickened, often to a disabling degree. Over a period of years the bone will slowly remodel.

Footwear

Whilst wheelchair-bound children have a wide variety of footwear available to them, difficulties can arise for walking children. These are usually the result of weak musculature around the foot and ankles. Often the foot is over-pronated, which particularly increases stress on the ankle. Other joints and bones of the leg are also affected. Splintage can be difficult as it tends to transfer a stress area to the site at the top of the splint. Soft insoles early in weightbearing or trainers or shoes with an integral arch support are more satisfactory.

Scoliosis

Scoliosis or kyphoscoliosis is an associated feature of OI and has proved difficult to manage. Some very young children show a tendency to lean to one side as soon as a reclined sitting posture is introduced. Alternative positioning and supporting symmetrically with foam blocks is important from an early stage.

As the child acquires sitting balance the spine should be monitored: a baseline radiograph is usually helpful, repeated at intervals as necessary (see Ch. 22).

Some children suffer backache, which is usually helped by a stretch, lying supine or prone, depending on the child's preference. Stable crush fractures are common and cause distress and pain. They respond well to simple support and analgesia. If the deformity progresses, a light plastazote jacket may be tried in an effort to stabilise, but is not entirely satisfactory as adequate pressure to control the scoliosis would compromise the child's breathing and could cause rib fractures.

Progressive spinal deformity is common, particularly in the more severe forms of OI. Surgery is difficult because of the soft porotic bone; methyl-methacrylate may be used to supplement screw and hook fixation (Benson & Newman 1981).

REFERENCES

Benson D R, Newman D C 1981 The spine and surgical treatment in osteogenesis imperfecta. Clinical Orthopaedics 59: 147

Lanting P J H, Borsboom P C F, Meerman G T et al 1985 Decreased scattering coefficient of blue sclerae. Clinical Genetics 27: 187

Lubb H A, Travers H 1981 Genetic counselling in osteogenesis imperfecta. Clinical Orthopaedics 159:36

McCall R E, Bax J A 1984 Hyperplastic callus formation in osteogenesis imperfecta following intramedullary rodding. Journal of Pediatric Orthopaedics 3: 361

Marini J C 1988 Osteogenesis imperfecta: comprehensive management. Advances in Pediatrics. 35:391–426. Year Book Medical Publishers, Chicago

Morel G 1971 Revue de chirurgie orthopédique et réparatrice. De L'Appareil Moteur 57: 409

Paterson C R, McAllion F, Miller R 1983a Osteogenesis imperfecta with dominant inheritance and normal sclerae. Journal of Bone and Joint Surgery (British). 65: 35

Paterson C R, McAllion F, Miller R 1983b Heterogeneity of osteogenesis imperfecta type I. Journal of Medical Genetics 20(3): 203–205

Pope F M, Nicholls A C, McPheat J et al 1985 Collagen genes and proteins in osteogenesis imperfecta. Journal of Medical Genetics 22: 466

Sillence D O, Senn A S, Danks D M 1979 Genetic heterogeneity in osteogenesis imperfecta. Journal of Medical Genetics 16:101

FURTHER READING

Cole W G 1988 Osteogenesis imperfecta. Balliere's clinical endocrinology and metabolism, vol 2(1): 243–256

Dean-McEwan G 1982 Scoliosis associated with osteogenesis imperfecta—results of treatment by Ken Yong Hing. Journal of Bone and Joint Surgery 64(1): 36–43

Kirks D, Morrish K, Shapiro J 1985 Vertebral bone mineral content in osteogenesis imperfecta. Calcified Tissue International 1985 (37): 14–18

Paterson C R 1974 Metabolic disorders of bone. Blackwell Scientific Publications, Oxford

Sillence D O (ed) 1981 Osteogenesis imperfecta: a handbook for medical practitioners and health care professionals. Osteogenesis Imperfecta Society of New South Wales

Thompson E M, Yound I D, Hall C M, Pembury M E 1987 Recurrence risks and prognosis in severe sporadic osteogenesis imperfecta. Journal of Medical Genetics 1987(24): 390–405

A database of literature on osteogenesis imperfecta is available from the Dutch Osteogenesis Imperfecta Society, from: Taco van Welzenis-Bunt, Luytelaer 1, 563 BE Eindhoven, The Netherlands

An annual update on osteogenesis imperfecta is available from: Dr C R Paterson, Department of Biochemical Medicine, Ninewells Hospital Medical School, Ninewells, Dundee DD1 9SY

22. Spinal deformity in the physically handicapped child

T.R. Morley

The term scoliosis is derived from the Greek meaning curvature, and is used to describe any lateral curvature of the spine. Scoliosis may be associated with exaggerations of the normal curve in the sagittal plane, producing either lordoscoliosis (forward curvature) or kyphoscoliosis (backward curvature).

CLASSIFICATION

Spinal deformities are either structural or non-structural.

Structural curves are characterised by loss of the normal flexibility and do not correct, either anatomically or radiologically, on side bending. In addition to the lateral curvature, the spine is rotated about a vertical axis into the convexity of the curve, producing rib prominence. The rib hump remains on forward flexion, and is the basis for the forward bending test.

Non-structural curves correct fully on forward flexion, and are not associated with vertebral rotation on lateral bending. (Fig. 22.1). The commonest causes for non-stuctural curves are:

- Poor posture—postural curves correct on forward flexion and there is no rib rotation. They also correct on lateral flexion (cf structural curves, Fig. 22.2). They can be overcome by active muscular effort.
- Pelvic obliquity—this causes a compensatory curve, which may be corrected by equalising leg lengths
- Pressure on nerve roots—either by adolescent discs, or by spinal tumours.

All these deformities become fixed with the passage of time and with growth. The differentiation between structural and non-structural curves is vital. Non-structural curves (which will not be discussed in this chapter) disappear when the underlying cause is corrected.

STRUCTURAL CURVES

Neuropathic causes

Upper motor neurone

- Cerebral palsy

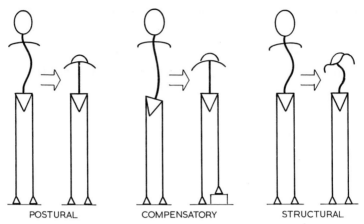

Fig. 22.1   Postural curves correct on forward flexion; there is no rib rotation. Compensatory curves are solely a response to pelvic obliquity and can be corrected by equalising leg length. In structural curves there are anatomical changes with rotation around the vertical axis, causing rib rotation and a rib hump on forward flexion.

- Syringomyelia
- Spinal cord trauma.

Anterior horn cell and lower motor neurone

- Spinal muscular atrophies: anterior horn cell degeneration
    —Werdnig–Hoffmann disease
    —Kugelberg–Welander syndrome
- Myelomeningocoele
- Poliomyelitis and other viral myelitides
- Hereditary peripheral neuropathies
    — Motor neuropathies

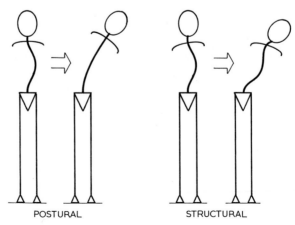

Fig. 22.2   Postural curves correct on lateral flexion. Structural curves do not.

— Peroneal muscular atrophy
— Degenerative disorders affecting peripheral nerves and spinocerebellar tracts, e.g. Friedreich's ataxia, Charcot–Marie–Tooth disease
- Dysautonomia (Riley–Day syndrome)
- Arthrogryposis: anterior horn cell damage in utero with static damage

Myopathic causes

- Muscular dystrophy: progressive degenerative myopathies
  — Duchenne muscular dystrophy
  — Limb girdle dystrophy
  — Facio-scapulo-humeral muscular dystrophy
- Congenital myopathies: specific structural abnormalities in the muscle, only occasionally progressive (Dubowitz 1978).

Other causes

Congenital scolioses are caused by failure of formation or of segmentation of the vertebrae. Congenital abnormalities are commonly seen in myelomeningocoele in addition to the laminar defects.

Typical *idiopathic* curves may also occur in the physically handicapped. Scoliosis has also been described as a feature in a large number of *genetic and metabolic disorders* associated with physical handicap.

GENERAL CONSIDERATIONS

Spinal deformity in physically handicapped children occurs as just one facet of a complicated whole; therefore physical examination and full assessment are of vital importance. Disaster attends treatment of these curves without a full understanding of all the complicating factors. Assessment as outlined in Chapter 3 is necessary, taking into account the child's general condition, his understanding of his disability and the family circumstances.

It is also important that the family and the child are fully involved in the treatment process so that they understand the need for bracing, the times when the brace should be worn, and when wearing can be relaxed. When surgery is planned the child and family need time to adjust to the idea, and to have some explanation of the actual process. This discussion is important in the final outcome as families who have been involved in this way have greater confidence during the period of stress surrounding the operation.

PHYSICAL EXAMINATION

There are three important areas to be recorded: the deformity, the aetiology and the complicating factors.

The patient is evaluated and the presence of abnormal body development such as dwarfism or excessive height noted, as well as any abnormal facies or evidence of generalised disease. Depending on these findings specific areas such as the heart, eyes, or other joints may need to be examined in more depth.

Examination of the spine includes:

a. The level of curve, i.e. thoracic, thoracolumbar or lumbar
b. The direction of convexity of the curve
c. The presence of abnormal kyphosis or lordosis.

Following this, clinical assessment of the mobility of the curve and the degree of rotation is made. Mobility is assessed by side-bending or suspension. The degree of rotation is measured—ISIS scanning is more accurate than conventional methods. Information must be recorded on the fixed deformities of other joints, particularly the hips, and also the degree of pelvic tilt. A full neurological examination should be carried out and also an assessment of mental ability and maturity.

An assessment of functional ability is necessary including information on the child's sitting ability, mobility and ability to transfer. A report from the child's home physiotherapist is also helpful.

Cardiopulmonary function is also important, and a general assessment can be made by such simple methods as singing and holding a note, and also by spirometry. If there is anxiety about cardiopulmonary function it is important to arrange for full assessment at a specialist unit. This is especially important in cases of Duchenne muscular dystrophy and spinal muscular atrophy.

Radiographic evaluation. The standard views, i.e. a standing anteroposterior (AP) and lateral view of the whole spine, may need to be supplemented. To assess mobility, if the child is unable to stand, radiographs may be taken sitting and in suspension, or even prone with passive bending or with traction.

Incidence and natural history

The incidence and progression of deformity in some of the more common conditions causing physical handicap will be discussed.

CEREBRAL PALSY

Approximately 40% of patients with cerebral palsy have a structural spinal deformity of more than 10°. Many of these curves are severe, i.e. 90–180°, especially in the non-ambulatory quadriparetic and in the more severe diplegics (Fig. 22.3).

Postural deformities, particularly kyphosis, are common in the very young, with loss of the normal truncal reflexes. The curves in cerebral palsy are typically long 'C' curves and may impair walking and sitting stability. The management may be complicated by the presence of athetosis or epilepsy.

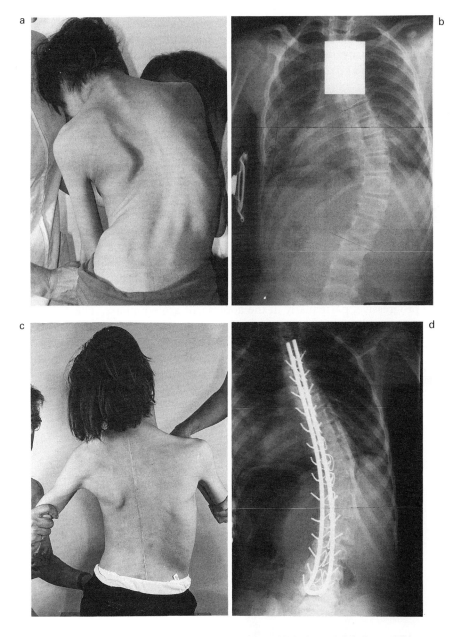

Fig. 22.3 a and b. Severe scoliosis in an athetoid quadriplegic. **c and d.** Same child following surgery.

RETT'S SYNDROME

This is an unusual condition occurring in girls, in which, after an apparently normal period of development in infancy, regression occurs with loss of speech and autistic features. Disordered motor control is evident with hypotonia predominating in infancy followed by variably progressive extrapyramidal signs, spasticity becoming manifest later. Not surprisingly the curve is associated with a typical neurological pattern of deformity and develops in 65% of cases.

MYELOMENINGOCOELE

Of all the causes of spinal deformity associated with physical handicap these are the most severe and difficult to treat. There are two separate types of deformity, which may well exist together: congenital and paralytic.

The congenital curves are due to failure of formation or segmentation of the spine and are present at birth. The paralytic curves are related to muscle imbalance and appear later. About 75% of patients with myelomeningocoele will develop a curvature, the majority being paralytic curves or mixed, with less than one-third being purely congenital.

The incidence of scoliosis is related to the level of paralysis and, generally speaking, one can expect a 100% incidence of spinal deformity with defects at T12 or above, reducing steadily to 25% at L5. All these curves are progressive, particularly in the adolescent growth phase. The congenital curves are particularly severe, and never respond to bracing.

The paralytic curves are usually 'C' curves from the mid-thoracic region to the sacrum, frequently with pelvic obliquity. Many are associated with deformity in the sagittal plane, i.e. lordoscoliosis (Fig. 22.4) or kyphoscoliosis (Fig. 22.5).

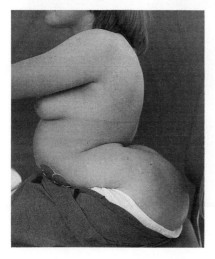

Fig. 22.4   Child with myelomeningocoele showing gross lordoscoliosis.

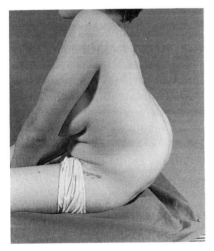
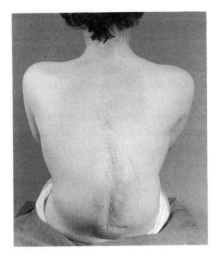

Fig. 22.5   Child with high spinal lesion showing typical collapsing kyphosis.

In a case where there is wide open spina bifida there is a loss of posterior stability and kyphosis tends to occur. Where the laminae are partly formed, there is posterior tethering and the lordosis occurs in association with a scoliosis (Fig. 22.6).

Deformities in the sagittal plane alone may occur, producing kyphosis (Fig. 22.7). Congenital deformities present at birth may complicate closure of the myelomeningocoele. These curves are severely progressive, unresponsive to conservative treatment and require early surgical intervention.

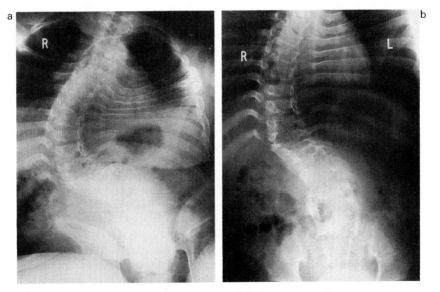

Fig. 22.6   Radiographs showing a mixed congenital–paralytic curve producing lordosis, scoliosis and kyphosis. **a.** Sitting. **b.** Suspended.

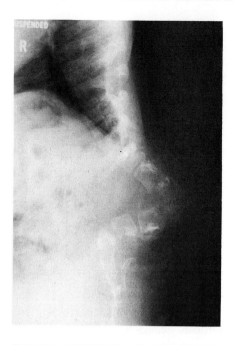

Fig. 22.7   Lateral radiograph showing gross kyphoscoliosis.

SPINAL MUSCULAR ATROPHY

Spinal muscular atrophy produces a wide spectrum of clinical manifestations. Scoliosis is more common in the less progessive types, i.e. in those children living into adolescence. Only about 20% of children with spinal muscular atrophy have scoliosis before the age of 5, increasing to 85% in those over the age of 12.

These curves are collapsing and are associated with respiratory problems. Early bracing is important but braces are often poorly tolerated and careful adjustment is necessary.

Surgical tratment should be considered early when the curve is not more than 30–40°, because if the scoliosis remains easily correctable then surgical techniques can be used that allow the child to sit up immediately postoperatively without the use of bracing. If the opportunity to correct the spinal deformity is missed, rapid progression may occur in adolescence with loss of sitting balance and death from respiratory failure. The anaesthetic risks are formidable when respiratory function falls below 20% of predicted normal.

DUCHENNE MUSCULAR DYSTROPHY

Spinal deformity develops commonly in boys with Duchenne dystrophy, usually after loss of ambulation. Early bracing is important with the aim of increasing the lumbar lordosis in order to lock the posterior facets and try to prevent lateral collapse. Attention to seating is also important: a firm base to the seat and well placed back-rest will reduce the tendency to asymmetry.

Surgery can offer important benefits to these boys in whom a rapidly progressive curve is likely to impair respiration. However, it is also important to evaluate cardiac function as a significant number have involvement of cardiac muscle and arrhythmias and heart failure may occur postoperatively.

MANAGEMENT OF SPINAL DEFORMITY

Conservative management

- Observation
- Bracing
- Electrical stimulation
- Plaster correction
- Seating.

Surgical management

- Minor localised fusion
- Anterior fusion
- Posterior fusion
- Anterior and posterior fusion.

Where possible, treatment should always be conservative. Operative treatment involving fusion of the spine in a corrected position is a traumatic undertaking for both child and parents, and has the disadvantage of halting spinal growth.

In order to have any hope of treating these deformities without operation they need to be diagnosed early and referred to a specialist clinic. Most physically handicapped children are already under medical supervision but despite this *deformities are regularly ignored* until they are too far advanced, making any form of treatment impossible and missing the opportunity to achieve surgical correction and stability.

Children are often not referred, either because of a mistaken desire to protect them from more forms of bracing, or a lack of understanding of what can be achieved by treating small curves before progression.

CONSERVATIVE MANAGEMENT

Observation

Small curves under 20° can often be treated by observation alone, particularly if the child is nearly at maturity. It is not true that curves stop progressing at the end of growth, but the rate of progression does dramatically decrease. Neuropathic and myopathic curves particularly progress in adult life because the imbalance causing the deformity persists.

Most curves are observed initially' in order to develop an overall picture of the child in relation to the deformity, and also to develop a picture of the individual natural progression. Not all curves behave predictably.

Bracing

Aggressive bracing is the mainstay of nonsurgical treatment. Bracing is not a new invention; indeed apparatus was described by Hippocrates! Ambrose Pare was the first to describe body shells in 1579; these were made by armourers. The landmark in effective bracing control was the Milwaukee brace, originally described by Blount and Schmidt in 1946 (Blount & Moe 1973). More recently, underarm orthoses such as the Boston have been developed.

The principle of bracing is to exert force, either lateral or distractive, to the spine. The force is indirect and is transmitted via the pelvis, ribs and the paraspinal muscles. The force over the apex of the curve is opposed by two other forces in the opposite direction. The correction is both active and passive, but where possible should be active, the child coming away from the brace and correcting his own spine. In cases where there is paralysis of the paraspinal muscles, only passive correction is possible. Although normal skin sensation is desirable, lack of this should not exclude the use of braces.

Modern braces tend to avoid the neck rings associated with the Milwaukee; these rings are much disliked and are often a considerable disadvantage to the physically handicapped. Underarm braces can be used, either taken from a mould of the child or 'off the shelf'. An example of the latter modular brace is the Boston brace, which is widely used with idiopathic scoliosis but is of less value in the physically handicapped.

Whichever form of brace is used, careful follow-up is necessary in collaboration with an orthotist, physiotherapist and occupational therapist, together with the cooperation of the nursing staff if the child is in hospital. It is quite wrong to believe that a well-fitted brace disturbs the development of a handicapped child. On the contrary it may enhance developmental potential significantly by allowing the child to hold up his head and use both hands instead of using them for support. The brace can easily be removed for prone lying and physiotherapy.

The general *indications* for bracing are: (a) a small curve, under 40°, which remains flexible; and (b) in a child with remaining growth potential.

Relative *contraindications* for bracing are: (a) a large curve, over 50°, which is stiff; and (b) where growth has ceased. Special care must be exercised where sensation is abnormal.

Since many of the curves in the handicapped result form an imbalance that persists, the indications for bracing may continue into adult life. In this situation the aim is to prevent a slow downward progression.

Bracing the physically handicapped has been associated with poor results, mainly because braces have been used inappropriately. There is no hope of holding a progressive congenital curve or a stiff neuropathic curve of over 90°. In certain situations a brace may be used as the only realistic method of control in the severely handicapped, in which case the predicted result and outcome must be modified.

Usually the brace is applied having corrected the lumbar lordosis in order to control rotation. In some specific situations, such as Duchenne muscular dystrophy, the lordosis may be increased to lock the posterior facet joints and prevent spinal collapse.

In all situations one must be prepared to be flexible and to listen to the views of all caring staff as well as to the child and his parents.

Electrical stimulation

The indications for electrical stimulation are very much the same as for bracing. A small electrical stimulus is applied to the paraspinal muscles in order to 'pull' the spine straight. So far the results are very much the same as for bracing, and there is very little experience in the physically handicapped. This is partly due to the problems of control and acceptance, and partly due to the fact that abnormal muscles cannot be stimulated. The idea remains theoretically attractive.

Plaster casting

Plaster corrective techniques were first described in the latter part of the 19th century. The techniques have become more sophisticated, combining both distraction and lateral pressure. Plaster correction is called 'localising' and involves correcting the curve maximally, often under sedation, and then holding the corrected position for 6–12 weeks before repeating the procedure. This is often done in conjunction with a bracing policy. Localising is particularly effective in the young child with a mobile curve, but may also be useful and acceptable in long 'C' curves such as in cerebral palsy.

Seating

Specialised seating should not be considered a method of spinal control. All that seating can do is to contain the child in the optimum position for function; it cannot alter the progress of deformity, although by anchoring the pelvis and hips it may reduce the risk of deformity. In the severely handicapped this aim may be a justification in itself, if no active treatment is possible or acceptable (see Ch. 25).

SURGICAL MANAGEMENT

General considerations

Respiratory function is often limited due to a collapsing spine and/or abdominal muscle paralysis. Careful evaluation is required, both to try to prevent respiratory failure and also in patients being considered for surgical intervention.

In the presence of a neuropathic bladder, intercurrent infection and renal hypertension may complicate surgical treatment; therefore renal function should be fully assessed. The presence of urinary tract diversion may also make bracing difficult and can interfere with any surgical treatment by the anterior approach.

If the child has hydrocephalus the function of the valve must be considered. Treatment of the spine can affect the relative length of the catheter and produce obstruction postoperatively. Excision of the cord may cause acute hydrocephalus.

Spinal fusion is a crude concept: it indicates that the deforming forces are out of control and that the only way of stabilising the situation is to fuse the spine.

The spinal surgeon dealing with these deformities in the physically handicapped should first be experienced in the treatment of idiopathic scoliosis. When surgery is contemplated children are best managed in centres well versed in the competent care of the problems of physical handicap as well as of spinal surgery. The decision to operate should be taken only after careful consideration of all the interrelated factors, and where possible should include a team approach.

Having made the decision to treat a curve operatively, the general condition should be re-evaluated, particularly in relation to cardiovascular, respiratory and renal function. Complications during surgery and the immediate postoperative phase are common, but with careful planning they can be predicted and in most cases avoided. In some instances, minor surgery may prevent serious progression. Attempts to modify spinal growth on one side (usually the convex) have been tried without notable success. These operations to modify spinal growth must be done very early, as half the spinal growth has been achieved by the age of 2½ years. There are situations where these operations are indicated, particularly in congenital curves with a localised area of uneven growth. In such cases, by fusing on the side with normal growth potential the uneven growth can be neutralised.

More extensive fusion procedures must wait for greater spinal growth, or a very short trunk may result. In order to avoid this complication, attempts are being made to use extendable rods. At this stage the problems, both of repeated surgery and biomechanical failure, remain considerable.

Spinal corrective procedures are usually carried out between the ages of 10 and 13, but may have to be performed earlier if control is lost. In neuropathic and myopathic curves, because the deforming force will continue into adult life, the fusion procedures must be based on the principle of achieving a correction that is as straight as possible, and then producing a really strong fusion. This usually involves both anterior and posterior surgery.

The most common and well-tried form of posterior surgery is to use a

Harrington rod to distract the spine and then to fuse the spine posteriorly by excising the posterior joints and laying on graft (Harrington 1962). This technique has been developed to include segmental wiring, or multiple rods as developed in France with the Cotrel–Debusset system. In cases with a significant degree of kyphosis, failure is almost inevitable if posterior fusion alone is carried out, particularly where the spinal deformity is 'collapsing' and is associated with neuropathy or myopathy (Fig. 22.8).

Where the curve is small, but remains easily correctable and is of the collapsing type, the technique described by Luqué in Mexico may be used — two steel rods are laid up either side of the spine and the laminae are wired at each level to the rods. This is a technique that is particularly applicable to the neuropathic collapsing spines such as poliomyelitis and spinal muscular atrophy. The great advantage is that there is no need for postoperative bracing and the child can be sat up immediately.

The alternative is to do both anterior and posterior staged surgery. Initially the spine is approached from the front by a transthoracic, retroperitoneal or combined thoraco-abdominal approach. The spine is exposed and the discs are excised at each level within the curve. Following this the spine may be instrumented by using screws and a cable, a technique developed by Dwyer & Schaffer (1974). This technique has also been improved by using solid rods such as the Zilke or Webb–Morley

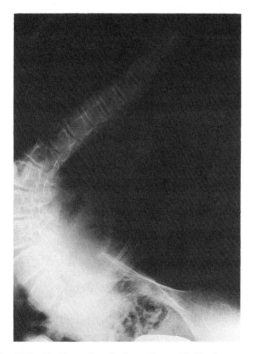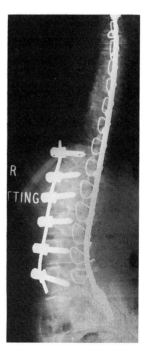

a   b

Fig. 22.8 Radiographs of spine of boy with Duchenne muscular dystrophy before and after anterior and posterior surgery.

(W–M) system. The spine may be left mobile with bone chips inserted, and then put on traction in preparation for a second stage procedure. Anterior instrumentation is indicated if there is an element of lordosis, but is contraindicated if there is kyphosis as this tends to increase the deformity.

If the spine is to be treated by traction, then, at the same time, a halo is applied and fixed to the skull, and traction is applied through this and through pins inserted through the lower tibia. At a second stage the spine is approached posteriorly and is instrumented in the normal way. This method of anterior release, followed by posterior instrumentation and fusion, gives an excellent correction and firm fixation, but remains a very big procedure, and its indications are limited.

The most difficult area to achieve fusion is at the lumbosacral junction. The problem is to achieve firm fixation into the pelvis, where the stresses are high in the postoperative phase. The most successful techniques involve cancellous pedicular screws.

The risks of damage to the spinal cord must always be borne in mind. Preoperative assessment of the spinal cord by myelography is indicated where there is any possibility of cord tethering. During the operation the integrity of the cord can be monitored electrically using a modified electromyogram, or so-called spinal cord monitor.

Despite understandable reticence to operate on mentally and physically handicapped children they tolerate these major procedures very well and are remarkably cooperative. It is very rare for behavioural problems to be a contraindication.

Postoperative treatment

Postoperative treatment is simplified as far as possible. In the immediate postoperative period no form of spinal brace is used, and where possible the child is allowed to get up after a period of 1 week. At the end of this time the child is mobilised either unbraced or wearing a plastic removable brace, which is maintained until fusion is solid. The brace is worn when sitting, except for washing (Fig. 22.9). Solid fusion may require 6–12 months for the treatment of neuropathic deformity.

Great advances continue to be made in the treatment of scoliosis. These techniques can now be particularly applied to the physically handicapped, where surgery has always been daunting because of the severity of the deformity and other associated problems. The rewards of spinal surgery and correction may be even greater in these children than in others, as correction and stabilisation improves function, sometimes dramatically. The future lies in being able to isolate the cause of these curves and hopefully to prevent them. Meanwhile we must rely on early detection and more aggressive conservative measures, always with the aim and hope of avoiding major surgery in children who cannot be expected to cooperate fully in these procedures.

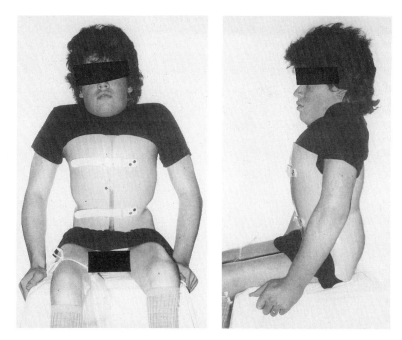

Fig. 22.9   Postoperative bracing following anterior and posterior fusion.

REFERENCES

Blount N P, Moe J H 1973 The Milwaukee brace. Williams and Wilkins, Baltimore
Dubowitz. V 1978 Muscle Disorders in Childhood. W B Saunders, Philadelphia
Dwyer A F, Schaffer M F 1974 Journal of Bone and Joint surgery 56B: 218
Harrington P R 1962 Correction and internal fixation by instrumentation in scoliosis.
   Journal of Bone and Joint Surgery 44A: 591

FURTHER READING

Moe J H, Winter R B, Bradford D S, Lenstein J E 1978 Scoliosis and other spinal
   deformities. W B Saunders, Philadelphia
Nash C C 1980 Scoliosis bracing. Journal of Bone and Joint Surgery 62A: 648
Watts H G 1976 The Boston brace. Children's Hospital Medical Centre, Boston,
   Massachusetts

23. Orthotics

J. Florence

FOOTWEAR AND INSOLES

Wherever possible the physically handicapped child should wear shoes that are similar to those worn by normal children. Ordinary shop-bought shoes can be modified and adapted in numerous ways to accommodate abnormal feet or to attach to orthoses. With modern adhesives the majority of soles can be raised, sockets can be fixed and inserts moulded to fit in the shoes or to reinforce the uppers.

For the less fortunate who cannot be accommodated in normal shoes, there is a range of specially constructed footwear in stock sizes with different width fittings and depths, and these are available on the NHS. Insoles for correction of deformities can be made in a variety of materials today, ranging from man-made plastics to rubber, leather and cork. The expanded polyethylene (Evazote, Plastazote, Texlon) can be purchased in varying densities and used for correction and pressure problems.

The child with grossly abnormal feet will need custom-made surgical footwear to a specially built cast. Care in selection of style of uppers can greatly enhance the appearance. Anaesthetic feet, for example in spina bifida, need to have boots that lace low for easy access so that toes can be straightened out when they are applied. It is far easier for the boots to be made from a plaster of Paris (POP) cast where there is a severe deformity such as equinus.

Non-weightbearing feet may be accommodated in soft boots lined with lambswool, or these can be moulded in expanded polyethylene and covered with stretch plastic or gloving kid. Even when special shoes or boots have to be made, it is possible to copy the style of a standard shoe upper to make the wearing of these more acceptable. Raises to accommodate shortening can be made in cork, microlite or high-density expanded plastic.

ANKLE–FOOT ORTHOSES (AFOs)

These are below-knee bracing for correction of ankle–foot deformities or stabilisation of ankle and foot. They are made of conventional steel or aluminium alloy, and may be either single or double sided.

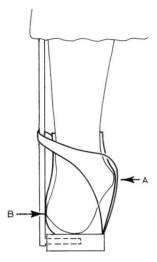

Fig. 23.1   Adapted boot for an AFO (viewed posteriorly). Unless the boot is reinforced at B, the corrective force A will distort the upper, and the foot will turn inside the boot.

Single medial or lateral strut with calfband and round spur.   This is used in conjunction with a T or Y shaped strap for the correction or stabilisation of a varus or valgus condition of the ankle. It is important that shoes should be adapted correctly and reinforced where necessary with inserts, otherwise the foot will turn inside the boot or shoe (Fig. 23.1).

Double medial or lateral struts with calfband and round spurs.   This is used for the same condition as the single AFO. This double AFO can control both varus and valgus, and stabilise the heel of a shoe.

Both single and double AFOs can be used with dorsi-plantar flexion stops, either with round spurs or ankle joints. Toe-raising springs can be fitted either to the AFO ankle joints or attached to the toe of the shoe. Springs should never be used on a spastic limb as this will only antagonise and increase the spasticity. This will not be effective unless the sole of the shoe is reinforced. Better control of the ankle and foot can be achieved by fixing the angle of dorsi-plantar flexion. With the small child or infant, steel AFOs attached to footplates can be used. As the weight of the individual increases, the sole-plates tend to break due to the leverage on the foot-pieces. All conventional steel AFOs rely on the footwear for stability.

With the availability of high density plastics, much better control of ankle–foot deformities can be achieved. Polypropylene is the most adaptable plastic currently in use. A cast is taken of the leg below knee with the child seated and the knee flexed. In this way the orthotist can hold the foot in the correct position controlling varus or valgus and angle of dorsi-flexion and plantarflexion. This cast is removed from the leg and filled with POP to form the positive cast of the limb. Careful rectification of the cast is needed, emphasising any prominences such as the malleoli, and reducing soft tissue areas. Polypropylene is heated to 190°C and can be drape-formed or vacuum-formed over the cast. This should be left on the

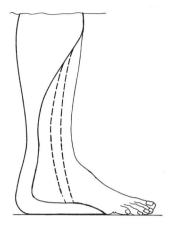

Fig. 23.2 Shell orthosis showing how it can be trimmed to either eliminate or allow dorsiflexion or plantarflexion.

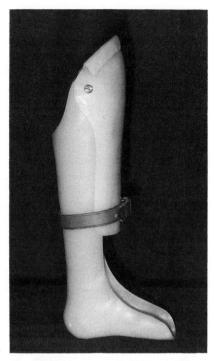

Fig. 23.3 Patellar tendon bearing AFO.

cast for 12 hours before removing. The trim-line can be varied either to eliminate ankle–foot movement or to allow dorsiflexion and plantarflexion (Fig. 23.2).

The fixed ankle AFO is used extensively for a low spina bifida lesion (below S1–2) where there are no active plantarflexors. The child is unable to stand still and dorsiflexion gives rise to knee flexion. Accurate positioning of the feet can enable the child to stand still and can influence knee control. This fixed ankle orthosis is also useful for spastic hemiplegia and quadriplegia, and muscle disorders, and can be worn both day and night. However, reaction to a rigid splint may be more difficult with spastic children, and spasm may produce more problems with pressure sores.

A modification of the polypropylene AFO is the patellar tendon bearing orthosis (Fig. 23.3). This can be used in two ways:

1. A reinforcement to the standard AFO which gives both stronger anterior support and can extend to take a bearing on the femoral condyles. This is particularly useful for the heavier child with a lower spina bifida lesion, to help control genu valgum.

2. A suspension orthosis for relief of weight from the tibia or fibula or for relieving pressure from the plantar surface of the foot has been used very successfully in the treatment of ulcers under the heels of children with vertical talus and absence of plantarflexors.

Contraindications for the use of polypropylene AFOs are oedema and severe spasticity.

KNEE–ANKLE–FOOT ORTHOSES (KAFOs)

KAFOs (Fig. 23.4) are above-knee bracing for correction of knee–ankle–foot deformities or stabilisation of knee, ankle and foot. KAFOs are an extension to the thigh of AFOs, the ankle and foot being controlled as described with AFOs. Knee deformities may be flexion, recurvatum, varus and valgus. With conventional steel or aluminium alloy construction these are corrected with slings at the knee using the medial lateral struts for correction.

Knee joints may be fitted and can be used to allow flexion, but resist hyperextension or lock at 180° to eliminate movement when weightbearing, unlocking to allow the child to sit with the knees flexed. These locking joints can be either locked or unlocked by hand or can be spring-loaded to lock automatically when the leg is straightened. All knee locks are difficult to operate under load and where flexion spasm is present. It is almost impossible for the child to operate knee locks. A useful aid to make this easier has been designed by the Rehabilitation Engineering Unit at Chailey. This is a boss added below the ring of a standard ring-catch joint. It works on a

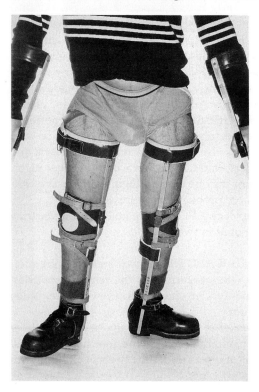

Fig. 23.4   KAFOs.

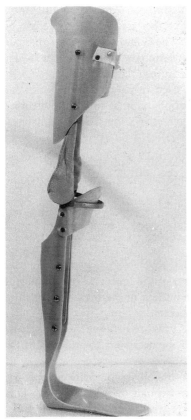

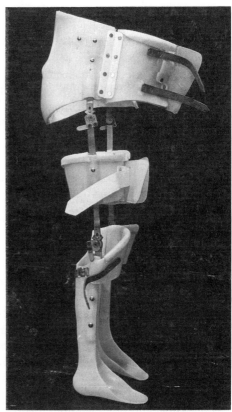

Fig. 23.5 Polypropylene KAFO with cantilever knee lock.

Fig. 23.6 Polypropylene TLSO and KAFOs.

cantilever principle (Fig. 23.5) and can be used on each individual joint or can be connected by an anterior bar to operate both joints in unison. It is useful for children with weak hands, for example those with muscular dystrophy or arthrogryposis.

If recurvatum control only is needed, it may be possible to have an extension to the thigh on the lateral side only with a free joint allowing flexion, but resisting hyperextension by stopping the joint at 10° of flexion. This is particularly useful for children with spina bifida at the level of L4–5 where the quadriceps are active and the hamstrings weak.

Steel or aluminium constructions are heavy and, apart from mass production of joints facilitating speedier construction, little has been done to improve the design, which has not changed for over 100 years. In the late 1960s experiments were carried out using high density plastics for shell construction and carbon fibre to replace steel or alloy side-members. One significant factor to emerge from this research was that half the weight of a conventional KAFO was leather! Replacing side members with lightweight materials did not alter the weight of the complete orthosis significantly. Considerable advances have been made over the last decade in the use of high density plastics for shell construction. The Stanmore cosmetic caliper highlighted the use of high density polyethylene (Ortholen) (Tuck 1971), and polypropylene vacuum-formed shell orthoses (Yates 1971).

Polypropylene shell KAFOs are widely used in paediatric orthotics for poliomyelitis, spina bifida, muscular dystrophy, spinal muscular atrophy and arthrogryposis. Some of the advantages over conventional construction are listed below:

- Lightweight
- Easy to take off and put on (doff and don)
- Speedy construction
- Easy to adjust
- Long lasting
- Normal footwear can be worn
- Cosmetically more acceptable.

Skill is required in taking an accurate cast of the limb and techniques of rectification of the positive cast and the moulding of the orthoses are time consuming, but the end result is so much better.

Contraindications for the use of shell KAFOs are oedema, severe spasticity, and gross deformity of the knee. It may be necessary to attach KAFOs to some form of body orthosis (Fig. 23.6).

Reciprocal gait is difficult and almost impossible in complete paraplegia. The only method of ambulation is swing-through or jump-to gait. This involves high energy consumption and consequently nearly all children requiring stability at this level become wheelchair-bound when they reach adolescence. Strong shoulders and arms are required for this method of ambulation (see Fig. 12.10).

The same orthoses with thoracic and pelvic bands are used as standing frames for muscular dystrophy and spinal muscular atrophy, but ambulation is not possible. Recent advances in design of the hip joints and rigid thoracolumbar bracing have made reciprocal gait more possible (Rose & Stallard 1979). Polypropylene can be used as the thoracolumbar brace and attached to KAFOs with hip joints. This reduces the weight of the orthoses, but does nothing to improve the problem of high-energy-consumption ambulation.

Reciprocal gait has been the subject of considerable discussion over recent years with a design of orthoses from the USA utilising Bowden Wire cables. The lower limbs are connected at hip joint level to thoracolumbar orthoses with hip joints allowing flexion and extension. A cable system is incorporated connecting the lower limbs on a parallelogram system. It should be clearly understood that this system does not have any external power source: the power still has to come from the patient. This parallelogram system was in use at Chailey Heritage from 1969–1974 without any significant success. A rigid TLSO with strong side members, and hip joints allowing 10° flexion and extension with built-in thrust races on the articulating surfaces has proved to be successful in many cases where reciprocal gait is considered to be appropriate. The rigid TLSO and side members hold the limbs in abduction, which will prevent the legs from impinging on each other when walking (Fig. 23.7). To achieve ambulation in high levels of paraplegia where bracing is necessary, strong arms, shoulders and latissimus dorsi are required.

a

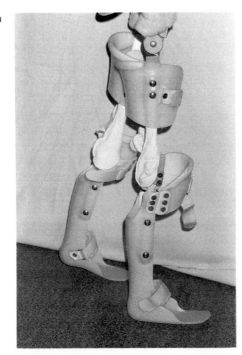

Fig. 23.7 a and b. Reciprocal gait orthosis for a child with a high spina bifida lesion. Note the hip and knee locks.

b

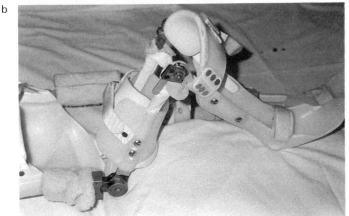

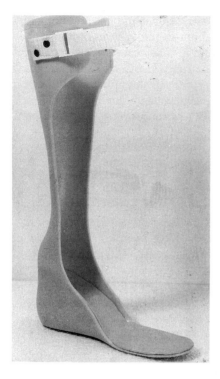

Fig. 23.8 Equinus deformity accommodated in an AFO.

EXTENSION PROSTHESES

Extension prostheses are widely used in paediatric orthotics for congenital limb deficiency, as compensation for shortening, and as an aid to diminutive height.

Ultra-lightweight construction using polypropylene has led to a higher acceptability of extensions for limb deficiency. Joints at knee level facilitate sitting and can be added to enable patients to use public transport.

Compensation for shortening can be made more cosmetically acceptable. Equinus deformity of feet can be used to good effect to replace unsightly block raises on surgical footwear (Fig. 23.8). Extensions can be incorporated in AFOs and KAFOs to accommodate shortening from as little as 1 cm to a gross shortening of 20 cm or more. In many cases this will enable children with one normal limb and one disabled limb to wear ordinary footwear (Fig. 23.9). Feet that have resisted cooperative correction, as is frequently the case with arthrogryposis during growth, can be accommodated comfortably and cosmetically in bilateral extensions attached to KAFOs or AFOs. These can also be used as an aid to diminutive height.

The child with achondroplasia, although able to walk on his feet, has many disadvantages as compared with people of normal height. Inability to reach normal-height electrical fittings, water taps, shelves and even door

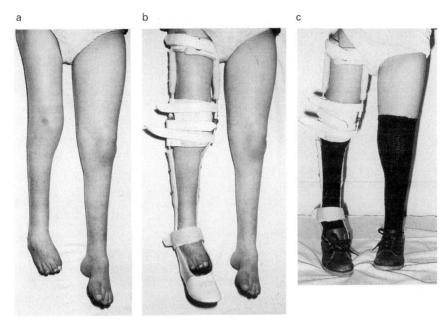

Fig. 23.9 a, b and c. Extension orthosis incorporated in KAFO accommodating a short leg to match the normal leg.

handles restricts the activities of daily living in the normal community. Short limbs also mean short length of step and the child is consequently slow in ambulation. Bilateral extensions can both enhance appearance and provide a better chance of acceptance in the community.

THORACO-LUMBO-SACRAL ORTHOSES (TLSO) AND CERVICAL THORACO-LUMBAR ORTHOSES

With the advance in moulding thermoplastics conventional steel spinal orthoses are rarely used in paediatric orthotics. Accurate casting techniques and correct postural seating methods have led to a better, understanding of the correction of the spinal deformities.

The spinal orthosis invariably used is the total contact moulded plastic TLSO. Polythene or polypropylene can be used, although the former in lower density will need reinforcing for stability. The orthosis is the same for all thoracic and thoracolumbar support. Cast rectification and trimlines will vary depending on whether the child is ambulant or chairbound. The aim is always to achieve the maximum tolerable degree of correction, and comparison of radiographs is needed so that the orthotist can see what the orthosis is achieving.

The spine extends from the pelvis, and therefore it is important with all spinal orthoses to have a firm grip on the pelvic structure, otherwise it is like a house without a foundation. Bearing this in mind, the lower edge

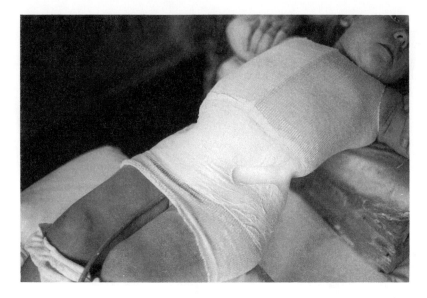

Fig. 23.10 Casting a TLSO. Note the emphasised anterior superior iliac spines.

must extend below the anterior superior iliac spines anteriorly, fit close to the greater trochanters laterally and extend to the level of the coccyx posteriorly. The upper limits will depend on the extent of the spinal abnormality.

The best method of casting for the majority of conditions is to lay the patient supine on two blocks, the shoulders resting on one and the seat on the other. By varying the angle of hip and knee flexion, the amount of lordosis can be accurately controlled. The cast should be started round the pelvis at trochanter level and extended to the waist. As this sets, a firm grip over the iliac crests should be maintained, emphasising the anterior superior iliac spines (Fig. 23.10). The cast can then be extended up to axilla level, correcting any scoliosis manually as the bandages are applied.

If there is a gross degree of lateral pelvic obliquity with a compensating scoliosis, it may be necessary to extend the TLSO to rest on the chair seat to give more stability. Casting by this method will give a clear indication of the limits required. Casting supine has advantages over casting under traction:

- The maximum degree of tolerable correction can be achieved
- The rectification of the positive cast is assisted as the abdomen flattens naturally
- It is more comfortable for the patient
- Seating posture can be checked before removal of the cast
- Where there is poor muscle tone, as in muscular dystrophy and spinal muscular atrophy, traction is incompatible with casting an orthosis.

The negative cast should be sealed immediately after removal to avoid distortion. The positive cast needs careful rectification, which should be supervised by the orthotist. The trim-line of the orthosis should be marked clearly on the cast. In the case of Duchenne muscular dystrophy it is wise to fit a TLSO as soon as the child becomes non-ambulant. Experience has shown that if a good lumbar lordotic posture can be maintained this will prevent lateral pelvic obliquity and discourage the onset of scoliosis. The first TLSO need therefore only be extended to mid-thoracic level. Lumbar kyphosis must be avoided as this results in unacceptable pressure over the thighs and makes the wearing of a TLSO impossible. The higher the curve, the higher the orthosis must be carried. It is important to note that axillary pressure for spinal distraction is rarely, if ever, acceptable. There is no point in carrying the support high above the apex of the curve (see Ch. 22).

The more complex the shape, the more difficult it will be to spring open, and a hinge may be necessary. Where a hinge is added, the cast is examined to find the flattest area to place the hinge, as it will only work in one plane. A low density lining is first moulded, and a flat area created to place the hinge (Fig. 23.11).

Where there is a high cervical thoracic curve, or where head support is needed, the orthosis will need to be extended to chin and occiput. This can be achieved either by a standard Milwaukee brace, or by moulding a plastic extension (Fig. 23.12). The principle of the Milwaukee brace is one of self-traction: the patient must be able to lift his head away from the neck ring. Where there is muscle weakness in the neck, the TLSO should be carried high to make this possible. In some cases of spinal muscular atrophy or

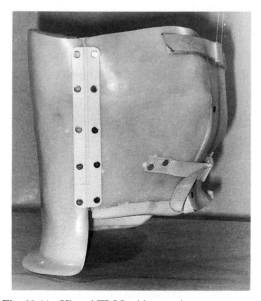

Fig. 23.11 Hinged TLSO with extension to rest on seat.

a 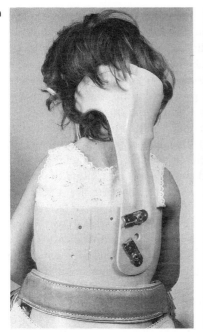 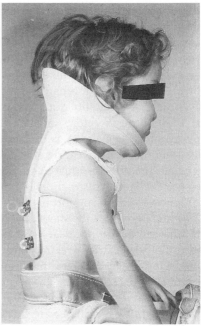 b

Fig. 23.12 a and b.   TLSO with a specially designed neck piece to correct head tilt.

congenital muscular dystrophy, the head piece may not need to be worn continually or may only need to support posteriorly. This can be made detachable and need only be worn when necessary .

No matter how careful the orthotist may be, some scoliosis will progress, and, with rotation, gross rib abnormality may occur, which will make the wearing of a plastic orthosis impossible. In these cases moulded leather is the best alternative as it is more tolerable to wear. The disadvantages are mainly hygienic as it is not possible to clean and will absorb perspiration. Plastic orthoses can be perforated for ventilation. It is important not to perforate in areas that are taking the most pressure, as sores may develop. The perforations should be not less than 6 mm in diameter and not more than 9 mm. Plastic TLSOs may be lined with low density expanded polyethylene, but wherever possible this should be avoided as this makes the orthosis very hot to wear.

REFERENCES

Rose G, Stallard J 1979 The principles and practice of hip guidance articulation. Journal of Prosthetics and Orthotics International 3: 37–43
Tuck W H 1971 Recent advances: 2. Lower extremity. In: Murdoch G (ed) The advance in orthotics. Edward Arnold, London, pp. 187–193
Yates G 1971 Recent advance: 3. Modular orthotic systems. A modular system of exoskeleton bracing. In: Murdoch G (ed) The advance in orthotics. Edward Arnold, London, pp. 211–217

24. Rehabilitation engineering including microelectronic and computer technology

R.L. Nelham   A. Brown   C. Thornett

INTRODUCTION

Rehabilitation engineering is defined as the appropriate clinical application of engineering principles together with existing and emerging technologies in collaboration with the physical and life sciences to restore or elevate a person to an optimal level of physical, mental and social function, and wellbeing. As there are many different definitions of rehabilitation, so there will be different definitions of rehabilitation engineering. This one illustrates the broadest of applications of engineering to the generally accepted principles of rehabilitation.

Engineering has been applied to the process of rehabilitation for many years. In 1976 in the USA the application of engineering to solve problems in rehabilitation was recognised as rehabilitation engineering. In 1978 the US government funded the establishment of 10 rehabilitation engineering centres across the USA.

In the UK similar applications of engineering had been taking place under different titles in established centres, including Chailey Heritage, since the early 1960s. Many other establishments now provide rehabilitation engineering services under a range of titles including bioengineering, clinical engineering, medical engineering, medical physics and disablement services as well as rehabilitation engineering. There are in fact at least 17 different titles by which an engineer or technician may be employed in providing these services.

THE ROLE OF THE REHABILITATION ENGINEER

The successful practice of rehabilitation engineering involves an interdependent multidisciplinary team effort by a number of people of different disciplines including engineering. The rehabilitation engineer is part of the clinical team concerned with the rehabilitation process and it is essential that the engineer is involved at the earliest possible stage, which is usually assessment As well as providing an engineering perspective on the process of assessment and problem identification, the engineer learns from his other colleagues about the implications of various approaches and the aims and objectives that each team member is attempting to identify for each particular child. The engineer will thereby be aware of the significance of the engineering input in relation to achieving these rehabilitation goals and the fact that time scales are all important in the delivery of the service.

Traditionally engineers work from a specification of the problem to be solved and the performance to be attained within the solution. This principle applies as much to the field of rehabilitation as it does to other engineering problems but the process is perhaps subject to a greater degree of modification through the intimate involvement of the individual child. In general it is not often possible to derive a specification and the engineer has to identify from the medical and paramedical objectives the precise nature of the rehabilitation engineering input required. The rehabilitation engineer's colleagues will also need to be made aware of the various engineering options that are available in order that a compromise may be reached. There is rarely a well defined, single solution to a problem and reaching a compromise is perhaps the most difficult aspect of the assessment process with regard to the provision of rehabilitation engineering.

For this process to be successful it is essential that the rehabilitation engineer is able to communicate with colleagues in other disciplines and is also able to understand the influence and implications of the engineering input to the overall rehabilitation process. This will apply at all levels of technology from the simplest aid to daily living to more complex postural control equipment and microcomputer and microelectronic applications to communication, mobility and environmental control.

THE REHABILITATION ENGINEERING PROCESS

It may be helpful to understand the stages by which a rehabilitation engineering service is provided to solve a particular problem. These will vary according to the specific problem but are generally as follows:

- Carry out an assessment of the child with other members of the clinic team and parents as appropriate to identify the problem or problems required to be solved
- Discuss various solutions in order to reach a compromise acceptable to all concerned
- Derive a specification from the agreed compromise
- Identify the particular commercially available item or service required to meet the specification
- Design the particular device according to the specification (if not commercially available)
- Develop the one-off item of equipment
- Reconvene the original assessment team to carry out trial fitting and use
- Finalise the production of the item
- Instruct all who need to know in the use of the item
- Ensure that the performance of the device comes up to expectations and record baseline data for future monitoring of progress or otherwise

- Identify potential for wider application and, if appropriate:
  — Design for production
  — Evaluate production prototypes
  — Proceed to manufacture using subcontract companies as appropriate
  — Market the product as widely as possible.

It will be apparent from the above that until some of these stages have been completed, the child and those who are treating him will be unable to progress in the rehabilitation programme that has been planned and which may be dependent upon the piece of equipment concerned. Accordingly, formal engineering design and development procedures will not very often be possible and the skill of the rehabilitation engineer is in the balancing of performance, safety, aesthetics and cost for what might be a one-off piece of equipment for relatively short duration use. There are times when it is essential to carry out the formal engineering procedures in order to produce the most effective device at the lowest cost for a large number of children but this will not become apparent until the later stages of the above procedure.

The above procedure outlined for the rehabilitation engineering process will serve to identify gaps in knowledge There may be insufficient information to derive a solution to a problem, or the solution that can be derived requires a great deal of further investigation to optimise the design for efficient use and function. These are just two examples by which research projects can be identified and it is the rehabilitation engineer's responsibility to undertake the planning of research projects and to obtain the funding for these to pursue the improvement of rehabilitation engineering knowledge, equipment and services. The paramedical nature of rehabilitation will necessitate close cooperation between rehabilitation engineering, medical and paramedical disciplines in both the planning and execution of the research projects as well as the delivery of the service.

Examples of the areas of activity, services provided and subjects of research undertaken by departments of rehabilitation engineering are as follows:

— Wheelchairs and special vehicles including controls
— Specialised prosthetics
— Specialised orthotics
— Seating
— Communication systems for the speech and language impaired
— Environmental control
— Functional electrical stimulation.
— Assistive devices for all activities of daily living in domestic, educational, vocational, recreational, social and institutional environments
— Gait analysis
— Applications of computer aided design and manufacture
— Research, design, development, production and marketing.

Rehabilitation involves various levels of therapeutic input from the initial, highly intensive therapy to monitoring and reviewing progress. Whatever the level of input required the child is unlikely to obtain the ideal amount of time from the relevant therapists concerned with the current programme. Accordingly all concerned with the management of the child should be carrying over the therapy aims and objectives in the daily activities. It is therefore essential that rehabilitation engineering services, particularly the equipment for daily living, also carry over the techniques and philosophy that the therapists are implementing. In this way, maximum benefit can be derived from therapy and a fully integrated service of rehabilitation engineering can be provided. This again serves to emphasise the need for rehabilitation engineers and the paramedical staff to work as closely as possible in the delivery of the rehabilitation engineering service. Chapter 25 further demonstrates the need for this.

The publication *Assistive devices* provides the reader with information on a large number of assistive devices or aids to daily living together with a brief description of research projects carried out in the rehabilitation engineering unit and publications produced. This is available free of charge from the Rehabilitation Engineering Unit, Chailey Heritage.

DISABILITY RELATED PROBLEMS

Each child is an individual and each problem to be solved requires a somewhat individual approach but the following generalisation may be of assistance.

Cerebral palsy

Over 70% of children who require the services of the Rehabilitation Engineering Unit at Chailey Heritage have one or more forms of cerebral palsy. The more able of these children may require specialised walking aids to overcome difficulties experienced with the commercially available devices, and some require individually designed aids to improve functional ability in the classroom or in daily living activities. Adapted cutlery and specially designed feeding aids are examples of such equipment. The children who need to use a wheelchair will always need special attention to their seating requirements, and the seating components that they require—from the simplest to the most complex systems—will need to follow the biomechanical principles described in Chapter 25. Such equipment can play a significant part in encouraging development of ability but, if wrongly provided, can impede this development. Microelectronic equipment to enable participation in educational programmes to permit communication and environmental control may also be required and will need to be operated by special designs of switches. The same switches may be used for the control of powered wheelchairs for those who need them. For those with a reasonable degree of hand function, the powered wheelchair controls need to be accurately sited and symmetry of posture maintained during mobility.

Arthrogryposis

Modified cutlery and aids to dressing and personal toilet are the main requirements of this group. Sometimes these children can manage with commercially available equipment, but purpose-made designs are often needed to overcome the particular difficulties that each child experiences. Assistance with mobility may also be required, particularly in the design of special crutches for instance to overcome a child's inability to grip.

Spina bifida

A major problem experienced by children with spina bifida and which requires the input of rehabilitation engineering is in tissue trauma prevention and management. Special cushions and, sometimes, backrests are required to offload pressure from vulnerable parts of the body to more tolerant areas. Incontinence can also be a problem requiring rehabilitation engineering intervention by way of specially designed or modified urine collection devices and the materials they are made from.

Muscular dystrophy

Orthotic intervention at the early stages of this condition will maintain boys with muscular dystrophy on their feet for as long as possible. Rehabilitation engineering may provide an input to the design of these special orthoses and later with standing frames as appropriate. More intensive involvement will arise as the boys come off their feet and become wheelchair dependent. Spinal jackets should be provided at this stage if not already worn, and integrated with special seating. The need for special seating will increase as the disability progresses. Although the biomechanical principles described in Chapter 25 will be applicable here, the boys themselves are the main guide in the provision of appropriate equipment. The objective is to maintain function, comfort and head control for as long as possible.

MICROELECTRONIC AND COMPUTER TECHNOLOGY

The microelectronic and computer revolution of recent times has made as much impact on rehabilitation engineering as it has on the other professions and on daily life in general. It has been responsible for a dramatic real and potential improvement in the capabilities and expectations of physically disabled people of all ages. Even severely multiply handicapped individuals can now be offered the prospect of useful and gainful employment on an equal footing with the able-bodied workforce in an increasingly technology-dependent society. Educational prospects need no longer be limited, and the previously insurmountable barriers—to communication, self-expression, independent mobility and intellectual development—that confronted multiply handicapped people such as those with cerebral palsy are rapidly being demolished.

It is one of the tasks of the rehabilitation engineer to ensure that optimal access to the 'new technology' in all aspects of daily living can be made available to the disabled user, and that full use is made of all residual physical and intellectual abilities in the rehabilitation process.

Microcomputer technology has made it economically possible to compensate reliably and effectively for highly specific individual disabilities. Equipment design allows an aid to be tailored to the exact needs and abilities of the user. It also allows flexibility to accommodate changing progressive or regressive conditions. In addition, the rehabilitation engineer has been provided with a wide range of tools for the effective assessment of aids and users, design of equipment, monitoring of physical and physiological characteristics and user and equipment performance. Illustrated below are some of the specific contributions of this technology to the rehabilitation engineering process.

Powered independent mobility

Children normally acquire the ability to move independently within the first 2 years of life, and subsequent development—both intellectual and physical—is being shown to be highly dependent upon this early achievement and experience. If a physically handicapped child can be assisted to master a means of exploring his environment at a comparable age, perhaps with appropriate technological assistance, then his chances of attaining independence in other spheres such as communication, feeding and education can be considerably enhanced. The technology is now available to make this possible, and it is one of the tasks of the rehabilitation engineer to ensure that this can be provided.

There are some children who are unlikely ever to achieve mobility without technological assistance, and it is often the case that they are offered powered mobility only as a last resort. A physically handicapped child who has failed to walk with or without walking aids will have had little opportunity to experience any sort of active play alone. Eventually a powered wheelchair may be suggested, but this may happen after years of failure and frustration with the attendant destruction of morale and motivation. This will make success in independent powered mobility much more difficult to attain. Almost always the powered wheelchair will have a conventional joystick control and for a child with limited hand function, various techniques may be tried to allow some control over the powered chair. The position of the control box and thus the integral joystick may be adjusted, or the shape of the control knob modified. Often all of these attempts achieve limited success and by this time the child may be in his teens without having experienced any real achievement.

Current developments

A series of research projects at Chailey Heritage, funded by the Spastics Society, has achieved considerable success in meeting the needs of the young people described above. Multiply handicapped children and young adults, identified nationwide, were referred to the projects when their needs could not be met from established channels for the supply of a wheelchair control system or computer switches. The projects were able to provide special switch systems, software and technical support to meet individual requirements.

A switch bank consisting of a wide range of special switches was developed (Fig 24.1). Many of these were multipurpose switches, which could be used with a variety of electronic assistive equipment such as communication aids and computers as well as powered chairs.

The switch systems are worn on the body rather than mounted on a tray or wheelchair. The former method is chosen in the majority of cases because the switch system can move with the person and does not require frequent adjustment as the seating position changes.

Some of the special switch systems produced are described below.

Necklace switch system. Switches in the form of beads are mounted on a thin collar, which is worn around the neck (Fig. 24.2). The diameter of the beads can be chosen from a range to suit the user.

Chin switch system. Up to four chin operated switches are mounted on

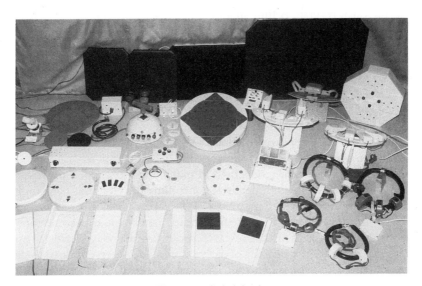

Fig. 24.1 Switch bank.

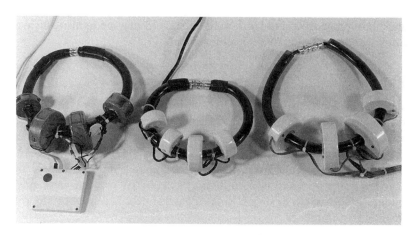

Fig.24.2 Necklace switch system.

an arc supported by a chestplate (Fig. 24.3). The switch system is attached to the user by a leather strap. The chestplate rests on the chest with the ends of the arc lightly resting on the shoulders to provide stability to the switch system. The switches are worn on the body to ensure that they move with the person and are highly adjustable to accommodate the user's ever changing needs. The switches can be adjusted to any position around the arc and may be moved inwards, further under the chin or further away as required. The arc can be raised or lowered on a screw adjustment.

The young boy in Figure 24.4 was provided with a set of four chin switches for wheelchair driving and computer use. When driving a powered chair, each switch corresponds to one of the four directions—left, right, forward, reverse. A fifth small on/off toggle switch is on the left side of the arc. This is normally added to the switch system when the user becomes a confident driver. The toggle switch allows the boy to deactivate the switches so that he can drive himself into his classroom or school hall and then relax without fear of accidently hitting one of the switches. It may also be used to switch between wheelchair driving and, for example, control of a communication aid or an infra-red link to a variety of devices.

A simple infra-red link used with a computer avoids the need to unplug the switches from the powered chair. The on/off switch is then used as a changeover switch between wheelchair driving and computer use.

Children of all ages have benefited in many areas as a result of powered mobility when a satisfactory means of controlling the chair has been found.

The provision of powered mobility to very young physically handicapped children at the same age as their able-bodied peers would become mobile has been the subject of further research projects at Chailey Heritage. Elsewhere research into the benefits of early mobility has been confined to children who are able to operate a conventional joystick control (Butler 1986). Previous research projects at Chailey Heritage have indicated that success-

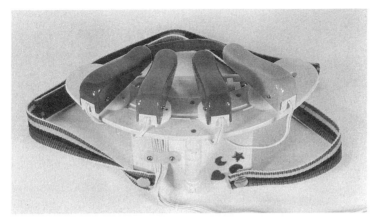

Fig. 24.3 Chin switch system.

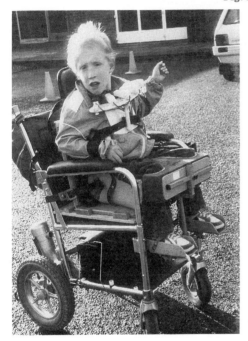

Fig. 24.4 Control of fast outdoor powered chair through use of chin switches.

ful switch use at a young age provides benefits in many areas of development, particularly for severely multiply handicapped children with minimal useful hand function. A similar range of switches of a size appropriate to the very young child has been designed and produced as part of the early mobility project and forms part of the switch bank. Young children learn by exploring their environment and frequently are highly motivated to find out for themselves 'what's going on'.

A small powered platform has been constructed. It is possible to mount a wide variety of seating systems on the platform to enable a child to

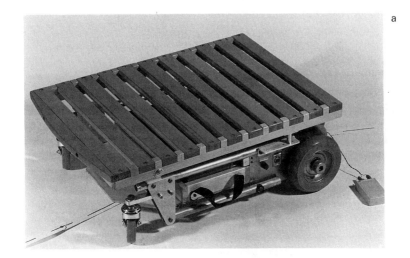

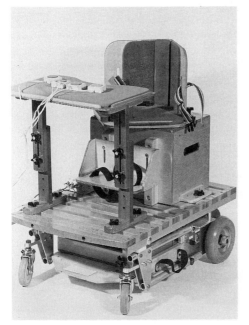

Fig. 24.5 a and b. Powered platform to allow young children in a variety of seating systems to experiment with powered mobility.

experiment with powered mobility from within his or her existing seating system (Fig. 24.5). Appropriate controls—usually small, highly adjustable switch systems—are provided from the switch bank. Some intelligence is being built into the platform so that the degree of control given to the child can be increased as the child becomes more proficient. Track following, where the child operates a single switch to enable the platform or a wheelchair to follow automatically the route of a wire stuck to the floor, can be used as an introduction to mobility or as an aid to meaningful and safe

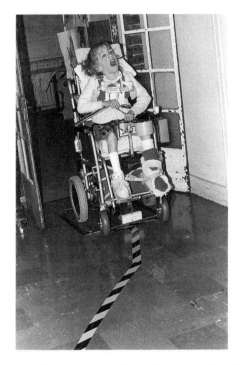

Fig. 24.6   Child with visual handicap using powered wheelchair with track-following system.

mobility for the blind physically handicapped (Fig. 24.6). For 4–5-year-olds, powered chairs (supplied by Disablement Services Centres & wheelchair services) can be used with the special switches or other control systems provided by the project. Powered mobility for this group of children is discussed in more detail in the section on powered chairs.

Communication

A communication problem is frequently only one of a number of interrelated and interacting difficulties experienced by a multiply handicapped individual throughout life. For the person with a nonprogressive but changing disability such as cerebral palsy there can never be a single and final solution to his communication or other needs. There is a continual requirement for the assessment, prescription, training, follow-up and reassessment throughout all aspects of development, education and guidance along the path towards independence, and a fruitful and fulfilling adult life.

This process can often only progress successfully in an environment where all the physical, emotional and intellectual needs and changing conditions are continuously monitored and served. In particular, since the problems and factors influencing them are so diverse, it is usually essential for this process to be carried out in a multidisciplinary environment where medical, paramedical and educational professionals work together in consultation with each other, and with the child, parents and carers making compromises where necessary to ensure the optimal solution. It is also vital that the child and parents accept the device and understand the need for it, and so should be included fully in the decision-making process if success is to be achieved.

Adequate follow-up and effective training of the carers and staff involved with the client, in all aspects of the disability and the solutions applied to relieve it, are also necessary. It is an unhappy fact that poor provision of medical, educational and social resources seldom allows this to be practised effectively, and the situation is likely to get worse with the integration of the physically disabled population into the community and mainstream education.

In the context of communication, the contribution of the rehabilitation engineer or rehabilitation engineering technician covers an extremely broad field. Although he could be, and often is, involved in the design and construction of a particular aid, a major contribution should be in ensuring that any aid can be operated reliably by the user, and that it should offer a significant functional enhancement of his residual communicative ability. In particular, communication using the aid should be faster than the user's existing communication rate, be more reliable than using his existing method, or allow him to communicate on a different level from the one on which he normally operates. Essential factors governing the ultimate acceptance of a communication aid are therefore: (a) an effective matching of the aid to the user's physical and intellectual capabilities; (b) the provision of an appropriate mounting and a reliable physical input device and selection strategy; and (c) adequate training of the user and his helpers in the setting up, use and maintenance of the device.

Communication encompasses not only speech but other media and should be examined in a much wider context. Modes of expression and creativity such as the written word, music and art are now heavily influenced by recent developments in microelectronics and computer technology. Disabled people who are already heavily dependent on this technology in their normal lives are able to make as much use of this progress as are the able-bodied, and note should be taken of this in the design and provision of electronic communication aids.

Conversation, writing and computer access are the three basic requirements of a general purpose communication aid. A number of distinct modes of output need to be incorporated:

1. Synthetic speech output (ideally with a user's characteristic 'voice').
2. Visual display for messages that are only temporary, and for which there is no requirement for hard copy.
3. Hard-copy printed output when used as a writing aid.
4. Computer-compatible electronic communication channel to allow access to general purpose information technology equipment and digital electronic communication over telephone lines.

SWITCH ASSESSMENT

It is essential that the user of a communication aid or other electronic assistive device be provided with a means of controlling it efficiently. It is therefore necessary to assess the user's physical capabilities in operating any switches or other transducers available, preferably in isolation from the aid in the first instance. This is to ensure that the user's ability to use the switches can be monitored free from any intellectual burden which could be imposed in mastering the aid itself. This is often effectively achieved using a computer running some motivational switch-operated program, or by means of simple switch-controlled toys that provide immediate feedback and require minimal intellectual involvement. More elaborate computer programs can allow the automatic monitoring of switch use by the client during this process, and so furnish the assessor with useful information on the appropriate choice and mounting of user switches.

The number and reliability of all controllable anatomical sites on the individual should be investigated, and the most suitable of these selected for further tests to determine the most appropriate type and placement of a switch or other transducer system, and the electrical and mechanical characteristics necessary for ensuring an optimal match between the user and the aid. Although readily available switches should be investigated in the first instance, it is frequently necessary for switches to be specially constructed, modified or mounted in some unusual way to ensure reliable operation. Since the physical capabilities of the user may vary over a period of time, it is essential that any switch design takes this into account so that future changes can be accommodated, either automatically or by means of a relatively simple setting up procedure.

There is a wide variety of special switches available to enable physically disabled people to have access to assistive equipment. In addition to hand-operated mechanical or touch switches, there are eye-blink switches, eye-movement switches, long-range head-mounted light pens, head, chin and foot switches, proximity switches, breath switches (operated by blowing or sucking on a tube), myoelectric devices and many other transducers. A publication describing many of these devices is available from the Aids to Communication in Education Centre (ACE Centre 1989). With some disabilities the interface between the person and the equipment will depend on those actions that remain under voluntary control. However, for severely physically disabled children with cerebral palsy, there may be involvement of all limbs and few, if any, wholly reliable control sites.

Once appropriate switches have been selected and provided, care should also be taken to ensure that adequate training is given to the user as well as all helpers, teachers or other staff concerned, in the use and setting up of the equipment and switches. Adequate follow-up should also be provided to prevent the rejection of the aid or input controls by the user as a result of some trivial fault or incorrect setting-up procedure. Particularly important is regular cleaning, adjustment and checking of equipment to prevent problems caused by the spillage of food, drink or saliva, which can cause malfunctioning of electronic equipment.

The widespread introduction of microcomputers into special schools has provided considerable impetus to switch design and the development of switch assessment strategies. Assistive equipment such as a microcomputer or an environmental control system may be controlled adequately with a single switch. However, the identification of a reliable movement for the operation of a single switch has significant limitations when a severely handicapped young person also requires independent mobility. Additional interfacing circuitry will be necessary if a single switch is to be used to control a powered chair. The solution most frequently adopted is to design a scanning controller (Fig. 24.7 a–c) in which each direction of movement is scanned at a pre-selected rate and the operation of the switch halts the scanning and selects the direction of movement for as long as the switch remains activated.

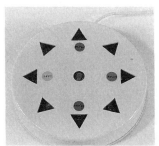

Fig. 24.7 a, b, and c. Scanning wheelchair controllers.

a

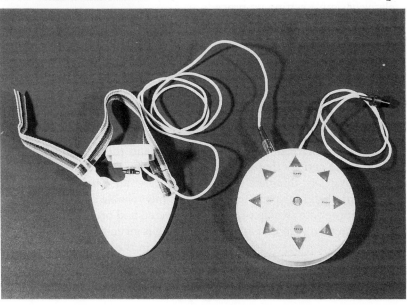

b

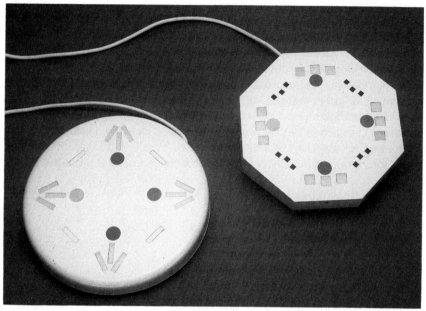

c

Scanning controllers are desperately slow when compared with conventional joystick operation, and to manoeuvre a powered chair by this means requires considerable skill. The anticipatory nature of any form of scanning which is not directly controlled by the user can be very tiring. Experience has shown that inability to comprehend a scanning system does not mean that the person will be unable to achieve independent powered mobility.

Switch system design for the multiply handicapped

The response of multiply handicapped young people to powered wheelchair driving has proved particularly interesting. The desire to move to a position where more is happening, or to seek a familiar person, appears to be present even in the profoundly mentally handicapped. Thus a pertinent factor in the design of a wheelchair control system must be the intellectual ability required to operate the switch system. It is essential that this is appropriate to the child's developmental level. For example, a system which requires the user to look in the direction in which he or she wishes to go and to lower the head onto an appropriately positioned chin-operated switch does not require an understanding of the concepts of direction in terms of left/right and forward/reverse. The physical movement of a switch cover under pressure, and the click resulting from the mechanical activation of a microswitch beneath, provide feedback that appears to be essential.

NHS supplied wheelchairs: range and limitations

In the UK powered wheelchairs are provided through District wheelchair services and Disablement Services Centres (DSCs). All currently supplied powered wheelchairs are intended for use indoors, in the school playground, or in the garden. An attendant-operated power-assisted wheelchair can be prescribed for indoor or outdoor use where the attendant is not strong enough to push a standard manual chair or the district is hilly.

A limited selection of DSC-supplied powered chairs will accommodate a wide range of physical disability when used in conjunction with a wheelchair insert or seating system. There has been some standardisation of control boxes in recent years, and the Penny and Giles proportional controller with integral or remote joystick (i.e. the joystick is connected by a length of cable to the control box) is a standard feature both on many commercially available powered chairs and on DSC chairs. Standardisation of wiring looms and 12/24-volt motors on chairs permits the exchange of control boxes to suit the type of control system used.

For the very young child able to operate a simple switched joystick the DSCs will supply a BEC Bambino or Bec Fireball. The latter is in the process of being replaced by the Barrett Jewel and Newton Badger. A BEC switched joystick is hard-wired in the Bec Bambino and consequently this chair cannot normally be chosen where limited hand function precludes reliable operation of a joystick control. The Bec Fireball and Barrett Jewel both have a seat width of 38 cm; therefore, when used with a very small child, they will require some form of seating insert and modified foot rests. The Jewel is not a direct replacement for the Fireball with respect to size. It has a deeper seat canvas (40 cm rather than 30 cm) and the batteries are positioned further forwards; these differences have implications for stability when used with special seating inserts. The Badger has a seat width of 38 cm and a depth of 43 cm; the seat and backrest cushions can be replaced with a seating system and interface board.

For the older child and young adult the Vessa 110JX and 110X, (with seat canvas dimensions of 38×40 cm and 43×43 cm respectively) are the most commonly supplied powered chairs. The 110JX has a seat canvas of similar size to the Jewel but has rear tyres more suited to the playground or garden paths. The 110X can be supplied with a longer wheelbase where stability may be a problem. All DSA-supplied wheelchairs must be tilt tested in a static situation with the client and seating system in position on a 16° ramp. This is a static test and does not make allowances for the dynamic performance of the wheelchair over uneven ground and on a camber.

Commercially available powered wheelchairs for children

The majority of powered chairs from commercial manufacturers available for children are scaled down versions of adult chairs; for example, the BEC

Horizon and the Vessa Vitesse chairs are manufactured with a 35 cm width wheelchair canvas for young children. There are a few notable exceptions. The Ever Active, previously Everaid Turbo, and Joncare Hi/Lo Rider provide a manoeuvrable indoor/outdoor chair which includes a user-controlled elevation mechanism. The Turbo will accommodate a made-to-measure seating system and a variety of controls and special switches is available.

Switches and wheelchair control systems

The range of switched controls provided by the DSCs for handicapped people who are unable to operate a conventional joystick is manufactured by Dudley Controls of Milton Keynes and is intended for use with the Dudley Limited Acceleration control box. The range includes:

1. *Puff/suck switches.* Operated by blowing or sucking on a tube. Switches of this sort are seldom used.

2. *Head switches.* Shaped around head as headrest; 'forward' switch behind head, 'left' and 'right' on appropriate sides of head, 'reverse' at front end of side supports.

3. *Head switches with scanning control.* Switches form headrest as above; 'left' and 'right' switches rotate scanner clockwise or anticlockwise, switch behind head moves the chair in the chosen direction. Can include on/off switch behind head to one or other side.

4. *Chin operated joystick.* Small, light, eight-way joystick with mounting bracket for attachment to wheelchair.

5. *Foot or chin operated swash plate.* Tilting a small disc provides eight-way selection from an arrangement of microswitches.

All joysticks intended for use with the Dudley Limited Acceleration Control box incorporate microswitches. If the joystick is pushed forward, this operates an arrangement of microswitches so that the chair moves forward at a speed predetermined by the setting of a separate toggle switch or knob on the control box. This differs from the Penny and Giles proportional joystick, where the degree of movement of the joystick affects the speed such that the greater the movement, the higher the speed. The Penny and Giles control box includes a speed control knob to adjust the speed range. A remote but hard-wired version of this joystick is available, which can be operated by the chin or positioned midline or within a wheelchair tray.

The limited acceleration feature of the Dudley control box provides the chair with a slow acceleration from rest to avoid jolting the occupant as the chair gets underway.

Commercial manufacturers providing alternatives to joystick control for powered chairs are limited, since well over 90% of commercially available chairs are supplied with joystick control. BEC provide the following:

a. Light touch joystick—requiring only 3 ounces (85 g) of pressure
b. Touch sensors—requiring little muscle strength
c. Tilting plate—for hand or foot use
d. Slot control—five separate switches including on/off for hand or foot use.

Other manufacturers providing special switches or other control systems include Ever Active, and Fortress Scientific.

Combined communication and powered mobility

While a communication system based on a word board can be an effective system in a sympathetic environment such as the home or special school, many non-speaking teenagers develop an increasing need for a portable communication system appropriate for conversing with strangers in more adult environments.

Wheelchair-based universal interfacing device

The technology exists to allow severely physically disabled people to lead a far more independent lifestyle than many handicapped people enjoy today. To use an ever increasing range of sophisticated domestic equipment without special modifications, an individually tailored control system and a universal accessing device are required.

A prototype multipurpose interfacing device for disabled people has been constructed at Chailey Heritage (Fig. 24.8). The equipment is based on an IBM-compatible portable microcomputer and uses, where possible,

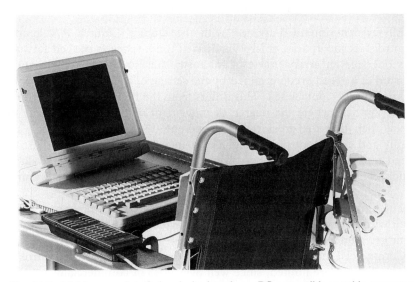

Fig. 24.8   Multipurpose interfacing device based on a PC-compatible portable computer.

commercially produced modules available at mass market prices. The device provides a severely physically handicapped user with access to a wide range of standard, unmodified domestic infra-red controlled equipment, such as compact disc players, televisions, video recorders, cassette and record players through a programmable infra-red controller. In other modes the device provides a means of communication through the medium of computer–computer communication over telephone lines access to commercially available IBM-compatible software packages such as word processors and will interface to a powered chair for independent mobility. Through a specialised adjustable multipurpose switch system and the universal control device the handicapped person should be able to enjoy the independence afforded by the intelligent home of the future.

Commercially available systems for multipurpose access include the Elfin Multiscan, which allows interaction with up to 12 devices (e.g. television, video recorder, lamps or heaters) or features of the devices (e.g. channel changing or volume control). An additional module, Elflink, provides an infra-red link between switches and switch operated equipment.

Many of the multiply handicapped young people at Chailey Heritage have become highly proficient switch users. These switch skills, when applied to daily living, should bring a better quality of life to young adults when they leave Chailey. The intelligent home of the future will include many remote controlled devices, not only domestic appliances but security cameras and access to devices from outside via telephone lines. Prospects for greater house security can contribute significantly to the peace of mind of severely disabled people wishing to live alone with daily support provided through community services. We need to ensure that young handicapped people are suitably prepared for this lifestyle. Such preparation should include an appropriate intelligent man–machine interface between the user and standard commercially available equipment, and a graded ongoing training programme.

MICROCOMPUTERS IN EDUCATION

The economic availability of microcomputers as writing aids in the classroom has made it possible for those unable to hold a pencil to participate in normal writing activities. Physically handicapped children benefit in the same way as their able-bodied peers from word processing facilities, which allow mistakes to be corrected easily and a neat copy to be printed out (Fig. 24.9). The use of a personal computer for written work can expedite the integration of a moderately physically disabled child into the majority of classroom activities in a normal school.

Special software has been written for physically handicapped people who are unable to operate a keyboard and therefore rely on switches or some other input device to interact with the computer. To enable switch users to operate standard software requiring conventional keyboard access, a

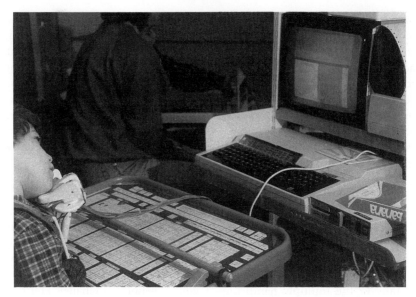

Fig. 24.9 Simple word processor operated by a switch user.

variety of keyboard emulators are available. Using one or two switches and various scanning algorithms, individual letters and numbers or strings of alphanumeric characters can be selected and are fed into the computer as if they had come from the keyboard. Emulators can be implemented in software or additional hardware. The use of keyboard emulators in special education has been limited by speed of access to standard software. Programs not intended for switch users can require many superfluous key presses and are thus frustratingly slow to use when each character must be read in by scanning and selecting. Many keyboard emulators will allow phrases to be stored for later recall.

For the non-speaking child the ability to read and write words or symbols plays an essential part in the acquisition of communication skills. All communication aids require the user to access speech by symbols, letters or words, and thus require some scanning skills and appropriate cognitive abilities. A computer system with specially tailored software provides a handicapped child with the means to practise these skills by himself (Fig. 24.10).

Software for special needs covers a wide range of ages and abilities. For the preschool child and those with more profound learning difficulties there are simple cause-and-effect programs where operating a switch or pressing a single key on the keyboard gives the reward of a sound or a picture on the monitor screen. In a similar way a picture can be built up on the screen with music or sound effects being provided as a reward. A useful publication is *Tiny Tech* from the Spastics Society, which suggests a graduated series of programs for acquiring and building on new skills for the preschool child. Colour matching, picture matching and simple programs

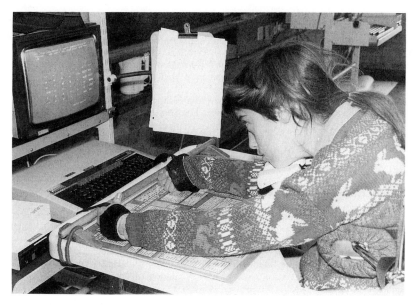

Fig. 24.10 Simple scanning practice.

involving choices are available, and many make good use of the motivational aspects provided by colour and sound. Much of this software allows the child to experiment, with minimal supervision.

The majority of switch user software is operated by either one or two switches. In making choices a scanning technique is normally used. With a single switch the options are auto-scanned at a predetermined scan speed and the user operates the single switch to make a selection. The most common method implemented with two switches uses one switch to scan and the other to select. Many handicapped people, particularly those with cerebral palsy, find the latter technique easier since it provides full control of the scan speed and the user may pause during the scanning without losing his place or making an unwanted selection.

The computer also has a role to play in leisure activities. A limited selection of games are available for switch users and, if matched to intellectual skills, they can be self-motivational and provide many hours of pleasure.

An increasing amount of written material, including complete books, is available in computer readable format. Excellent graphics facilities can be provided through video disk systems, but at a price.

As more young handicapped people are leaving residential placement and moving into the community, computer communication via the telephone system can provide a vital link with other disabled people in the community. Files such as letters can be prepared in advance at the user's own pace and then sent at high speed through a modem attached to the computer. Similarly, a disabled person working in his own home can communicate with his place of work, sending information, software, etc.

REFERENCES

ACE Centre 1989 Switches and Interfaces, 2nd edn. Ormerod School, Waynflete Road,
    Headington, Oxford, OX3 8DD
Butler C 1986 Effects of powered mobility on self-initiated behaviours of very young
    children with locomotor disability. Developmental Medicine and Child Neurology
    28:325–332
Spastics Society. Tiny Tech: microtechnology and preschool children with learning
    difficulties. Microtechnology Support Service, The Spastics Society, 16 Fitzroy Square,
    London, WIB 5HQ

USEFUL ADDRESSES

BEC Mobility, Sunrise Medical, Fens Pool Avenue, Brierley Hill, West Midlands, DY5 1QA
Dudley Controls, 10 Peverel Drive, Granby, Milton Keynes, Bucks., MK1 1NL
Elfin Systems Limited, Llanthony Road Trading Estate, Llanthony Road, Gloucester,
    GL1 1SB
Ever Active Ltd, Ermine Street North, Papworth Everard, Cambridge, CB3 8RH
Fortress Scientific, 3750 Chesswood Drive, Downsview, Ontario, Canada. UK Distributors:
    Samson Products, 239 Alder Road, Parkstone, Poole, Dorset, BH12 4AP
Joncare, 7 Ashville Trading Estate, Nuffield Way, Abingdon, Oxon., OX14 1RL
Vessa, Paper Mill Lane, Alton, Hampshire, GU34 2PY

25. Postural management

T.A. Fearn   E.M. Green   M. Jones   C.M. Mulcahy
R.L. Nelham   T.E. Pountney

Postural management is a total approach to the facilitation of correct positions in all postures. The aims are to:

- Encourage development of physical and functional ability in all postures.
- Prevent tissue trauma.
- Prevent deformity.
- Enable the child's maximum potential to be realised (or achieved).
- Provide comfort.

Much attention has recently been given to various aspects of sitting posture resulting in many different seating systems and therapeutic approaches. Equal attention has to be paid to positions of lying (including while asleep), standing and walking. This will result in an integrated system of appropriate therapy and equipment that can easily be managed both at school and, especially, at home where most of a child's time is spent.

This chapter covers the total approach that is being advocated and developed at Chailey Heritage. The total approach is being incorporated into a 24-hour management programme for children with a motor handicap but is readily applicable as appropriate to all disability groups—children and adults—including those who already have deformities.

NEUROLOGICAL ASPECTS OF POSTURAL CONTROL

Posture control appears to arise from three areas:

1. *Central*—from the brain.
2. *Segmental*—from the spinal cord.
3. *Environmental*—from the external forces present.

Changes in spinal segmental organisation have been investigated developmentally (Grillner 1975, Thelen 1986, Thelen & Cooke 1987). Several studies have demonstrated short-term reduction in tonic stretch reflex responsiveness by voluntary control (Wolpaw 1985, Neilson & McCaughey 1982, Harrison & Kruze 1987a,b) and changes of orientation in space have been shown to affect tonic muscular activity in cerebral palsy, tilting of the seat causing extensor spasm (Nwaobi 1986). Segmental and supraspinal influences may be modulated by the spinal interneurone (Harrison 1988), which is thought to play an important role in coordinating activity in different muscles (Harrison et al 1983). Nashner et al (1983) have suggested that the exaggerated stretch reflexes present in spasticity may be the consequence of abnormal coordination patterns rather than vice versa.

Feedback from the environment has been shown, from studies of the visual system (Wiesel 1982), to be essential for growth and differentiation of the nervous system. Correct positioning equipment may mimic normal experience, provide feedback and improve the biomechanical properties of the body; for example, Thomas et al (1989) have shown that when an ankle–foot orthosis stabilises the ankle, reduced abnormal muscle activity is shown on EMG, as well as increased velocity and stride length.

THE LYING POSTURE

The lying posture is highly significant in postural management. If a child does not achieve postural ability in lying, deformity is likely to begin to develop. Acquisition of competence in the lying position also establishes a foundation for the development of postural ability in sitting and standing. Pountney et al (1990) showed that until a child achieves a symmetrical lying posture with an ability to shift weight longitudinally and laterally he has inadequate postural control to sit independently.

Development of lying ability

Six levels of lying ability in both prone and supine have been established and described (Table 25.1). The normal sequence of lying abilities is based on the following:

a. Weightbearing, i.e. which areas of the body are in contact with the supporting surface.
b. Position of the trunk (including shoulder girdle and pelvis), head and limbs relative both to the floor and to one another.
c. Ability to move in the position (Hare 1984).
d. Ability to move into and out of position (Hare 1984).

Table 25.1 shows the child's progression from an asymmetrical non-conforming position through a symmetrical fairly static position to a variety of mobile active positions.

At levels 1 and 2 the child is asymmetrical with the pelvis posteriorly tilted and shoulder girdle retracted. In supine the pelvis, trunk, shoulder girdle and head are all weightbearing (although only momentarily at level 1) and dissociation of head movement from the trunk and pelvic movement is therefore very difficult. Thus an inability to move the head without concomitant pelvic movement is observed. In prone the pelvis is unable to make contact with the floor due to its posterior tilt; thus weightbearing is through the knees, upper trunk and head. Head raising is therefore difficult as the pelvis has no fixation and a great deal of weightbearing is through the upper trunk.

Progression to levels 3 and 4 results in a symmetrical posture as the shoulder girdle becomes more protracted and the pelvis more anteriorly tilted. The resultant weightbearing in supine is through the shoulder girdle and pelvis, and in prone is through the abdomen and thighs with hands or arms used to prop the upper trunk. This increase in girdle control allows dissociation of movement between upper and lower trunk and the beginning of limb movement dissociation from the limb girdle. The ability to vary the position of the pelvis and shoulder girdle also begins at level 4.

On reaching levels 5 and 6 the infant displays no predominant positions. A full range of movement in the shoulder girdle and the pelvis allows the baby to adopt a variety of positions. As he achieves this he is able to move in the position, i.e. pivoting or moving backwards, and into and out of position, e.g. rolling or crawling.

THE SITTING POSTURE

For the physically disabled child the sitting posture is likely to be the posture adopted for most of the day. If immature sitting postures are not supported or controlled, postural deformity will occur.

Development of sitting ability

Seven levels of sitting ability have been identified and described (Table 25.2). From early infancy (level 1 lying ability) a normal child can be cradled in a sitting position and can anchor his bottom when pulled to sitting (Shumway 1986), i.e. he weightbears through his bottom adequately for his trunk to be brought forwards over it and to be maintained upright (level 2 sitting ability). The lateral profile of this infant shows a rounded spinal curvature (Fig. 25.1). Note his posteriorly tilted pelvis and his need for trunk and shoulders to be maintained forwards over his base in order to balance.

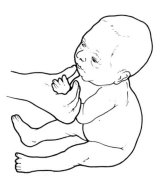

Fig. 25.1 An infant pulled to sitting showing a rounded spinal curvature in lateral profile with posteriorly tilted pelvis.

Table 25.1   Levels of lying ability in supine and prone positions.

LEVEL 1
PLACEABLE, BUT
UNABLE TO
MAINTAIN

LEVEL 2
ABLE TO MAINTAIN
POSITION WHEN PLACED

LEVEL 3
ABLE TO MAINTAIN
POSITION.
BEGINNING
LONGITUDINAL
WEIGHT SHIFT

LEVEL 4
ABLE TO MAINTAIN
POSITION.
BEGINNING LATERAL
WEIGHT SHIFT

LEVEL 5
CONSISTENTLY MOVING
OUT FROM LYING
POSITION. BEGINNING
TO ATTAIN LYING
POSTURES

LEVEL 6
CONSISTENTLY MOVING
BETWEEN LYING
POSTURES AND INTO
SITTING

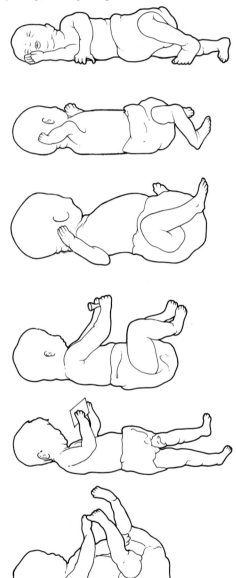

SUPINE

Unable to maintain supine when placed except momentarily and then very asymmetrically. Body follows head turning in a total body movement and therefore rolls into and maintains side-lying. Weightbearing through lateral aspect of head, trunk and thigh. Neck extended with chin poke.

LEVEL 1
PLACEABLE, BUT
UNABLE TO
MAINTAIN

Settles on back when placed. 'Top heavy'. Weightbearing through upper trunk, head. Pelvis tilted posteriorly. Shoulder girdle retracted. Asymmetrical posture—head to one side, difficulty in turning it side to side—bottom moves laterally as the head is turned giving 'corkscrew' appearance.

LEVEL 2
ABLE TO MAINTAIN
POSITION WHEN PLACED

Maintains supine position with neutral pelvic tilt, hip abduction, shoulder girdle neutral. Symmetrical posture but top heavy. Chin tucked, not retracted— head in midline and able to move freely side to side without lateral movement of bottom. Able to track visually and make eye contact. Weightbearing through pelvis and shoulder girdle giving general curvature to trunk—with 'pot belly' lateral profile. Beginning of unilateral grasp to side of body and takes fist and objects to mouth. Longitudinal weight shift begins. May roll into prone due to lack of lateral weight shift.

LEVEL 3
ABLE TO MAINTAIN
POSITION.
BEGINNING
LONGITUDINAL
WEIGHT SHIFT

Symmetry of posture and midline play is seen at this level. Pelvis anteriorly tilted, shoulder girdle protracted. Chin retracted. Shoulders flexing and adducting allowing midline play above chest with hands together; feet also together. Symmetrical posture. Weightbearing through upper trunk and pelvis. Definite lordotic curve. 'Free' pelvic movement beginning, allowing child to touch knees with hips flexed (but not toes). Alternatively can extend hips and knees; rests in crook lying. Beginning unilateral leg raise—independence of limbs from trunk. Adept finger movements towards end of this stage.

LEVEL 4
ABLE TO MAINTAIN
POSITION.
BEGINNING LATERAL
WEIGHT SHIFT

'Free' movement of shoulder girdle and pelvis on trunk. Pelvis has full range of movement allowing child to play with toes with legs extended and rolls into side-lying. Side-lying functional. Can return to supine. Weightbearing either on shoulder girdle and pelvis or on central trunk only and playing between these postures. Efficient limb movement—hand play and prehensile feet—crossing midline.

LEVEL 5
CONSISTENTLY MOVING
OUT FROM LYING
POSITION. BEGINNING
TO ATTAIN LYING
POSTURES

Pelvic and shoulder girdle moving freely. Consistent ability to roll into prone by achieving sidelying as in level 5 and then anteriorly tilting pelvis on trunk and extending hips.

LEVEL 6
CONSISTENTLY MOVING
BETWEEN LYING
POSTURES AND INTO
SITTING

PRONE

LEVEL 1
PLACEABLE, BUT
UNABLE TO
MAINTAIN

Top heavy. Unstable with tendency to topple.
Weightbearing through face, shoulders and chest.
Pelvis posteriorly tilted. Hips and knees flexed.
Shoulder girdle retracted, shoulders flexed and
adducted. Asymmetrical posture and head to one
side.

LEVEL 2
ABLE TO MAINTAIN
POSITION WHEN PLACED

Settles when placed. More generalised
weightbearing than Level 1. Weightbearing through
chest, upper abdomen. Pelvis posteriorly tilted.
Shoulder girdle retracted, shoulders flexed and
adducted. Head to one side but beginning to lift it
from floor with 'flat back' profile but not sustaining.
Asymmetrical posture, bottom moving laterally as
head turns side to side.

LEVEL 3
ABLE TO MAINTAIN
POSITION.
BEGINNING
LONGITUDINAL
WEIGHT SHIFT

Maintains prone position with neutral pelvis,
shoulder girdle beginning to protract. Symmetrical
weightbearing through abdomen, lower chest and
knees and thighs. Maintains head lift from floor
with total trunk curvature—head in line with spine.
Rocking longitudinally. No lateral weight shift and
therefore often topples into supine when lifts head
and chest up.

LEVEL 4
ABLE TO MAINTAIN
POSITION.
BEGINNING LATERAL
WEIGHT SHIFT

Pelvis anteriorly tilted but not 'anchoring'. Shoulder
girdle protracted, weightbearing through abdomen
and thighs, varying between forearm and hand
propping with shoulders elevated. Head and upper
trunk movement dissociated from lower trunk
allowing lateral trunk flexion with lateral weight
shift = beginning of pivoting. Angular lateral profile
of upper chest and bottom. Unilateral leg kicking.
Hand and foot play is midline.

LEVEL 5
CONSISTENTLY MOVING
OUT FROM LYING
POSITION. BEGINNING
TO ATTAIN LYING
POSTURES

Pelvis anteriorly tilted. Shoulder girdle protracted—
hand propping with extended elbows and lumbar
spine extension. Weightbearing through iliac crests
and thighs and lower abdomen. Pelvic anchoring
and upper body movement (extension and rotation)
upon it. Deft pivoting with lateral trunk flexion and
moving backwards on floor. Purposeful roll prone
into supine.

LEVEL 6
CONSISTENTLY MOVING
BETWEEN LYING
POSTURES AND INTO
SITTING

'Free' movement of pelvis and shoulder girdle.
Beginning to weightbear on all fours—anteroposterior rocking on all fours.

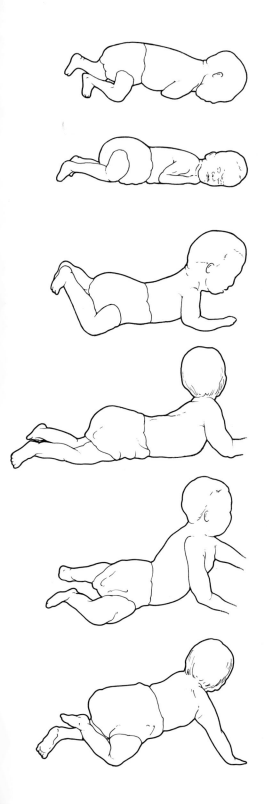

LEVEL 1
PLACEABLE, BUT
UNABLE TO
MAINTAIN

LEVEL 2
ABLE TO MAINTAIN
POSITION WHEN PLACED

LEVEL 3
ABLE TO MAINTAIN
POSITION.
BEGINNING
LONGITUDINAL
WEIGHT SHIFT

LEVEL 4
ABLE TO MAINTAIN
POSITION.
BEGINNING LATERAL
WEIGHT SHIFT

LEVEL 5
CONSISTENTLY MOVING
OUT FROM LYING
POSITION. BEGINNING
TO ATTAIN LYING
POSTURES

LEVEL 6
CONSISTENTLY MOVING
BETWEEN LYING
POSTURES AND INTO
SITTING

Table 25.2 Levels of sitting ability

LEVELS OF SITTING ABILITY

With an individual placed on a flat box of the correct height, feet on floor.

LEVEL		DESCRIPTION	
1	UNPLACEABLE	Wriggles and slides and cannot be placed in a sitting position	
2	PLACEABLE, NOT ABLE TO MAINTAIN POSITION	Can be placed in a sitting position but needs holding to stay in position - at best can balance momentarily	
3	ABLE TO MAINTAIN POSITION BUT NOT MOVE	When placed in a sitting position can just keep balance as long as there is no movement	
4	ABLE TO MAINTAIN POSITION AND MOVE WITHIN BASE	Once placed in a sitting position can sit independently and can move trunk forward over sitting base but cannot recover balance after reaching to one side	
5	ABLE TO MAINTAIN POSITION AND MOVE OUTSIDE BASE	Can sit independently, can use either hand freely to the side of the body and can recover balance after leaning or falling to either side	
6	ABLE TO MOVE OUT OF POSITION	Can sit independently and can transfer weight across the surface of a seat but cannot regain a correct sitting position	
7	ABLE TO ATTAIN POSITION	Can regain sitting position after moving out of it	

As the infant improves in his ability to weightbear symmetrically when lying (lying ability levels 1–3), his ability to assist in being pulled to sit improves. In lying he develops the ability to weightbear through a neutral pelvis and shoulder girdle; therefore in ring sitting he becomes progressively more able to stabilise his trunk and head in an upright posture above his weightbearing base (i.e. bottom and legs). When parents hold a child they naturally withdraw support from their infant's head and upper trunk as he develops this ability. They eventually feel able to prop him sitting in an armchair or sofa, surrounded by cushions.

The general arch of the spine seen in lying ability level 3 prone and supine can also be witnessed as the child is pulled up to a sitting position, and he can appear to be throwing his trunk backwards. Just prior to sitting independently he may get stuck in a jack-knife position when placed in ring-sitting on the floor. His legs adopt a diamond-shaped base and he can maintain sitting with very little support, but when this support is released he is top heavy, his hips flex, head and arms touch the floor and he ceases to weightbear through his bottom. He has inadequate stability of his upper trunk and shoulder girdle to push himself upright and regain a sitting position.

Independent sitting is only achieved after the infant is able to anteriorly tilt his pelvis and protract his shoulder girdle and, when lying, efficiently transfer his weight longitudinally (lying ability level 4). In sitting he now has adequate pelvic and shoulder girdle stability to weightbear through his ischial tuberosities and arms in a forward prop position.

As the infant masters the ability to shift weight laterally when lying (lying ability 5) so he develops the ability to move outside his sitting base and maintain his balance. It is at this time that we see a straight back posture prior to the development of a lordotic curve in an upright posture. The child counterpoises laterally before being able to recover his balance when his trunk weight is behind his sitting base.

As the interplay between pelvic and upper trunk stability and movement becomes efficient the infant becomes increasingly proficient at weight transference in an upright position. He becomes efficient at counterpoising in a variety of sitting postures including long-sitting, eventually developing control of his movement from sitting to lying and from the prone position to sitting (in a variety of ways).

STANDING

Development of standing ability

Before a child learns to stand and walk he may have learned to lie symmetrically, sit independently and to move in a variety of different ways. To stand unaided a child needs the ability to support his own body against gravity. Postural fixation of head on trunk and trunk on pelvis is necessary.

For weightbearing to be practical, counterpoising must be developed. This is acquired by holding onto a support at about 9–12 months, followed by the ability to counterpoise without holding a support.

A child will first develop a standing posture by slightly flexing his upper trunk forwards over his base and propping with his hands. The pelvis is slightly posteriorly tilted, with the lumbar spine flexed. As the child becomes more able the pelvis tilts anteriorly and the hips extend, giving a more upright posture. During this period the infant learns anteroposterior and lateral counterpoise as a precursor to walking. Tilt reactions, along with saving reactions, develop in standing as a child begins to stand and walk unaided.

Importance of weightbearing in standing

Walking is an emotional milestone for all parents; the hope of parents of disabled children is to see them develop to as near normal standing and walking as possible.

If it is possible for a child to stand and walk, even with aids, then his management at home is much easier. Children can acquire independence as wheelchair users at home but the ability to stand and move around enhances this independence.

Correct standing can help prevent soft tissue contractures and, together with walking, can also improve development of the joints, particularly the hip joints. As the hip joints are especially vulnerable to deformity, it is important to get good weightbearing as early as possible. Standing is also important for physiological reasons, e.g. bladder function, bone formation and blood pressure control. Psychologically it is advantageous for a child to experience being at the same height and eye level as his peers.

It is important to give the right support for each child; some children with poor head and upper limb control when seated, even with good support to give correct positioning, have better control when correctly supported in standing.

Correct standing also helps increase tone in the antigravity muscles. If a child has not developed sitting ability, it is still important to support him in a standing position when mature enough. All infants experience weightbearing through their feet during normal play and handling, before they develop the ability to sit and stand.

ASSESSMENT

The child's assessment should be comprehensive, considering the total child and his normal environment and identifying treatment and equipment needs for management in all postures. *For equipment to be prescribed and used most effectively everyone involved with the child, including parents, care staff, therapists, doctor, rehabilitation engineer and technician, orthotist, teacher and nurse, needs to understand the reasons for its use.* The assessment should:

- Identify a child's abilities, and a means of capitalising on these
- Identify (and if possible measure) any present or potential postural deformity and define the treatment, including equipment, required to control and improve this where possible and to prevent the development of fixed deformity.
- Establish and record a baseline as a reference for later reviews and assessments

• Provide a means whereby the performance of the prescribed equipment can be monitored, i.e. the child's ability within his prescribed equipment should be better than his ability with no postural support.

ASSESSMENT PROCEDURE

The assessment procedure is in three stages:

1. Establish the child's abilities without postural support.
2. Observe the child's posture in his current equipment
3. Examine the equipment without the child.

Photographic and written records are kept of all assessments.

First stage of assessment

The first stage of assessment begins with the observation of how easy the child is to handle; for example, has the posture been reinforcing an extensor pattern of movement or encouraging a postural deformity?

It continues with a full assessment of the child's abilities in the positions of lying: supine, side and prone; during pull to sit; in long-sitting; sitting on a flat box; sitting on a ramped cushion; and standing. The following are observed in all positions:

a. Symmetry and weight distribution.
b. The child's ability, with minimum support, to conform to positions, to maintain positions, to move within positions and to move into and out of the positions.
c. Any present or potential deformities or contractures.

The hamstrings, back, hips, knees and ankles are checked to establish whether any contractures present will physically interfere with the child attaining different postures.

Any poverty of hip and trunk control will be reflected in the child's difficulty in coordinating his body and weightbearing through his base of support in each posture. The ability to align his trunk or his head and limbs once his pelvis is organised is observed. The effect of aligning his pelvis and trunk on the organisation of his head and limb movements is also noted.

The minimal support required to improve the child's abilities and to correct any possible deformities is simulated by hand, and the effect of this simulated support upon the child's abilities is studied. The child's ability in each position is recorded.

Lying

Assessing and identifying a child's level of lying ability gives a positive indication of how much the child can achieve physically. A child with motor handicap may take many years to reach the major milestones identified in standardised motor assessments such as Milano-Comparetti, Sheridan, etc. The levels of lying ability provide a more detailed method of assessing improvements in postural ability during early development.

The six levels of lying ability observed in normal infants can be used as a model on which to base assessment and prescription for the child with motor handicap although some adjustments may need to be made for fixed deformities and the child's acquired use of trick movements to achieve motion. A clear picture of the child's motor development is obtained together with identification of the skills required to achieve the next level of ability (Table 25.3), e.g. a child at level 2 needs to progress to a more symmetrical posture with his shoulder girdle and pelvis in a neutral position and his head in midline.

The level of lying ability for the child with motor handicap is established by observing *what the child can do* in each position rather than noting his disabilities. Neurological signs such as tone and reflexes are disregarded as they often vary with position and the child's state of awareness and give little objective prescriptive information for treatment and postural management.

Sitting

Pull to sit.   From supine, the child is pulled into a long-sitting position. The ability of the child to anchor his bottom is noted, that is, whether he is able to dissociate his trunk movement from the lower part of his body. If he anchors his bottom, he should be placeable in a sitting position.

Long-sitting.   This is a very important position because it accentuates any contractures and potential deformities that may not have been so pronounced in other postures, and emphasises any need for correction through treatment and postural control.

Sitting on a flat box.   The height of the box (which is adjustable) allows the child to place his feet flat on the floor with his femur supported throughout its length. The ease with which he can be placed on the box and his ability to maintain that position is noted, as is his stability once placed with minimal or no support. Symmetry of posture in the antero-posterior and lateral planes, and from head to toe, is observed and noted. The child is considered, literally, from all points of view, that is, front, sides and back.

Sitting on a ramped cushion (see p. 426). When sitting on the ramped cushion on top of the boxes, a check is made that the femora are horizontal and supported through their entire length, and that the feet are on the floor. The ischial tuberosities must be on the flat rear portion of the cushion. The effect of the ramped cushion is to bring the upper body weight forwards over the sitting base. The stability and symmetry of the child and the effect of the cushion on his ability to maintain sitting posture is

Table 25.3 Skills achieved at each level of ability in lying in prone and supine positions

	Level 1		Level 2	
	Supine	Prone	Supine	Prone
SYMMETRICAL POSITION (CAN MAINTAIN)				
Weightbearing				
Head	Only w. b. momentarily w. b. in side lying	√	√	√
Shoulders		√		
Arms		√		√
Hands		√		√
Thorax		√	√	√
Abdomen				√
Pelvis			√	
Thighs				
Knees		√		√
Feet		√		√
Shoulder girdle				
Retracted	√	√	√	√
Neutral				
Protracted				
Pelvic girdle				
Post. tilted	√	√	√	√
Neutral				
Ant. tilted				
Head movement				
Trunk follows head movement	√	√		
Head mvt, followed by pelvic mvt, in opposite direction			√	√
Turns head freely				
Lifts head				
Lifts head and shoulders				
Lifts head, shoulders and thorax				
Chin				
Poke	√	√	√	√
Tucked				
Retracted				
Limb movement				
Random	√	√	√	√
To side				
To midline				
Bilateral				
X-midline				
Weight shift				
Uncontrolled			√	√
Longitudinal				
Lateral				

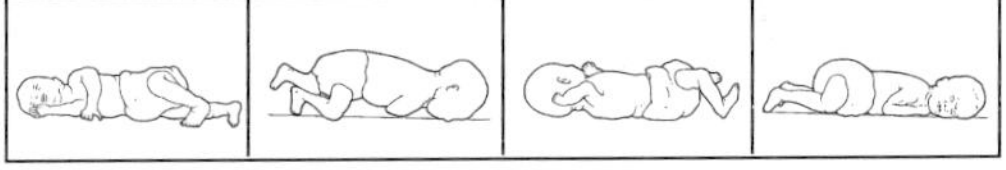

Table 25.3   Contd.

	Level 3		Level 4	
	Supine	Prone	Supine	Prone
SYMMETRICAL POSITION (CAN MAINTAIN)	√	√	√	√
Weightbearing				
Head	√		√	
Shoulders	√			
Arms		√		√ or
Hands		√		√
Thorax		√	√	
Abdomen		√		√
Pelvis	√		√	
Thighs		√		√
Knees		√		
Feet				
Shoulder girdle				
Retracted				
Neutral	√	√		
Protracted			√	√
Pelvic girdle				
Post. tilted				
Neutral	√	√		
Ant. tilted			√	√
Head movement				
Trunk follows head movement				
Head mvt, followed by pelvic mvt, in opposite direction				
Turns head freely	√		√	√
Lifts head		√	√	
Lifts head and shoulders				√
Lifts head, shoulders and thorax				
Chin				
Poke				
Tucked	√	√		
Retracted			√	√
Limb movement				
Random				
To side	√	√		
To midline			√	√
Bilateral			√	
X-midline				
Weight shift				
Uncontrolled				
Longitudinal	√	√		
Lateral			√	√

Table 25.3 Contd.

	Level 5		Level 6	
	Supine	Prone	Supine	Prone
SYMMETRICAL POSITION (CAN MAINTAIN)	√	√	√	√
Weightbearing				
Head	√		√	
Shoulders	√		√	
Arms			√	
Hands		√	√	√
Thorax	or √		√	any of
Abdomen		√		
Pelvis	√	√	√	
Thighs		√	√	
Knees				√
Feet	√		√	
Shoulder girdle				
Retracted				
Neutral				
Protracted	√	√	√	√
Pelvic girdle				
Post. tilted				
Neutral				
Ant. tilted	√	√	√	√
Head movement				
Trunk follows head movement				
Head mvt, followed by pelvic mvt, in opposite direction				
Turns head freely	√	√	√	√
Lifts head				
Lifts head and shoulders	√			
Lifts head, shoulders and thorax		√		√
Chin				
Poke				
Tucked				
Retracted	√	√	√	√
Limb movement				
Random				
To side				
To midline				
Bilateral				
X-midline	√	√	√	√
Weight shift				
Uncontrolled				
Longitudinal	√	√	√	√
Lateral	√	√	√	√

observed from all sides and noted. The ability of the child to rise from the cushion to stand up is assessed.

Standing

The child is placed in the standing position or, if he is able, allowed to achieve it independently. The child's ability to take up and maintain the position either with or without human assistance or aids is noted. The ability to move into and out of standing, and to walk, is assessed. This will indicate whether the child is able to assist with transfers or to transfer independently. This is important when deciding the height of a seat and an appropriate seat base (wheeled or free standing).

In standing, weight should be taken evenly through both plantigrade feet with the line of gravity passing through the hips and ankles. If a child can stand unaided, observe his ability to maintain the posture and to move anteroposteriorly and laterally.

If a child requires assistance, assess how much support is required to help the child maintain a good standing posture. This is defined as one in which the feet are controlled horizontally at floor level; the ankles are slightly dorsiflexed to bring the shins forward over the feet; the knees are supported in a slightly flexed position to bring the femora close to vertical; and the hips are symmetrically abducted and slightly flexed to bring the trunk forward over the feet (Fig. 25.2). The degrees of flexion at each joint will need to be carefully assessed for each child. As a child's ability in standing improves he will be able to move from this position to a more upright posture.

Lateral pelvic and thoracic supports, together with a well designed pommel and shoulder girdle control, may be required to give support and help maintain symmetry and function. Note how any joint deformity affects the posture and the postural control required to alleviate this.

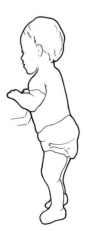

Fig. 25.2 An infant demonstrating a good standing posture.

Second stage of assessment

The second stage of assessment defines the reasons for the child requiring postural support equipment; for example, is he growing and, if so, is he maintaining his ability with his growth? Are his abilities changing? Does his treatment and postural support meet his changing needs? A note is made of the child's use of his existing posture and movement to eat, operate his wheelchair or computer and any obligatory patterns that might need re-education when his equipment is altered.

Third stage of assessment

The third stage of the assessment looks at the existing equipment to provide information about its use. The areas where it is most worn are noted, as these indicate where the child has borne most weight, and can confirm his preferred (or obligatory) postures in this position.

PRESCRIPTION

Each child's baseline level of achievement and his needs are recorded both for treatment and for postural support adequate to maintain his abilities and control his posture throughout the day and night. The levels of ability in both lying and sitting describe the ease with which a child can be placed in a position, how he can maintain that position and how he adjusts his body to move within and out of position. These levels of ability form the basis of prescription for postural management.

LYING

By taking the child through the normal developmental sequence using treatment and equipment, the use of normal automatic and volitional movement can be encouraged rather than movement that requires gross body movements and associated reactions. Normal head and limb movement can only be achieved in lying if the trunk is correctly positioned and stabilised to provide the basis for movement. Attempts to gain normal movement on an unstable or ill-positioned trunk will be unsuccessful.

A close resemblance can be seen between the normal infant at level 2 lying ability, and lying posture of the motor handicapped child with a windswept deformity (Pountney et al 1990). If the progression of deformity is to be arrested it is vitally important that the child progresses beyond the asymmetrical levels 1 and 2, i.e. the child needs to be capable of maintaining a symmetrical posture independently or else be provided with equipment to maintain symmetry.

The surface upon which the child is lying can affect ability. A hard surface can adversely affect a child of low ability, i.e. below level 3 lying ability, but can assist postural fixation for the child with greater ability.

Both therapy and equipment must aim to improve the child's ability and prevent the progression of deformity.

Therapy

Individual or group therapy can be given to improve lying ability. Both are important methods of treatment. Individual therapy allows the child to practice his lying skills at this own pace, working with skilled therapists to correct any minor postural problems. Therapy time, however, is limited and group work allows the child more time to practice, although a need to conform to the group programme may mean that it is difficult for him to achieve the quality of performance possible in individual therapy.

The aims of group therapy should reinforce the aims of individual therapy and vice versa. Both should be based on the normal developmental sequence, encouraging the children to move through the levels of ability. Ideally, therefore, the children in the groups should be of similar levels of ability. Each child should be assessed individually and a clear programme of his goals for a period of time outlined. Imagination is required to prevent treatment becoming tedious and repetitive. Activities should be appropriate to each child's level of ability, e.g. bilateral limb movement for a child at lying ability level 3. The child's family and all staff involved with the child should be aware of the treatment aims in order to encourage appropriate movements and development of skills. Each child should be regularly reassessed during individual therapy sessions so that his programmes can be progressed as appropriate. Progression can consist of specific movements to be encouraged, graded therapeutic techniques, specific equipment or a change of surface that the child is lying upon (soft or firm mat, or a hard surface at floor level or at a raised height).

Although the child receives therapy in lying, therapy in other positions is not excluded as the experience of a variety of positions is vital to the overall development of any child.

Equipment for postural control

Equipment which provides postural support and control in lying is used to reinforce the therapy programme. It should be designed to help the child achieve and maintain a symmetrical position, thereby aiming to prevent deformity as well as improving his lying ability. A child should be more able in his equipment than he is out of it.

The provision of equipment for a child to use when lying falls into two categories: (1) night lying boards; and (2) equipment to facilitate posture and movement during treatment.

Night lying boards provide an ideal opportunity for the child to experience a long period of correct posture and to improve his biomechanical efficiency. Night-time positioning aims to maintain the child in a sym-

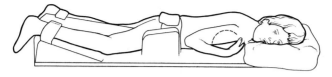

Fig. 25.3 Prone positioning to maintain symmetry at night.

a   b

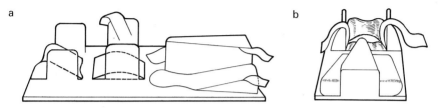

Fig. 25.4 Two views of the prone lying board showing the small wedges in place to support the chest and pelvis.

metrical position by abducting the hips and providing lateral pelvic and thoracic support (Fig. 25.3). At levels 2 and 3 lying ability, small wedges under the chest and pelvis may be added (Fig. 25.4) to allow the child to experience weightbearing through these areas of the body. Generally the child is positioned in prone, but occasionally a lying board has been provided for use in supine and this can incorporate wedges to achieve weightbearing appropriate to a higher level of ability.

Problems with tissue trauma may occur when night lying boards are first used and checks should be made for red areas of skin. Care should be taken to ensure that the design and materials used provide adequate weight distribution to avoid localised areas of pressure (Fearn & Tutt 1990).

Equipment for use in therapy

Equipment to facilitate posture and movement during treatment assumes the child's active contribution to obtain his optimum lying ability. At level 2, small chest and pelvic wedges are used to encourage weightbearing in prone and help the child prop on his forearms and lift his head from the floor (Figs 25.5 and 6). In level 2 supine, a curved piece of foam under the shoulders may encourage protraction of the shoulder girdle, and a foam support for the lower thoracic and lumbar region can assist a longitudinal curve to the spine (Figs 25.7 and 8).

At level 3 prone, a chest wedge can be adequate to encourage head raising and weightbearing through the pelvis onto the floor. In supine, again a curved supporting surface should be provided under the shoulders to encourage shoulder girdle protraction. A small wedge can support a lordosis or can be used under the sacrum to facilitate an alternative posture of hip and knee flexion towards the chest.

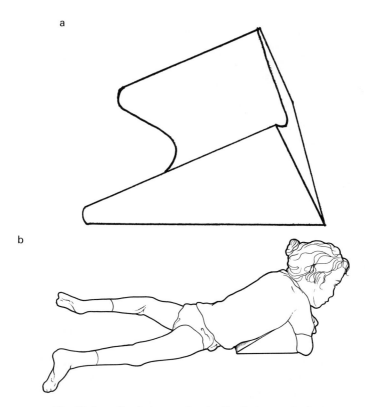

Fig. 25.5   **a.** Small chest wedge. **b.** Small chest wedge in use.

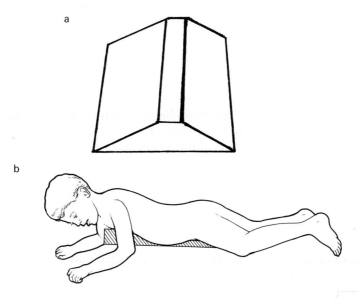

Fig. 25.6   **a.** Small pelvic wedge. **b.** Small chest and pelvic wedges in use.

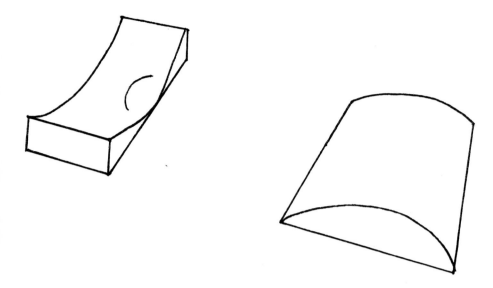

Fig. 25.7 Curved piece of foam to be placed under the shoulders, and a foam support for the lower thoracic and lumbar region.

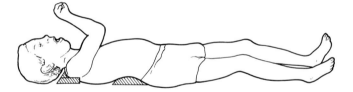

Fig. 25.8 Shoulder and lower thoracic and lumbar supports in use to promote protraction of the shoulder girdle and longitudinal curvature of the thoracolumbar spine in supine.

At level 4 prone, a small wedge at the lower end of the chest will facilitate the level 5 position and fixation of the pelvis. In level 4 supine, a curved supporting surface placed under the shoulder can assist increased dexterity, and a small wedge tipping the pelvis posteriorly will encourage further flexing at the hips and knees. Interplay between the positions of posterior and anterior tilt of the pelvis should be experienced.

For the child at lying ability 5 or 6, equipment providing specific postural assistance during therapy is not necessary, as he needs to learn his own control of movement into and from the lying position. It may, however, be desirable to use a firm curved support surface.

SITTING

Physically handicapped children spend a long time sitting and receive only comparatively short periods of therapy. Adaptive seating together with other positioning devices should therefore reflect and reinforce therapeutic principles, thus encouraging the child to maintain his ability throughout the day and, in the long term, improve his postural control. For the child with motor handicap, therapeutically correct seating should improve ability to sit and should limit the progression of deformity.

The following describes problems encountered with certain designs of seating and some solutions to overcome these problems.

Intimately moulded seating

During the last decade the most frequently prescribed supportive seating system has been the intimately moulded seat (Nelham 1985), of which the Chailey moulded seat, the Derby moulded seat and its derivatives and the individually contoured Matrix seat are examples. This type of seating has major disadvantages:

1. In the sagittal plane (Fig. 25.9) the curved base of the moulded seat is shaped to the fleshy contours of the buttocks. The trunk weight causes the pelvis to slide round the curved contours of the base and this leads to sacral sitting. Sacral sitting is undesirable from two points of view:

a. There is potential for the development of tissue trauma in the sacral region—an area that is not capable of sustaining high pressures (Motloch et al 1979).

b. It is a reclined posture and infants develop the ability to sit from a position of forward prop (Illingworth 1974), their trunk weight well forward over their sitting base. To achieve a position of forward prop from a reclined posture requires mature postural reactions, i.e. at least sitting ability level 5. A child who has not developed an ability to forward prop will not have achieved the ability to recover sitting balance from a position of recline, and the development of sitting ability will be compromised by reclined or sacral sitting postures.

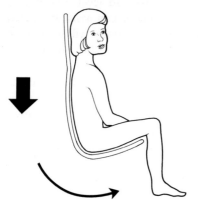

Fig. 25.9 Effects of sitting on a surface curved in the sagittal plane.

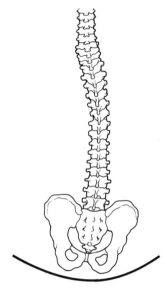

Fig. 25.10 Pelvic instability arising out of sitting on a surface curved in the coronal plane.

2. In the coronal plane (Fig. 25.10) the base of the moulded seat is also curved to fit the fleshy contours of the buttocks. This shape does not provide the stabilisation required to prevent the pelvic obliquity caused by asymmetrical muscle tone or the way the child is placed into the seat. If pelvic obliquity is not counteracted by the base of support, a compensatory scoliosis is likely to develop. If uncorrected, this postural deformity is likely to increase and become a fixed deformity (Bell & Watson 1985, Bell 1987, Fulford & Brown 1976).

Posture accommodation and posture stabilisation

It is convenient to divide the biomechanics, and equipment that achieves biomechanical support, into two categories: posture accommodation and posture stabilisation.

Posture accommodation. Posture accommodation involves the accommodation and support of an existing posture, for example a severe fixed deformity or extremely complex problems. Invariably the children themselves determine the approach that needs to be taken to maximise comfort and function, and there is often little potential for improvement. Included in this category are those who have severe disability due to spina bifida, or advanced stages of muscular dystrophy and similar conditions. The priorities are comfort and the avoidance of tissue trauma. The posture presented is not greatly modified by the equipment produced. The biomechanics associated with the design of the posture accommodating seating must, however, be compatible with the biomechanics associated with posture stabilisation, even though the final result may be a considerable compromise, i.e. a well designed moulded seat.

Posture stabilisation. Everyone needs a stable base in order to function. Every seat therefore has to provide postural stability to be of benefit.

Posture stabilisation is a pro-active approach that involves using the appropriate biomechanical principles to produce the seating systems that will be compatible with therapy programmes, facilitate and improve function, meet orthopaedic requirements and encourage improvements in ability.

It is necessary to be fully aware of the objectives of treatment and equipment and to constantly review performance against these objectives. It will also be necessary to revise objectives according to the child's changing needs.

Once the correct principles have been adopted and the appropriate equipment provided, short and long term improvements in posture and function are indicators that postural stability has been achieved. If these improvements are not forthcoming, then the design of the equipment or its adjustment needs to be reviewed. *It should be noted that while the child is becoming accustomed to a new posture, previously achieved activities used for eating and operating switches for a powered chair or computer may initially deteriorate.* For instance, if the child has been using obligatory patterns of movement that necessitated asymmetrical posture and movement, he will need physical and emotional support and re-education of these skills once he is symmetrically seated.

The seven levels of sitting ability are used to determine the prescription for seating, to measure the effectiveness of the equipment in use and to measure the long-term gains achieved by the individuals through the appropriate therapy and the use of this equipment. All children should be able to function at a higher level of sitting ability when in the seat, compared with sitting on the floor, on a box or in a basic wheelchair.

Biomechanics of the upright sitting posture

The upright sitting posture is defined as one where the hips and knees are flexed at right angles, the femora are horizontal and the ankles are in the plantigrade position (0° of flexion/extension).

Problem

The upright posture is not achieved on a right-angled upright chair. In order to reduce the discomfort if the ischial tuberosities are the only area of weightbearing, the seat surface must also support the thighs. On a flat seat, this results in the femora sloping towards the front of the chair. (Fig. 25.11) Equally, in this position, postural control is required to retain the pelvis in the neutral plane. Without postural control the pelvis is posteriorly tilted with a correspondingly slumped posture (Fig. 25.12). This poor posture will progress and the child may slide off the chair onto the floor. Frequent repositioning is needed. In an effort to prevent the pelvis from posteriorly rotating, the child is often placed in the chair so that the pelvis is held in the neutral position by the backrest (Fig. 25.13). Unfortunately, dimension *a* (Fig. 25.13) is less than dimension *b*, and the vertical backrest therefore pushes the trunk forward into a forward slumped posture. In order to sit up, the child has to push his bottom forwards thus allowing the pelvis to posteriorly rotate and hence enacting a vicious circle.

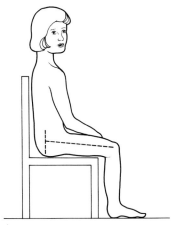

Fig. 25.11   Sloping femora on a flat seat of right-angled chair.

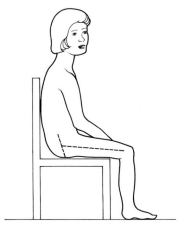

Fig. 25.12   Right-angled chair, sloping femora, posteriorly rotated pelvis and slumped posture.

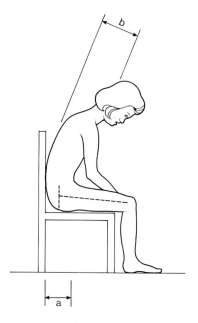

Fig. 25.13   Pelvis in neutral position against vertical backrest, showing slumped posture arising from difference between dimension **a**—anteroposterior pelvic depth, and dimension **b**—anteroposterior thoracic depth.

Solution

The femora must first be stabilised in the horizontal plane. There are various ways in which this can be achieved. At Chailey Heritage, the ramped cushion (Mulcahy & Pountney 1987) is used to provide a flat, horizontal support for the ischial tuberosities and a 15° ramp to support the underside of the thigh (Fig. 25.14). The feet must be supported at the appropriate height. The 15° angle has been found to be appropriate for a wide range of anatomical sizes. Individual adjustments may be necessary, adults usually requiring a larger angle than infants.

Postural ability is still required on this cushion to hold the pelvis in the neutral plane as the posteriorly tilted pelvis described above can occur on the ramped cushion (Fig. 25.15). In order to accommodate the different anteroposterior dimensions of the pelvis and the trunk (dimensions *a* and *b* Fig. 25.13), it is necessary to have a basic understanding of the relationship between the spine and the pelvis.

In order for the spine to adopt its natural curvature in the upright position, the pelvis has to be in the neutral plane and this is best achieved when in the standing position (Fig. 25.16). When seated, tension on the hamstrings and general relaxation lead to posterior tilting of the pelvis, flattening of the lumbar curve and a generally slumped posture (Fig. 25.17). There are seating systems designed to overcome this such as the Balans or Mandal type of seating, where the user sits with slightly extended hips to relax the hamstring tension. This allows the pelvis to adopt the neutral position more easily (Fig. 25.18) but does not induce it. It is therefore likely that handicapped children will required a lot more support than the traditional kneeling seat provides, and straddle or saddle type seating should be evaluated (Stewart & McQuilton 1987, Pope et al 1988).

In 'right-angled' seating the traditional method of achieving the lumbar lordosis is to use a lumbar pad (Fig. 25.19). Since the spine can only adopt its natural curvature when the pelvis is in the neutral plane, the lumbar pad

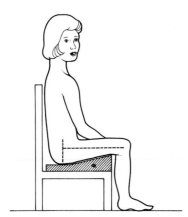

Fig. 25.14   Horizontal femora on ramped cushion.

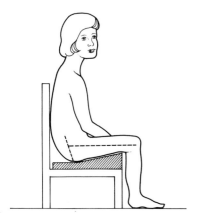

Fig. 25.15 Posteriorly tilted pelvis on ramp cushion.

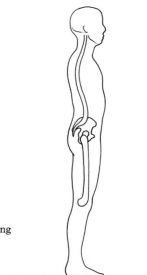

Fig. 25.16 Standing posture showing neutral position of pelvis and natural curvature of spine.

applies a force to the spine to use it as a lever to bring the pelvis into this position. This will cause high shear forces on the L5/S1 joint and can lead to a great deal of discomfort or low back pain.

In addition, the child with immature posture will not have developed a lumbar lordosis and the use of a lumbar pad may cause the child to extend against it or be pushed into a flexed posture.

It is more appropriate to apply the force direct to the pelvis by the use of a sacral pad (Mulcahy & Pountney 1986), which extends no higher than

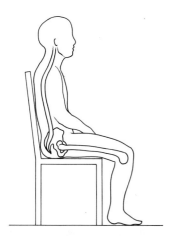

Fig. 25.17 Sitting posture showing posteriorly tilted pelvis and flattening of the lumbar curve.

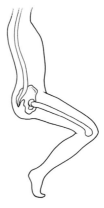

Fig. 25.18 Sketch of posture adopted on a Balans or Mandal type of seat.

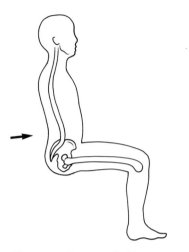

Fig. 25.19   Force applied by lumbar pad in sitting.

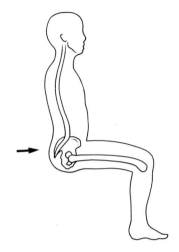

Fig. 25.20   Force applied by sacral pad in sitting.

the L5/S1 joint and is placed across the width of the pelvis at the back of the seat (Fig. 25.20). The sacral pad serves two purposes:

- It applies a force to the posterior aspect of the pelvis to bring it into the neutral plane.
- It compensates for the difference between the anteroposterior dimensions of the pelvis and the trunk.

The sacral pad should be curved, as should the backrest of the seat to which it is fitted, so that it more appropriately aligns with the natural body contours to avoid point or line contact with the spine, which will occur if the backrest or sacral pad is flat. The thickness of the sacral pad should be related to the difference in the anteroposterior dimensions of the trunk and pelvis in the upright posture.

If the sacral pad is used on its own with the ramped cushion, there is still a tendency for a child to slide his bottom forward and adopt a sacral sitting posture. A pelvic strap pulling back and down at 45° is an essential part of any seating system but it is unlikely to prevent the posterior tilting of the pelvis. As the pelvis begins to rotate into a posteriorly tilted position, the posterior iliac spines are in contact with the sacral pad and cannot move backwards (Fig. 25.21). The ischial tuberosities must therefore move forwards and the pelvis tends to move in an arc. In so doing, the anterior superior iliac spines move down and forward causing the pelvic strap to ride up and back onto the waist. The pelvic strap cannot therefore prevent this rotation without exerting excessive, intolerable force.

The solution is to apply an equal but opposite force to the pelvis so that a torque is applied to resist the rotation. This is achieved through a kneeblock, which pushes posteriorly along the femur to the hip joint. The

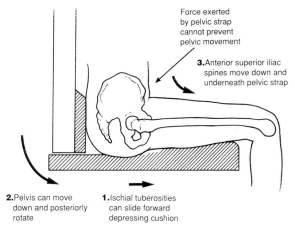

Fig. 25.21 Movement of the pelvis around the pelvic strap in sitting.

hip joint lies below the top of the posterior iliac spine, and this arrangement of forces applies a restoring torque to the pelvis to maintain it in the neutral position (Fig. 25.22).

The sacral pad, kneeblock, ramp cushion, correct height footplates and the pelvic strap act together as a total system to stabilise the lower part of the body and achieve anchoring of the pelvis on the seat surface. (Fig. 25.23) With this arrangement the child is able to function with the top half of his body, which can begin to act in a dissociated manner; that is,

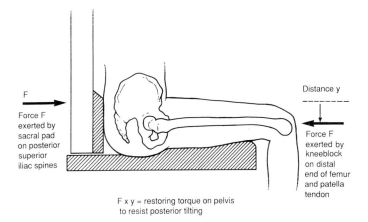

Fig. 25.22 Knee block and sacral pad restoring torque on pelvis. Note: the more posteriorly tilted the pelvis is, the more distance y is reduced and force F is high. As the pelvis reaches the neutral position, so y reaches a maximum value and force F is minimum. Height of sacral pad, length of seat and position of knee block must be correct and frequently reviewed to achieve the desired result and avoid high forces on the pelvis and knees.

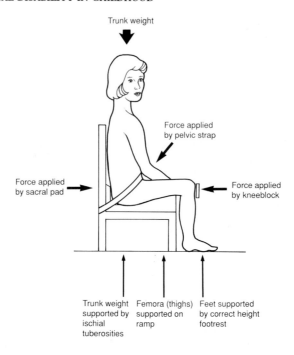

Trunk weight

Force applied
by pelvic strap

Force applied
by sacral pad

Force applied
by kneeblock

Trunk weight
supported by
ischial
tuberosities

Femora (thighs)
supported on
ramp

Feet supported
by correct height
footrest

Fig. 25.23   Forces to stabilise the lower part of the body.

it is learning to adjust over an anchored base. This encourages improved sitting ability and function. The degree of postural support required in this type of seating system to control the trunk is often a great deal less than would otherwise be required. For instance, it is possible to correct a mild, postural scoliosis with correct pelvic stability without any corrective forces being applied to the spine itself.

The force arrangement described and illustrated is that which is adopted for the Chailey Adaptaseat (Mulcahy et al 1988) and its successor, the CAPS II, and is the basis of many other seating systems supplied from Chailey Heritage. These biomechanical principles are also now applied elsewhere to many different seating designs. One of the most important aspects is the ability to adjust the seat length easily to allow frequent reviews during the first few days and weeks of use as the posture improves and the pelvis gradually adopts the neutral position.

It is unlikely that a child with cerebral palsy or similar condition will be able to tolerate positioning of the pelvis in neutral when sitting in the seat for the first time. As the child gets used to the seat, the position of the pelvis will improve towards the neutral plane. If the seat length cannot be shortened to accommodate this, a sacral sitting posture will continue and any further advantages of the seat will then be lost. By shortening the seat length, the gentle clamp exerted by the sacral pad and the kneeblock will be maintained and the pelvis will be brought progressively to the neutral position. Once in this position, normal development of the spine and the upright posture should follow.

Another application of the kneeblock is to correct asymmetrical postures and potential deformities such as the windswept hip posture (Fig. 25. 24a). The kneeblock arrangement can be used to push the abducted hip and pelvis against the sacral pad to derotate the windswept position. The previously adducted hip is then abducted to reduce the danger of dislocation (Fig. 25. 24b). If this previously adducted hip has already dislocated, great care has to be exercised in the degree of abduction that can be achieved. *No posterior force should be applied to a hip that is suspected of not being fully covered by the acetabulum, or which is already dislocated.*

Once stabilisation of the lower part of the body has been achieved, trunk support can be applied to correct asymmetry or scoliosis. It is essential that the support pads are capable of being aligned with the body contours so that the force can be applied along the line of the rib to the spine (Fig. 25.25). If this is not possible, then the pads will be very uncomfortable to the user and the corrective forces that can be applied will be severely limited.

It should be noted that if support or correction of scoliosis is the primary requirement it cannot be achieved by stabilisation of the pelvis alone. A spinal orthosis should be prescribed, before fitting the seat. Care has to be taken that the thoraco-lumbo-sacral-orthosis (TLSO) is sufficiently relieved over the anterior aspect of the iliac spine to allow the hips to be flexed to 90°. If this is not possible whilst maintaining the corrective forces of the orthosis, then a compromise must be reached on the degree of hip flexion that can be achieved and the ramp of the cushion modified accordingly. The action and position of the kneeblock will also require careful assessment.

Seating for different abilities

Children with sitting ability from levels 1 to 3 have poor postural ability. Without seating support they remain physically dependent and may even be unable to observe what is going on around them. When a seating system is used it is particularly important that the environment is adjusted to account for the child's position in space, i.e. the school work, the television or the visual display unit is positioned to allow for the line of vision.

Children with greater postural ability, i.e. level 4 and above, also require postural stability to encourage independence. This stability can be provided by ensuring their feet are supported at the correct height and by providing an orthogonal base (a horizontal seat base, ramped cushion, sacral pad and curved but upright backrest as in the Chailey Adaptaseat). This allows work and rest positions for the child. The dimensions of the seat cushion and sacral pad are critical, as wrong sizes may induce sacral sitting. The cushion is also secured, as a sliding cushion can induce a sacral sitting posture. Work heights are also considered along with the child's seating needs.

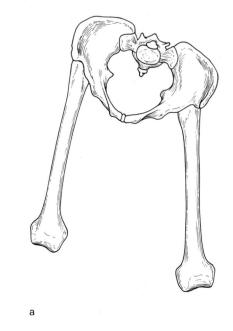

a

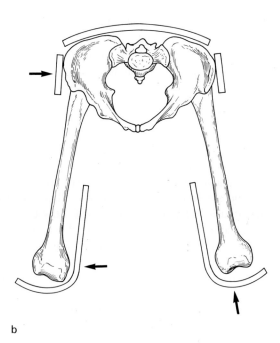

b

Fig. 25.24   Windswept hips and the correction applied by the knee block, sacral pad and lateral pelvic pads.

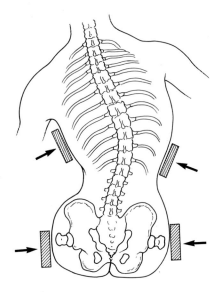

Fig. 25.25 Trunk support applied along the line of the ribs through pads aligned with the body contours.

Sitting ability level 1: the unplaceable child

When a child cannot easily be placed in a sitting position, this is recorded as a positive level of ability because it defines a major need for treatment and postural support. By definition the child cannot achieve or maintain a sitting posture, that is, he cannot anchor his bottom or dissociate his upper trunk from his lower trunk. Prescriptive seating must provide some postural fixation for him with particular emphasis on stabilising the pelvis. Such stability can be provided in a right-angled seat incorporating a ramped cushion, sacral pad, pelvic strap and curved backrest. An upright position with kneeblock to assist anteroposterior fixation should be introduced as soon as possible.

If a child remains at this low level of ability, he will become increasingly difficult to handle as he reaches adolescence and adulthood. It is therefore important that this child experiences frequent handling and changes of position if he is ever to improve his overall physical ability and become more manageable. Posture is dynamic and it is important to consider some alternative ways of introducing upright posture with symmetrical weightbearing. Pope (1985a, b) has had success with the adult population at the Royal Hospital and Home, Putney, in simulating the posture adopted by motorcyclists. This was achieved by stabilising the pelvis using a scooter saddle with kneeblock combination and supporting the trunk forwards over that base. Stewart & McQuilton (1987) have also shown preference for this type of posture for the lower ability child. The 'Symmetrikit' chair can also be a useful alternative seating support, particularly as its components can be varied to also offer comfortable and corrective support in the lying position. (The Symmetrikit chair is supplied by Symmetrikit Ltd, The Sherratts, School Lane, Tamworth Staffs B78 3AD.) If a child cannot achieve a symmetrical lying posture, he will not be easy to place or to manage in the sitting position.

Sitting ability level 2: the child who is placeable but not able to maintain position

This child will need a very supportive seat in which he can maintain an upright sitting posture. His pelvis needs to be supported symmetrically in a neutral position. Stability of the pelvis can be provided in the orthogonal base described in Figure 25.23; that is, anteroposterior control of the pelvis using a ramped cushion with sacral pad, kneeblock/pommel, pelvic strap and foot support. The seat needs to be horizontal.

In order to help the child learn to maintain an upright posture, trunk support—including anterior support—should be adjustable to provide stabilisation of the shoulder girdle. Lateral trunk support should align with the chest contours and a thoracic strap can give additional trunk security. A tray and grab bar at elbow height complement this posture, and arm gaiters can also assist the child.

Sitting ability level 3: the child who can maintain sitting balance but cannot move

This child is at borderline total dependency level. Although he may be able to forward prop, he would be totally dependent on his hands to maintain his sitting balance.

Seating for the level 3 child needs to provide adequate support to allow him to participate in life. A stable, symmetrical sitting base needs to be provided as described in level 2 above. From the forward position, the child should be able to regain an upright sitting posture and lateral supports should be spaced appropriately to facilitate this. Postural support needs to be varied throughout the day, limiting the use of a headrest and thoracic strap to when the child is driving a power chair or when he is in a vehicle.

Sitting ability level 4: the child who can maintain his sitting balance, move within his sitting base and recover sitting balance.

This child still has an immature, rounded spinal posture and he will not have adequate pelvic stability upon which to adjust his trunk and raise his arms to shoulder level. He cannot counterpoise efficiently and, in order to reach out to one side, this child will reach forward and down or might adjust his entire sitting base by swinging his legs to one side, thereby keeping his reaching arm over his sitting base. The most important feature of prescriptive seating for the level 4 child is a stable sitting base upon which he can feel secure enough to achieve a straight back posture and upper limb movement. A pommel that follows the contours of the medial aspect of the thighs as far as the femoral condyle may be necessary to widen the sitting base.

Sitting ability level 5: the child who can maintain his sitting balance, reach out from his sitting base and recover balance

It is important that this child has stability of his entire sitting base, which can be provided with the orthogonal base. His feet should be on the floor, if possible, to encourage him to reach further out from his base and eventually acquire the ability to transfer out of his seat. His working height is probably also a critical prop to his independence.

The child will probably find it easier to counterpoise to one side than the other and may initially need lateral support to allow side propping to either side, or a pommel as described in level 4. Armrests should be removable but may be needed for the child's security when he is mobile in his seat; for example, when being pushed in a manual wheelchair or driving a powered chair.

Sitting ability level 6: the child who can get out of his seat independently but cannot retain or attain sitting

A child who can get out of his seat by adjusting his trunk weight forwards or sideways over his sitting base will need a stable sitting base upon which he can develop a more mature sitting posture and from which he can transfer. An orthogonal base as described above can provide this. Ideally his feet should be on the floor to assist transfers and desk height needs to be appropriate for his manual and visual abilities, as well as to assist him reaching out of base and transferring.

Sitting ability level 7: the child who can retain or attain sitting

This child, although physically able, is not a normal child and is probably still learning to walk. His independence may still depend upon the height and depth of his seat, and on his work height. His seat will need to be stable and to have a rest position. He will need to be able to do up (as well as undo) his straps.

Orientation of a seat

It has been established that a few degrees of recline or tilt of a seating system can have a considerable effect on a child's posture and physical ability, delaying the acquisition of independent sitting. A *reclined seat* has only the backrest angled backwards, whereas a *tilted seat* is totally angled backwards. This, of course, has implications when fitting seating systems to wheelchairs, most of which have sloping seats that tilt a seating system. A levelling board may be fitted to a standard wheelchair to hold the seat and its occupant in the upright position. This will not, however, overcome the difficulty of driving a powered wheelchair up inclines. The reclined or titled posture may have the following effects:

1. It can promote extensor thrust as confirmed by EMG studies, which showed a significant increase in tone of both back extensors and hip adductors (Nwaobi 1986).

2. Hands become positioned in 'high guard', which is not a practical position for use—upper extremities cannot function with maximum efficiency (Nwaobi 1987).

3. Children with motor handicap feel that they are falling and often try to counteract this feeling by coming forward, (Hare 1987). This is often interpreted as flopping forwards and the child is given further restraints or is reclined or tilted further to stop this. For a child with poor protective reactions, this is not perceived as a position of comfort (Motloch 1977).

4. It alters the line of vision so that the child is looking upwards rather than horizontally (Nwaobi 1986).

5. It is difficult to eat and the risk of choking is also increased. Swallowing is neurologically a flexor activity (Guymer 1986, Siebens & Linden 1985).

6. A normal infant develops his ability to recover his sitting balance from a forward prop position before developing the ability to side prop and then returning to balanced sitting from a reclined position (Illingworth 1974).

7. An investigation into the effect of orientation upon cognitive ability showed that the tilted position had no significant effect on simple tasks but complex cognitive tasks were performed better in an upright position (Green 1987).

For the more able child, therapists may want to try seating solutions that have been developed for normal people suffering from back pain, such as forward sloping seats with or without knee pads (Mandal 1984). It is important, however, to realise that normal people can adopt an upright posture with lordosis. In providing a similar solution for the level 7 child, it is necessary to maintain his ability to get into the seat himself, and the seat may therefore need modification. When used for physically handicapped children, this type of seat will only facilitate the correct spinal posture if the child has the physical ability to attain it. The seat does not induce a lordotic posture if the child has not yet developed it.

STANDING

The standing position should be functional, i.e. the child must be able to undertake activities such as cooking, washing, use of switches, etc. A table or tray at the correct height should therefore be provided to encourage hand function and hand–eye coordination. Without a work surface a child will often hang over the front support of the standing frame.

Upright standing frames help to provide a dynamic posture for children who may soon be starting to walk. Prone boards or prone standing frames are less desirable because the child will not experience the desired orientation in space. If upright standing frames are unsuitable, however, prone standing frames may be the only alternative, but adaptations may be necessary according to each child's needs.

To assess the suitability of any equipment, the child will need a trial period of use. It is essential that the prescribers familiarise themselves with the wide range of equipment that is available; most manufacturers will respond to suggestions for improvement of their equipment and may carry out individual adaptations.

WALKING

Independent walking will only be possible once the skills of lying, sitting and standing independently are mastered. Many children who walk independently without aids do so using a variety of gaits to compensate for their disabilities. Such gaits may lead to deformity and painful joints in the future and careful attention should be paid to abnormal joint motion. Where possible, gait should be normalised (e.g. by the use of orthotics— see Ch. 23) to prevent contractures, although care should be taken not to decrease a child's independence and a compromise is likely.

Some children will be able to stand and walk with the assistance of walking aids ranging from a stick to adult assistance. Again, much care must be taken to encourage a normal reciprocal gait with a view to achieving independence and preventing the development of deformities. Walking aids that allow the child to push with the upper body and drag his feet behind are not recommended. The support that walking aids provide ranges from very supportive, including forward chest support with a grab bar for hands (Fig. 25.26), to very little for more able children in more upright positions using forearm and/or hand support only. Again a trial period of use of the equipment should be allowed at home and school to assess the practicalities of use and the degree of independence it allows the child.

To be able to walk is a desirable objective but if walking is slow and laborious it will only be practical for short periods and may not be possible during a child's busy school day. Other forms of mobility should then be considered.

MONITORING THE PERFORMANCE OF EQUIPMENT

It is important to monitor the effect of equipment on the child's ability using assessments of levels of ability and measures such as the Goldsmith Index for windswept hip deformity developed in Tamworth, Staffordshire. His postural ability should be better in his equipment than out of it. Additional support may be needed for some activities, e.g. driving a powered

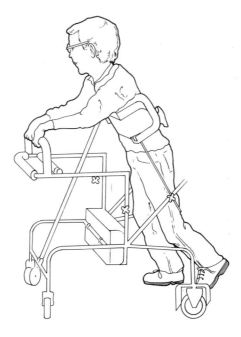

Fig. 25.26 Supportive walking aid providing chest support, a grab rail and additional pad to limit step length.

chair, when assistance is required to allow postural adjustment to the movement of the chair and joystick. At other times, reduced support may provide the child with the opportunity to contribute actively to his postural control.

Polaroid pictures and videos can assist with the monitoring of the effect of equipment upon the child, and the levels of ability can provide a written record of achievement.

DEFORMITY

Postural deformity in the physically handicapped child can lead to increasing discomfort and loss of function, including reduced lung and cardiac function, and problems with pressure distribution. We believe that long-term correct positioning can prevent the onset and progression of deformity. Although the mechanism of postural deformity is not fully understood, its sequence can be observed. The factors which appear to be important are immobility, growth and gravity.

In a child who does not achieve sitting balance, the deformities tend to progress in the lying position. The child takes up a progressively flattened appearance anteroposteriorly, with plagiocephaly, scoliosis, rib asymmetry, pelvic tilt and windsweeping of the legs. This windswept deformity can be assessed and measured using the Goldsmith Index. The upper limbs show reversed deformity with one arm externally rotated, and the other internally rotated and flexed at all joints. X-rays show that the acetabulum of the adducted hip fails to develop normally, with increasing subluxation and eventual dislocation of the hip.

Postural deformity can be disguised when the child sits in an ill-fitting chair (Scrutton 1978). Pope (1985a) described a population of physically handicapped adults with poor trunk stability, with one of two types of postural instability in sitting: (1) a characteristic C-shape; and (2) with the body arched backwards from coccyx to vertex. Sliding forward out of the seat is common to both postures adopted and the reclined body is subjected to a horizontal component of force acting to push the body in the direction of that force. Even if there is no movement at the interface, considerable deformation of subcutaneous tissues occurs and internal stresses are created resulting in damage and breakdown. The positive neurological signs of postural disorders can be exaggerated by imbalance (Traub et al 1980, Hare 1985, personal communication). The C-shaped and arched backwards postures described above result from instability and are therefore unbalanced in a situation which may correctly be considered to compound the neurological impairment further (Pope 1985a, Pope et al 1988). It is valid to consider that the converse is true, i.e. that a balanced, stable posture, produced by correct positioning, can reduce the progression of deformity.

The neurological aspects of the defective postural mechanism must be considered in addition to the effects of immobility, imbalance and gravity. Fixed deformity arises from postures produced by the forces of muscle power and gravity, compounded by the child remaining in static positions (Scrutton 1978). It has been postulated that the mechanisms of fixed deformity include abnormal disparity in muscle power in opposing muscle groups (Sharrard 1971) and further suggested that growth adapts in order to maintain the abnormal ratio of muscle length (Scrutton & Gilbertson 1975). It is the failure of the muscle to be put under normal loads, producing secondary failure of the growth of the muscle, which produces many fixed deformities (Brown 1985). This is important, as it suggests that it is not the brain damage which causes the deformity, but immobility or weakness of the antagonist. The latter—in normal postural reactions—co-contracts, so there is no muscle imbalance across the joint. Studies of deformities in children paralysed by poliomyelitis demonstrated that when there was muscle imbalance across the joint, it was always the normal and not the paralysed muscle that developed the contracture (Sharrard 1971).

Muscle contracture in cerebral palsy occurs because of a shortened muscle, not a fibrosed one (Bax & Brown 1985). There is a decreased number of sarcomeres, and a concomitant reduction in extensibility. Muscle growth control appears to be intact in cerebral palsy and contracture appears to be a response of the muscle to prolonged abnormal functioning. It has been demonstrated that no progressive contracture results when the soleus muscle was stretched for at least 6 hours per day, but progressive contracture results when the stretching time was as short as 2 hours (Tardieu et al 1988).

Our work on normal postural development before sitting confirms asymmetry in both prone and supine until lying ability level 3. In the normal infant of lying ability level 2, asymmetry is emphasised when he tries to turn his head. At this level of ability a head turn is accompanied by a total body turn in the opposite direction. The resultant posture resembles that seen in the 'squint baby syndrome' (Fulford & Brown 1976), and also in the individual with cerebral palsy and windswept deformities. The asymmetries decrease in normal children once they achieve sitting balance and rotation and increasing mobility. Increase in deformity is seen in immobile, severely handicapped individuals with cerebral palsy (Bell 1987). The posture seen at level 2 lying ability could well be the precursor to the development of deformities if the child does not progress to the symmetry of level 3 lying ability.

POSTURAL MANAGEMENT FOR CHILDREN WITH DEFORMITIES

The principles of achieving postural stability must be followed to provide the postural control required by children with deformities. Some improvements in posture can be expected as stability is achieved and some relaxation of the overriding muscle spasticity results. These improvements can be assessed and measured using the Goldsmith Index and other orthopaedic and clinical measures. The postural management equipment will probably be asymmetrical and adjustment of the support surfaces is essential during the initial fitting and first few days of use to achieve the control required and gradually produce the required support. Thereafter adjustment may not be as important although any changes in the child must be accommodated by adjustments of the equipment if improvements and comfort are to be maintained.

Accommodation and support for severe leg length discrepancy, asymmetrical seat height and severe windswept or rotated trunk postures are likely to be a requirement in most cases. Protection of a severe bony prominence may also be a consideration.

TISSUE TRAUMA

Tissue trauma or pressure sores will occur whenever excessive force, sufficient to cause tissue deformation, is applied to the skin for a prolonged period of time. Tissue trauma or damage results from the occlusion of the capillary blood supply and/or restriction of lymphatic drainage. Both the force and time of application of the force that can cause tissue damage will be different for different individuals and different parts of the anatomy. Tissue deformation will be caused by a combination of forces, mainly pressure and shear force, which often coexist. Pressure is caused when body weight is supported on a surface, and the degree of pressure is dependent on the body weight and the size of the area that supports it. Hence the sitting posture in which the body weight is supported by the buttocks, the thighs and the soles of the feet will create higher pressures than the lying posture, where the whole of the posterior, anterior or lateral aspects of the body support the body weight. In any posture there will be higher pressures over bony prominences than other areas that have a thicker covering of flesh or muscle.

Shear forces are created whenever friction forces are used to retain a person in a specific posture, or when someone is sliding out of position or is being moved by sliding or when a high pressure exists immediately adjacent to a low pressure, as when sitting on a slatted seat or plinth. Hence sitting up in bed, which usually results in a reclined posture, creates pressure and shear forces on the buttocks, the sacrum and the heels which are being used to prevent the reclined person from sliding down the bed. This is probably the quickest way to develop tissue trauma and should be avoided unless proper support and postural control can be provided to overcome the shear forces and distribute the pressures.

Temperature and humidity also play an important part: wet skin is very much weaker than dry skin and will therefore be more vulnerable to damage (Stewart et al 1980). An increase in skin temperature will result in an increase in metabolism of the tissues. This will require an increase in blood flow to maintain the higher rate of metabolism, and also an increase in lymphatic drainage to remove the build-up of waste products. If the tissues are sufficiently deformed to resist an increase in the blood flow and/or the lymphatic drainage, then the increase in metabolism is compromised and tissue damage or ischaemia can begin. The temperature rise alone can therefore be a major contributory factor of tissue trauma (Fisher et al 1978). A reduction in skin temperature may result in an increase in relative humidity at the skin surface due to condensation of atmospheric or perspiration vapour, and the inter-relationship between temperature and humidity requires a compromise in the choice of suitable materials and designs of postural support equipment.

Very tight or very loose, and hence creased, clothing and/or upholstery covers have a significant effect on the performance of any support system and may be the cause of tissue damage. Badges, clothing seams and contents of pockets can interfere with pressure distributing properties of support surfaces, and should be considered when assessing problems and solutions or choosing clothes.

There are no devices that are currently available for routine use in a busy clinic to enable shear forces, skin temperature or humidity to be easily measured, and some knowledge of how to control these factors is required by those who are prescribing and manufacturing solutions to tissue trauma problems. There are, however, pressure transducers that are commercially available; these give an indication of the pressure being exerted on the tissues but need careful placement to obtain realistic values. Pressure transducers should be used by all who are responsible for the provision of cushions and postural management equipment, particularly seating systems.

Since pressure is capable of being measured, it can also be modified; the problems and solutions of tissue trauma can be conveniently divided into (1) pressure distribution; (2) pressure redistribution; and (3) pressure relief.

Pressure distribution

In order to avoid tissue deformation it is desirable that the necessary forces to support a child in the sitting position are well distributed over the available area of support, thus keeping pressures to a minimum. This is usually achieved by the provision of a pressure-distributing cushion which may be constructed from foam, gel, or a combination of these and other pressure-distributing mediums. Developments are frequently bringing new cushions to the marketplace and it would be inappropriate to identify specific cushions here. The publications *Choosing the best cushion*, published by RADAR, and *Wheelchair cushions* (Summary Report, 2nd edn), published by the Department of Health Disability Equipment Assessment Programme, provide a comprehensive guide to the majority of the cushions that are available. It may, however, be helpful to discuss some of the properties of different materials in relation to temperature, humidity and pressure distribution.

All materials used in postural control equipment have to comply with the Statutory Instrument 1324, Fire and Furnishings (Fire Safety) Regulations 1988, and care must be taken by those who supply cushions or cushion covers infrequently, since everyone has a legal responsibility to comply with this legislation.

Combustion-modified foam fatigues with use; all cushions need to be checked for fatigue every 2–3 months, or more frequently for heavy or bony individuals. Fatigue is detected by permanent indentations in the cushion surface, which coincide with the bony prominences of the child using them. The foam may be looking 'tired' and be adopting the general shape of the user rather than the original shape supplied. As well as being permanently deformed, the resilience or 'springiness' of the material will also be reduced and therefore the pressure distributing properties may be compromised. Foam cushions should always be replaced as soon as fatigue is detected. A quick test of resilience is to manually press the cushion over the top surface to detect whether it is softer in the area of the bony prominences than it is elsewhere. Some cushions are designed to exhibit such properties when new to achieve pressure redistribution or pressure relief and care is required when deciding whether the foam is fatigued or not.

It is desirable that two-way stretch, water vapour permeable covers are used for combustion-modified foam in order not to mask the carefully selected pressure-distributing properties of the underlying material, and also to avoid accumulation of perspiration. If waterproof materials are required, then an extra cover should be used over the top of a waterproof cover to allow perspiration to be wicked away for evaporation. A cotton based material or sheepskin type material should achieve this, provided it complies with S.I. 1324. Inelastic covers will mask the ability of foam to conform to anatomical shapes and will increase both pressure and shear forces, creating a surface that resembles the canvas of a basic wheelchair. In the particular case of waterproof materials such as p.v.c., frequent soaking and drying, together with environmental ageing will result in hard and creased surfaces that could cause tissue deformation and hence tissue trauma.

Gel, as a pressure-distributing medium, does not generally have a significant effect on skin temperature (Stewart et al 1980, Fisher et al 1978) but the waterproof envelope required to enclose the gel often increases the relative humidity at the skin surface. This may be overcome by using additional appropriate covers such as two-way stretch, absorbent materials. Water absorbs more heat and conducts it better than gel; therefore water based cushions will have more of a cooling effect on the skin than gel cushions. As with gel cushions, the waterproof cover tends to increase the relative humidity at the skin surface, and the cooling effect of the water may further increase the humidity, resulting in a damp environment for the skin and consequent vulnerability to damage. Two-way stretch, water-absorbent, insulating covers may overcome this provided they do not mask the pressure-distributing properties of the cushion.

Air is also often used as a support medium. It is an insulator and may, therefore, raise skin temperature. The air-tight membrane in which the air is contained will also be impermeable to water vapour, which could lead to accumulation of perspiration and damp skin. The use of appropriate covers as described above may overcome this.

Cushions or mattresses using air as a support medium are either static or dynamic. Static cushions contain a reservoir of air that is distributed to maximise the contact surface with the body and thereby reduce the support pressures. A typical example of a static air cushion is the Roho balloon cushion, which is also efficient at reducing shear forces, since each of the individual balloons is able to follow body movements across the cushion. Active cushions are those that employ the rippling technique whereby alternate tubes or rows of balloons are inflated whilst others are deflated to provide high pressures for short periods of time. Ripple cushions, however, may not be as effective as ripple mattresses, since the support area on a cushion is much less than that on a mattress with consequently much higher pressures. The ischial tuberosities of a bony person may not be relieved of pressure, since they may protrude between the inflated tubes to the base of the cushion on the wheelchair canvas. It may be desirable to use the ripple cushion on top of a foam cushion to reduce this pressure.

Particulate or bead filled cushions are not very suitable for children who do not possess sensation, since these cushions rely on both body movement to distribute the contents away from high pressure areas and sufficient sensation to determine that this movement has been successful. Without a successful distribution of beads, very high localised pressures may result. Asymmetrical postures may also result from poorly distributed contents. Cushions that contain expanded polystyrene beads may cause an increase in skin temperature as a result of the insulating properties of expanded polystyrene. The beads can be contained in a water vapour permeable cover, which may help to reduce the accumulation of moisture.

Many cushions comprise a combination of the above materials. The performance of any cushion can be compromised by the use of an inappropriate cover. No cushion is able to obviate the need for frequent lift-ups since it is not possible to reduce the pressure over the area of support in the seated position to below capillary or lymphatic drainage pressures. It should therefore be stressed to all users of cushions that, although the cushion has been very carefully assessed and prescribed, lift-ups are required. For many children, this will require frequent reminders.

Pressure redistribution and pressure relief

These two subheadings are grouped together because the techniques used to construct the appropriate support surface are very similar. The aim is to redistribute pressures away from the vulnerable areas such as the coccyx, sacrum and ischial tuberosities to the more tolerant areas such as the thighs and subtrochanteric shelf. This is achieved by shaping a block of foam to the bony structure of the patient or combining different grades of foam to relieve pressure under bony prominences. Although due consideration should be given to the large range of pressure thresholds that exist from one individual to another, the following pressures have been established as guidelines (Motloch et al 1979):

Posterior thighs	80–100 mmHg
Subtrochanteric shelf	60 mmHg
Ischial tuberosities	40 mmHg
Coccyx/sacrum	14 mmHg

Although construction details vary, the shape of the cushion required to achieve this pressure redistribution is shown schematically in Figure 25.27. In order to avoid shear forces as a result of friction it is important that the support surfaces are constructed to provide postural stability and control as well as pressure redistribution. When used in a wheelchair, therefore, the cushion is either placed on top of a wooden board or the undersurface is curved to fit into the wheelchair canvas hammock and possibly tapered to overcome the reclined angle of the wheelchair seat canvas.

When a child has a scoliosis, a pelvic tilt will invariably also be present even if spinal bracing is worn. The same techniques for cushion construc-

Symmetrical profiled
surface to create
pressure redistribution
values, postural control
and stabilisation

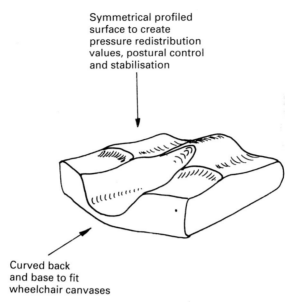

Curved back
and base to fit
wheelchair canvases

Fig. 25.27 Symmetrical contoured cushion shown schematically.

tion may be used to accommodate this pelvic obliquity but the excavated
shape will not be symmetrical (Fig. 25.28).

As a preventive device, the guideline pressures indicated above are used,
but once a sore has developed as a result of the pelvic tilt the pressure on
the area of damaged tissue is reduced to zero by ensuring that there is
clearance between the cushion and the user at this point.

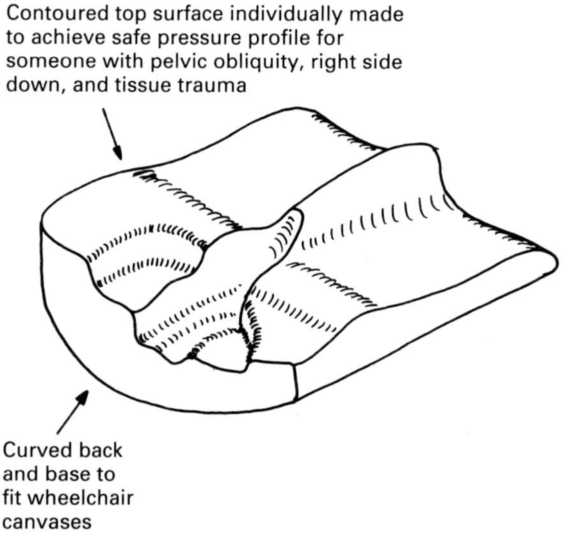

Contoured top surface individually made
to achieve safe pressure profile for
someone with pelvic obliquity, right side
down, and tissue trauma

Curved back
and base to
fit wheelchair
canvases

Fig. 25.28 Asymmetric contoured cushion shown schematically.

The simple act of elevating legs on wheelchair elevating leg-rests or a wooden wheelchair board may lead to excessive pressure or shear on the sacrum. It will be necessary to assess the need for a contoured cushion to prevent tissue damage in this area. It is essential that two-way stretch materials are used for covering contoured cushions in order that the pressure profiles so carefully established on the uncovered cushion are not altered.

Since pressure measurements can only give an indication of the suitability of any cushion design it is essential that skin inspection is used to establish that the choice of design is correct. No wheelchair cushion can distribute seating pressures sufficiently to reduce them to a tolerable level over a long period of time and it is therefore essential that all wheelchair users are encouraged to perform regular lift-ups to relieve pressures completely. The use of a firm foam or highly viscous material will be of help, since the slow response to movements results in frequent pressure relief as the user goes about daily tasks. If pressure relief cannot be obtained on a regular basis, a time limit for sitting must be established, based on pressure measurements and skin inspection.

WHEELCHAIRS

Many physically handicapped children need to use a wheelchair. A wheelchair is merely a means of mobility for those who cannot walk. Whilst it is an essential piece of equipment for those who need it, particularly for a young child who cannot be independently mobile to explore his environment, it should not be an initial or primary focus in the process of assessment of need. For example, no child should be expected to spend a long period of time (if any), sitting on the basic wheelchair support surfaces, which are usually of p.v.c. coated canvas. The prescription of an appropriate wheelchair—whether powered, occupant propelled or attendant propelled—should only be considered after the postural requirements of a child in the sitting position have been fully assessed, prescribed and supplied. A wheelchair is, after all, a 'chair on wheels', and the chair has to be correct for postural management before the wheels can be added.

The wheelchair that is finally prescribed must be able to safely and securely accommodate the postural support equipment supplied to the child without the need for modification of this equipment. The wheelchair may need to be larger than if the child had no equipment, and may need to be modified to accommodate the postural support equipment at the correct orientation, or to allow for the range of adjustments of the postural support equipment, or to provide the appropriate stability and safety.

PRESCRIPTION OF APPROPRIATE WHEELCHAIR

The wheelchair should look good, be easily manoeuvrable and not create a barrier between the child and his environment. The requirements of the family, of transportation and the size of the home are additional aspects that must be considered when choosing the correct wheelchair.

The child with inadequate postural control has particular difficulties in operating a self-propelled wheelchair. The movements required for propulsion and the momentum of the wheelchair cause postural disturbance and the child cannot then recover balance adequately to maintain his own stability or the chair's propulsion. The child will therefore be provided with a powered wheelchair and a joystick, switches or other interfaces to allow him to operate the chair. Whilst this will improve the child's independent mobility it does not inherently improve the child's physical ability.

A physically handicapped child's need for postural support may well increase if he is to react to the chair's momentum and maintain a balanced posture whilst driving. He needs to be sufficiently posturally secure to be able to maintain his balance to operate his controls and to compensate for the movement of the powered chair.

If a child needs postural support to maintain symmetrical weightbearing and posture, his controls will need to be positioned symmetrically: any asymmetrical positions of controls compound a child's preference for an asymmetrical posture. Complimentary, symmetrical postural control needs to be provided in order to prevent postural deformities occurring, e.g. a grab bar for the non-driving hand (or grab bars for both hands if using chin switches or other non-manual interfaces).

There is a wide range of wheelchairs available and more are regularly becoming available. Dual purpose indoor/outdoor powered chairs are also becoming available. Outdoor powered chairs are often heavier than usual due to larger batteries and motors and a more durable construction. They are also often larger to provide improved stability and are commonly fitted with lights and other auxiliary equipment. Dual purpose chairs, i.e. indoor/outdoor chairs, are often smaller than outdoor chairs but larger than indoor chairs. The dual purpose chair may therefore not perform as well outdoors and take up more room indoors; they also bring mud and other debris indoors. Care is therefore required when considering this type of wheelchair.

The wheelchair service has recently been reorganised and is now part of the National Health Service. There are resulting Regional and District variations in what is available and how it is supplied. A training package on assessment and prescription of wheelchairs has been produced by the Disablement Services Authority and is available to those with responsibility for these services. The centres and hospitals providing wheelchair and special seating services should be able to provide up-to-date information on the services available in each Health Region or District.

Wheelchairs and *Outdoor transport* are two publications produced by Mary Marlborough Lodge, Nuffied Orthopaedic Centre, Oxford, as part of the Equipment for the Disabled series. These are regularly updated and provide further, comprehensive and current information.

Acknowledgements

We wish to thank Action Research for their generous support for the research and development of the posture management programme.

The assessment procedure and prescription criteria are based on material previously published in the following paper:

Mulcahy C M, Pountney T E, Nelham R L, Green E M, Billington G D 1988 Adaptive seating for motor handicap: problems, a solution, assessment and prescription. British Journal of Occupational Therapy 51(10):347–352, and Physiotherapy 74(10):531–536.

Table 25.1 was previously published in Physiotherapy (Mulcahy & Green 1990).

Table 25.2 was previously published in the British Journal of Occupational Therapy, and the authors are grateful for permission to reproduce it here.

REFERENCES

Bax M C O, Brown J K 1985 Contractures and their therapy. Developmental Medicine and Child Neurology 27:423–424
Bell E J 1987 Management and prevention of certain deformities in cerebral palsy. Physiotherapy 73(7):368–370
Bell E J, Watson A 1985 The prevention of position deformity in cerebral palsy. Physiotherapy Practice 1(2):86–92
Brown K J 1985 Positional deformity in children with cerebral palsy. Physiotherapy Practice 1:37–41
Fearn T, Tutt P 1990 Prone lying night wedge for postural control. Physiotherapy 76(6):359–361
Fisher S V, Szymke T E, Apte S Y, Kosiak M 1978 Wheelchair cushion effect on skin temperature. Archives of Physical Medicine and Rehabilitation 59:68–72
Fulford G E, Brown J K 1976 Position as a cause of deformity in cerebral palsy. Developmental Medicine and Child Neurology 18:305–314
Green E M 1987 The effect of seating position on cognitive function in children with cerebral palsy. 59th Annual Meeting, British Paediatric Association abstract G158:108
Grillner S 1975 Locomotion in vertebrates: central mechanisms and reflex interaction. Physiological Reviews 55:247–304
Guymer A J 1986 Handling the patient with speech and swallowing problems. Physiotherapy 72(6):276–280
Hare N 1984 Ideas developed at Cheyne Centre 1969–1983. Friends of Cheyne Centre for Spastic Children, London
Hare N 1985 Personal communication
Hare N 1987 Children keep you thinking—interview with Dorothy Henham. Therapy Weekly (24 March): 6
Harrison A 1988 Spastic cerebral palsy—possible spinal interneuronal contributions. Developmental Medicine and Child Neurology 30:769–780
Harrison A, Kruze R 1987a Perturbation of a skilled action: 1. The responses of neurologically normal and cerebral palsied individuals. Human Movement Science 6: 37–65
Harrison A, Kruze R 1987b Perturbation of a skilled action: 2. Normalizing the responses of cerebral palsied individuals. Human Movement Science 6:133–159
Harrison P J, Jankowska E, Johannisson T 1983 Shared reflex pathways of group 1 afferents of different cat hind-limb muscles. Journal of Physiology 338: 113–128
Illingworth R S 1974 The development of the infant and young child: normal and abnormal. Churchill Livingstone, Edinburgh, p. 141
Mandal A C 1984 The correct height of school furniture. Physiotherapy 70(2): 48–53

Motloch W M 1977 Seating and positioning for the physically impaired. Orthotics and Prosthetics 31(2):11–21

Motloch W M, Pasillas R, Wright D, Ferdinand R, Le Blanc M A, Perkash I 1979 Seating systems for body support and prevention of tissue trauma. Progress Report II. Spinal Cord Injury Service, V A Hospital, Palo Alto, California

Mulcahy C M, Pountney T E 1986 The sacral pad—description of its clinical use in seating. Physiotherapy 72(9): 473–474

Mulcahy C M, Pountney T E 1987 Ramped cushion. British Journal of Occupational Therapy 50(3):97

Mulcahy C M, Pountney T E, Nelham R L, Green E M, Billington G D 1988 Adaptive seating for motor handicap: problems, a solution, assessment and prescription. British Journal of Occupational Therapy 51(10): 347–352, and Physiotherapy 74(10): 531–536

Nashner L M, Shumway-Cook A, Marin O 1983 Stance posture control in select groups of children with cerebral palsy: deficits in sensory organization and muscular co-ordination. Experimental Brain Research 49:393–409

Neilson P D, McCaughey J 1982 Self regulation of spasms and spasticity in cerebral palsy. Journal of Neurology, Neurosurgery and Psychiatry 45:320–330

Nelham R L 1985 Paediatric adaptive seating in the UK—present service and future developments. Adaptive Seating, proceedings of 1st International Symposium, Winnipeg, Manitoba

Nwaobi O M 1986 Effects of body orientation in space on tonic muscle activity of patients with cerebral palsy. Developmental Medicine and Child Neurology 28:41–44

Nwaobi O M 1987 Seating orientations and upper extremity function in children with cerebral palsy. Physical Therapy 67(8):1209–1212

Pope P M 1985a A study of instability in relation to posture in the wheelchair. Physiotherapy 71(3):124–129

Pope P M 1985b Proposals for the improvement of the unstable postural condition and some cautionary notes. Physiotherapy 71(3):129–131

Pope P M, Booth E, Gosling G 1988 The development of alternative seating and mobility systems. Physiotherapy Practice 4:78–93

Pountney T E, Mulcahy C M, Green E M 1990 Early development of postural control. Physiotherapy 76(12):799–802

Scrutton D R, Gilbertson M 1975 The physiotherapist's role in the treatment of cerebral palsy. In: Apley J(ed) Orthopaedic aspects of cerebral palsy Clinics in Developmental Medicine 52/53. Spastics International Medical Publications and William Heinemann Oxford

Scrutton D R 1978 Developmental deformity and the profoundly handicapped child. In: Apley J (ed) The Care of the Handicapped Child. William Heinemann, Oxford and Spastics International Medical Publications, 83–89

Sharrard W J W 1971 Paediatric orthopaedics and fractures. Blackwell Scientific Publications, Oxford

Shumway C 1986 Cerebral palsy—management. In: Cash's textbook of neurology for physiotherapists, 4th edn. Faber & Faber, London, p. 529–530

Siebens A A, Linden P 1985 Dynamic imaging for swallowing re-education. Gastrointestinal Radiology 10:251–253

Stewart P C, McQuilton G 1987 Straddle seating for the cerebral palsied child. British Journal of Occupational Therapy 50(4):136–138, and Physiotherapy 73(4):204–206

Stewart S F C, Palmieri V, Cochran G V B 1980 Wheelchair cushion effect on skin temperature, heat flux and relative humidity. Archives of Physical Medicine and Rehabilitation 61: 229–233

Tardieu C, Lespargot A, Tabary C, Bret M D 1988 For how long must the soleus muscle be stretched each day to prevent contracture? Developmental Medicine and Child Neurology 30(1): 3–10

Thelen E 1986 Treadmill-elicited stepping in 7-month infants. Child Development 57: 1498–1506

Thelen E, Cooke D W 1987 Relationship between newborn stepping and later walking: a new interpretation. Developmental Medicine and Child Neurology 29: 380–393

Thomas S S, Mazur J M, Wright N, Supan T 1989 Quantitative assessment of ankle foot orthoses for children with cerebral palsy. Developmental Medicine and Child Neurology, Supplement 59, vol 31(5): 7

Traub M M, Rothwell J C, Marsden C D 1980 Anticipatory postural reflexes in Parkinson's disease and other akinetic-rigid syndromes and in cerebellar ataxia. Brain 103: 393–412

Wiesel T N 1982 Postnatal development of the visual cortex and the influence of environment. Nature 299 (14 Oct 82): 583–591

Wolpaw J R 1985 Adaptive plasticity in the spinal stretch reflex: an accessible substrate of memory? Cellular and Molecular Neurobiology 5: 147–165

26. Augmentative communication

V. Moffat   A. Brown

Communication is among the most basic of human needs. The child with a physical handicap who is severely speech impaired may be unable to communicate by speech or gesture. He may be able at best to signal yes/no by nodding and shaking his head or smiling and frowning. His needs may be anticipated by parent or teacher, or the 'listener' may resort to a 'twenty questions' form of yes/no answer, which is exhausting for the child, time consuming for the questioner and frustrating for both.

Alternative methods of non-speech communication systems are being used by the severely speech-impaired to augment or supplement their speech. It is to be remembered that speech must always accompany any system, and that children are to be encouraged to vocalise or speak at all times.

ASSESSMENT

A multidisciplinary approach to assessment is essential, and often the child will need long-term assessment and training over a period of perhaps weeks rather than days to ensure that the most appropriate system is selected for his present needs; also some prediction and provision should be made for future requirements. (See Ch. 3 for further discussion on assessment procedures).

EARLY INTERVENTION

Communication is an exchange of information, feelings, needs and ideas between two or more individuals, and the young child learns to communicate by a process of interaction with his environment from birth. This communication can be achieved by a variety of means: body language, facial expression, eye gaze/pointing, reaching, pointing, vocalisation, gesture, sign language, pictures, symbols, and the written/printed word. Early intervention is therefore essential to look at the entire dynamics of interaction to influence the different environments of the child, e.g. home, school, clubs, and to prevent deviant patterns of communication from being established, e.g. passivity or learned helplessness.

451

DEVELOPING PREREQUISITE SKILLS

The most effective way to develop the necessary skills to acquire good communication patterns is to capitalise on the naturally occurring daily situations that will interest and motivate the child. Thus communication should not be limited to part of a therapy programme but be an ongoing process throughout the child's day (see Chs 1 and 6).

MOTIVATION

Motivation can be achieved by giving the child some control over his world. He should be allowed a choice, and have the opportunity to say 'no' or even to be naughty. He should be discouraged from becoming a passive watcher of the world (Moffat & Jolleff 1987).

DEVELOPMENTAL LEVELS

An understanding of the following levels of the child's development is necessary to encourage the skills needed for introducing an augmentative communication system or communication device:

- Attention control, both auditory and visual
- Imitation of gross and fine movements
- Symbolic development and play, including an understanding of cause and effect and the ability to imitate an activity
- Cognitive development. If the child is to be able to use a symbol system, he will need to:
  — Classify objects
  — Recognise pictures
  — Match picture to picture
  — Match picture to symbol
  — Match symbol to symbol
  — Additional skills to enhance system development
  — Colour recognition
  — Knowledge of size, spacing, direction and position
- Verbal comprehension
- Expressive language.

PHYSICAL ABILITY

Vision and hearing

Adequate visual acuity and perception is necessary to use a symbol system and hearing needs to be assessed to ensure that this does not affect language development (see Chs 4 and 5).

Seating and posture

The child needs to be posturally well-organised to maximise function (Carroll 1985) and may require a personalised seating system to achieve this (see Ch. 25).

Accessing skills

Assessment is needed of the child's physical capabilities for signing or accessing language boards, i.e. hand function; head, foot or eye control. This will include identifying a consistent and reliable movement that can be used for accessing, and looking at the range of movement possible to determine the amount and size of vocabulary display.

The selection of a suitable augmentative communication system will depend on the method of access. All but a few of the currently available electronic aids make use of one, or perhaps a combination, of three modes of user input. These are known as direct selection, scanning and encoding (Brown 1987).

Direct selection, by means of finger/fist pointing or the use of a headstick or light pointer, is the quickest and usually the most efficient method, but may be the most difficult for a child with a physical disability.

Scanning is the slowest method of access and requires a consistent, reliable movement of any part of the body to operate a switch. The switch activates a device that has a scanning light or cursor, and by pressing or releasing a switch the child can interrupt the scanning at an appropriate place to indicate his choices, which are displayed. Auditory scanning may be an easier option for children who are severely physically disabled and are unable to cope with the visual and motor demands necessary for visual scanning and simultaneous switch operation.

Encoding. The child may be able to use a code in order to make selection of a word or phrase. For example, by eye pointing to a number and letter for a grid reference, a word on a chart could be indicated. There are many ways of encoding; most require a reasonable degree of cognitive ability. The motor demands on a child vary widely and may be simple or complex.

Mobility

The ambulant child is often disadvantaged; his mobility will affect the portability of either an augmentative communication system display or device, since he will be unlikely to be able to use it while 'on the move'.

COMMUNICATION SYSTEMS

Communication systems show a developmental progression of cognitive function from recognising real objects to using the word or alphabet.

Signing systems

The young child will naturally use gesture and pantomime to communicate his wants before he is able to speak, e.g. pointing, reaching, hugging, and therefore the introduction of a signing system as an augmentative communication system to the severely speech impaired child may have hidden benefits. It may serve as a useful therapy technique for developing attention control, imitative skills and verbal comprehension. Signing may also be useful for children whose visual–perceptual problems make a symbol system inappropriate.

British Sign Language (BSL) is the naturally evolving language of the deaf population in Britain. It has its own grammar and word order so that signs have to be arranged into spoken word order and supplemented by finger spelling to be understood by the hearing population.

The Makaton Vocabulary was developed by Margaret Walker in the 1970s as a signing system for deaf adults with severe learning difficulties. The signs are taken from the 'British Sign Language' and consist of a specially selected vocabulary, considered to be most essential and useful in providing basic communication. It is structured in nine stages of increasing complexity following the normal developmental sequence of language concepts, and only key words are signed in spoken word order (Walker & Armfield 1982).

Paget–Gorman Signed Speech (PGSS). This system was devised by Sir Richard Paget in 1934 to help deaf people learn language. It is based on American Indian signs, of which each group of ideas has its own basic sign and each is further identified by additional gesture, e.g. 'animal' is a basic gesture, with the other hand adding further qualification to make a 'pig'.

All the grammatical features of English are included and signs are always accompanied by speech. There is a vocabulary of over 4000 words, which provides an accurate translation from speech or the written word, but the system requires good manual dexterity.

Cued speech was developed in 1965/6 as a tool to clarify spoken language for the profoundly deaf. Hand positions are used near the mouth during speech to provide detailed information to assist lip reading.

The manual alphabet. Finger spelling is a tool used by people who are deaf to support British Sign Language. Different finger positions are used to represent the 26 letters of the English alphabet. This system requires a high level of cognitive ability and motor coordination.

Morse code. Letters of the alphabet are encoded into a series of dots and dashes. This code could be used by severely physically disabled people who are able to perform two distinct movements to represent 'dots' and 'dashes', e.g. a single switch or a short eye blink for a dot and another switch or a long blink for a dash. A number of communication aids now provide for Morse code as an input option, but a high level of cognitive ability is needed on the part of the user.

Amer–Ind Gestural Code. This hand code, originally developed by the American Indians, is based on concepts, and 80% of the signs can be interpreted by the non-instructed viewer. It is not a language, having neither grammatical nor structural rules, and is determined by context.

Symbol systems

Symbols are sets of sensory (visual, auditory or tactile) images or signs that suggest or stand for something else by an association or simply by convention (Bennett 1987).

The symbols used reflect the cognitive development or visual acuity of the child, who will progress from conveying requests by indicating real objects to using symbolic toys, photographs, pictures or line drawings. The symbols can be used singly or displayed on language boards and are adapted easily to a variety of electronic displays or eye coding techniques.

Symbol systems can be used by both the child and the 'listener', as the word should normally be written above the symbol.

'Rebuses'. These are line drawings that visually represent objects, actions and attributes, and are usually readily recognisable. They can be used to communicate needs and ideas by indicating an individual symbol or sequence of symbols. Rebus systems include the following:

1. The standard Rebus glossary.

2. Makaton symbols—symbols for the Makaton vocabulary are based on developing vocabulary and can be used in conjunction with Makaton signs (Fig. 26.1).

3. Multi-meaning icons, as used with the Minspeak software in the 'Touch Talker' and 'Light Talker' (Fig. 26.2).

4. Pictogram Ideogram Communication (PICS) is a graphic symbol system based on language development of children. It has 400 symbols, which are semantically based and follow logical principles.

5. Picture Communication Symbols (PCS) provide over 700 clear line-drawings, which can be used for a wide variety of communication aids, environments and language training activities.

6. Sigsymbols are simple, bold outlines standing for a whole word. A Sigsymbol is either representational or conceptually linked with an established signing system, e.g. BSL.

'Blissymbols' enable more abstract and complex communication. The system originated from the work of Charles K. Bliss in 1949. Blissymbols are concept-related pictographs (they look like the things they represent) and ideographs (they represent ideas), and have the advantage that they are meaning-based and so can be used to expand language concepts. They are not restricted to the word written above the symbol, and can provide unlimited information by use of the various strategies; for example, symbol

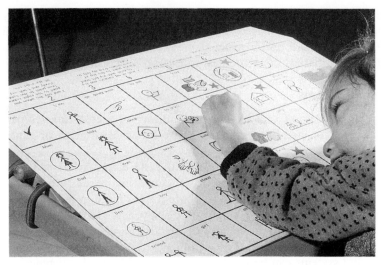

Fig. 26.1   Child using simple Makaton symbol chart organised to develop language structure and displaying clear information and instructions for the listener.

strategies and combinations can be used to create new ideas thus reducing the number of symbols required on the display. They provide flexibility of expression but require a higher level of cognitive development.

Alphabet/word systems

Traditional orthography refers to the written alphabet, which can be

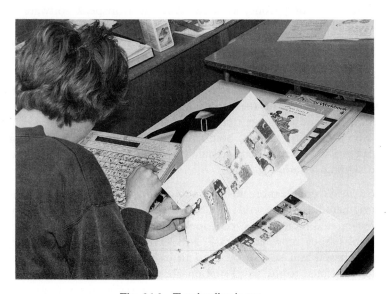

Fig. 26.2   Touch talker in use.

arranged and used in a variety of ways on spelling or word boards. This is the most acceptable system to the literate 'listener' as it is the one with which they are most familiar. It also gives the 'user' access to the range of typewriters and electronic writing devices available.

It is of course necessary to have good visual discrimination skills, since small differences between letters need to be noted; a high level of cognitive development for encoding of words; and a knowledge of language structure and spelling skills for formulating words and thus sentences (Bennett 1987).

Any of these systems may be used as an interim measure until speech is intelligible or until the severely speech impaired child has progressed to using the alphabet or word.

It has been found that the vocalisation of the child may be reduced initially while he is learning a new system, but more often it is discovered that, once the pressure of speaking is reduced by having an alternative method, the child relaxes and communication improves.

Further information on signing and symbol systems can be found in *Assistive communication aids for the speech impaired* (Enderby 1987).

INTRODUCING THE SYSTEM

Early skills in communication often need to be specifically enhanced or taught through everyday routines, interactive play or highly structured intervention.

Language awareness, both comprehension and expression, is fundamental to all aspects of the development of augmentative communication systems.

Careful assessment is required to highlight specific language difficulties, which are often associated with problems of symbolic representation (see Ch. 3).

The physical and cognitive skills of visual fixing and tracking, eye contact and referential looking will be particularly important for symbol display users. The knowledge of cause and effect will be vital for future switch users. Listening, attending, turn-taking, sharing, making choices and other 'people play' skills will be essential for social interaction and functional use of any communication system (see Ch. 1).

Vocabulary selection

Vocabulary selection is vital to the success of any augmentative communication system, whether it be graphic, or uses pictures, symbols, printed word or alphabet.

Vocabulary should never be static or restrict conversation to routine topics known to the listener, but should be based on previous knowledge of the child or on information provided in the daily home/school book.

Communication often relies on novel situations that occur naturally through the child's daily activities. New vocabulary needs to be added immediately the need arises; future requirements should be anticipated by producing 'topic' boards or 'theme' modes for outings or special events, or the user should have the facility to generate new vocabulary by using strategies and techniques, e.g. Blissymbolics uses a number of different strategies such as 'combine' and 'part of' to create new ideas or words.

Vocabulary needs to be functional allowing the user to open and close conversations, interject, ask or answer questions, give messages or pass on information and ideas.

In the young child, vocabulary needs to provide a framework to develop early language concepts; for example, the Makaton vocabulary provides a developmental introduction of vocabulary in stages for signing and symbols.

Motivation to communicate is encouraged by using vocabulary that will interest the *user*—not necessarily the parent, carer or teacher.

Language structure

Most language boards or communication devices, whether using symbols, icons, words or alphabet, need to be organised or programmed to generate sentences that can be used in a variety of situations.

A combination of symbol systems can be used to allow development beyond the limitations imposed by simple methods. Embellishment of symbols can be attractive as well as helping the child learn new vocabulary (Fig. 26.3).

1. Sets of symbols can be colour coded to help the child structure his expressive language; for example, using the Fitzgerald key (Fitzgerald 1937), where nouns/pronouns are yellow, verbs are green, adjectives and adverbs are blue, and other object nouns are red. This gives immediate reinforcement of the language structure for the young user who is developing the rules of language syntax.

2. The skill of scanning from left to right, which is fundamental in reading English, is taught by structuring the language board so that symbol sentences 'read' in this order. When accessing a language board, both user and listener are encouraged to indicate blocks or columns in this direction.

3. 'Topic blocking' can be used: sets of symbols are arranged in their category blocks, e.g. 'people' block, 'food block', etc. These blocks again need to be sequenced grammatically from left to right.

4. As literacy skills are introduced the layout of the language board may be altered so that words are sequenced in alphabetical order. Initially this could be displayed in topic blocks, but at a later stage alphabetical listing should be introduced in preparation for adult life.

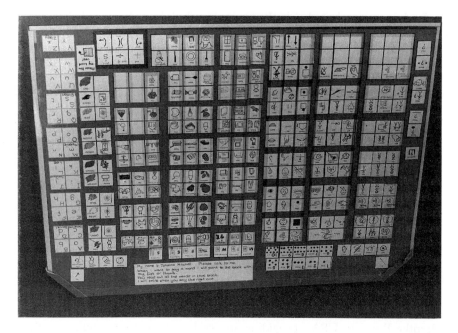

a

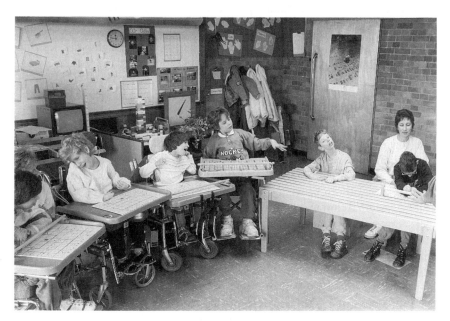

b

Fig. 26.3a. A chart organised in topic blocks showing a combination of systems being used to provide total communication. **b.** Language group using communication charts mounted on wheelchair trays.

5. A language board, whether using symbols, words or alphabet, may incorporate phrases or sentences. This will speed up the user's rate of communication so that he does not have to indicate a sequence of items for each communicative interaction

The augmented speaker needs to be encouraged to develop his own strategies for organising the information on his language board or communication device, so that he has the most effective and efficient means of communication.

Language function and use

The environment may have to be modified in order to teach the specific skills needed for language acquisition and use of an augmentative communication system.

a. Vocabulary can be introduced alongside a Language scheme, e.g. the Derbyshire Language Scheme.

b. The Minspeak Application Program (Interaction, Education and Play) has been devised for the Touch Talker or Light Talker devices (from Prentke Romich, USA), providing an overlay of a core vocabulary of 500 words, which have already been organised and coded for the user.

c. The Makaton vocabulary provides a developmental language programme for use with signs and symbols.

It may be necessary to insist on the use of correct language syntax during teaching sessions or while the child is developing language, but everyday conversation does not require this highly formal structure.

It is important that the child's language board should be readily available, especially while he is learning the system. The best way to ensure this is to have the system mounted on the wheelchair. This will not only encourage communicative interaction throughout the day but also provides an opportunity to reinforce vocabulary, language structure and literacy skills (Fig. 26.3). At a later stage the user may choose to have a more discreet display in an album or wallet, which can be brought out when necessary.

The system or aid must allow him to attract the listener's attention, interject, convey messages and use such social routines as greetings and closing, etc. It must enable him to ask questions and request objects, actions, information and clarification, as well as repair any breakdown in communication that has occurred.

The 'listener' must look for opportunities to create situations to encourage communication; learn to ask appropriate questions and not only expect, but wait for, a response. Questions should be asked one at a time and interaction expanded by not relying solely on yes/no answers. It may be necessary to admit that a message has not been understood and that it requires repeating or rephrasing. Each interaction should also create an opportunity to provide a correct model and expand the user's vocabulary and language skills.

The augmentative system may initially slow down the rate of communication between user and listener but will eventually give greater independence so that he can discuss and talk about a range of topics.

Reading skills can be reinforced by using a symbol system where the word is printed clearly above the symbol. Symbol systems are being widely used to develop reading skills. The Peabody Reading Programme is an example of a specially designed programme to teach reading through Rebuses.

The continual exposure to the printed word provides an opportunity for the child to read, and to learn specific literacy skills such as phonics and dictionary skills. A word board can also be used as a reference for spelling when using a computer or communication device. Conversely a communication device with a clear visual display and good auditory feedback helps reinforce language use and spelling. It has been found that auditory feedback has a positive influence on spelling accuracy (Koke & Neilson 1987).

The current trend is to use the more recognisable picture symbols for the benefit of the listener, especially as children become integrated into mainstream schools, making the training of carers and teachers more difficult. There is a danger that this might be to the detriment of the child's language acquisition and literacy skills.

ELECTRONIC AND COMPUTER BASED AIDS

The range of electronic communication aids and other electronic assistive equipment now available is very wide in terms of both capability and price. It is therefore vital that great care be taken in assessing the potential recipient in order to establish not only his present and future communication needs and ability and his literary skills, if appropriate, but also his physical capabilities and posture as they relate to the operation of a communication aid. The provision of a stable, functional and comfortable sitting posture is a fundamental requirement for the efficient and reliable use of a switch or other input device (Fig. 26.4).

The majority of electronic aids provide a painfully slow rate of communication—an often unavoidable drawback occasioned by the poor control ability of the disabled person. This is much less than the speed of output required for normal conversation, and can be a fundamental reason for the ultimate rejection by potential users of a communication aid. Happily, the inherent 'intelligence' offered by microprocessor technology can improve the situation significantly. The incorporation of features such as the ability to expand abbreviations or codes at the input, the provision of large word, phrase or sentence stores, and the ability to predict user input to reduce the number and rate of input selections required can all have a marked effect on communication output. Some machines are able to provide context sensi-

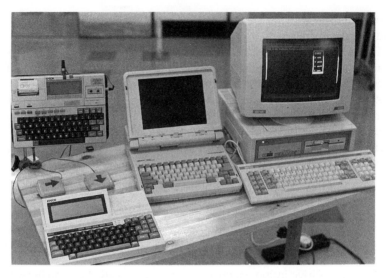

Fig. 26.4   A variety of portable tray or bracket mounted and desktop computers provide a choice of systems.

tive prediction and so reduce the number of choices that have to be scanned by the user before the appropriate selection is made.

SYNTHESISED SPEECH

Ideally an electronic communication aid incorporating synthesised speech should be capable of providing a substitute for voice communication at a rate consistent with normal speech. Unfortunately none of the currently available communication aids is yet capable of providing this function, although the quality and variety of electronically produced speech has improved dramatically in recent years. The essential characteristics of an effective aid are that it should provide a means of communication that is immediate, portable, fast and intelligible. It should also allow the use of a wide vocabulary and be suitable for a wide range of physical and intellectual abilities.

The rate of production of speech, or any other communication output for that matter, is limited mainly by the user's speed of access to the device and the techniques of internal storage, arrangement and selection of pre-prepared words, phrases or sentences provided in the design, and programming of the device. It is therefore extremely important that the user and carers are fully aware of the capabilities and limitations of any device proposed, so that expectations are not falsely raised and frustration is minimised.

An electronic communication aid can never cure a vocal disability but can enhance inherent communicative ability to a degree dependent on the physical capabilities of the person in using the aid and the limitations of the aids itself.

In the UK, the establishment of a network of Communication Aids Centres and other assessment units should ensure that the recommendation of an inappropriate aid is less likely to occur. It is hoped that sufficient resources will eventually be provided to allow adequate training in the use and setting up of an aid, and appropriate follow-up to ensure that the aid provided continues to match the user's disabilities and needs. Many new users of aids will rapidly 'outgrow' them as they become more proficient in their use, while others with progressive conditions may require aids more appropriate to their deteriorating abilities as time passes.

In some cases it may be more appropriate to provide a user with a computer system instead of a dedicated communication aid, and so fulfil a variety of different needs in a single, multipurpose device. The additional flexibility offered by this technology can also allow the aid to be adapted to changing physical and intellectual abilities.

Computers are already widely used in mainstream education for writing, mathematics, art, music and computer-assisted learning in all subjects, and physically disabled people should be given equal access to all of these where possible. There are now many ways of providing disabled users with a means of using unmodified general purpose computer programs, and these have offered them opportunities for education and employment previously unattainable.

Recent and continuing advances in microcomputer technology have allowed the production of extremely powerful, small machines which are completely self-contained, battery powered and portable. Improvements in standardisation have also meant that a growing amount of computer software will run on a variety of different machines. This allows the choice of equipment to be dictated much more by the physical requirements of the user as regards display legibility, keyboard size and layout, physical size and weight, and the provision of alternative input devices. It also allows an individual user to have a variety of machines such as a larger, desktop computer for home or classroom use, and a smaller portable machine for communication, with common software running in each (Fig. 26.4).

INTRODUCING A COMMUNICATION DEVICE

Other communication skills need to be considered by both the 'user' and the 'listener'. These will include accessing and a knowledge of how the system or communication device is operated, as well as what to do if communication breaks down for any reason.

Accessing skills need to be developed for the user who uses either direct selection or a scanning mode.

Direct selection. If the child is using a finger, fist, head/light pointer or mouthstick he will need to practise to improve the accuracy and speed of pointing. This can be attempted through games as well as locating symbols or letters directly on the language board or keyboard. A 'touch screen' with appropriate software can be very motivating to encourage accurate finger pointing.

Eye-pointing also requires careful training with emphasis on eye contact, visual fixation and referential looking (see Ch. 3).

Scanning is cognitively more complex than a direct selection method and the user will first have to learn a number of associated skills:

1. Visual fixation and tracking have to be developed in order that scanning an array of items displayed can take place both horizontally and vertically. This can be practised with a number of tracking toys or games designed for the computer.

2. The scanning mode has to be determined when selecting a communication device as to whether it will require linear or row/column scanning.

3. Whether the scanning rate is user controlled or autoscanned. Children with cerebral palsy often find the anticipation required in autoscanning difficult.

4. Cause and effect has to be understood and applied by the switch user. Young children are taught this concept by using switch operated toys. Older children learn to operate tape recorders, powered chairs or environmental control systems.

5. The user has to develop a reliable and consistent movement in order to be able to operate a switch successfully (see Ch. 24).

It is essential to introduce the 'idea' of a communication device to the augmented speaker when he has acquired the necessary ability and skills, i.e. developmental level, functional language, reliable use of an augmentative communication system and good accessing skills.

The 'listener', who may be family, carer, teacher or the general public will require some degree of information and training if he is to cope with the augmented speaker's non-verbal cues and alternative communication system.

Clear instructions need to be displayed on language boards as to how the augmented speaker communicates and how his system is accessed. Operational instructions should be clearly visible on a communication device itself, i.e. whether the message will be transmitted by synthetic speech or visual display unit and how the aid should be maintained.

The effective use of an appropriate device also requires a great deal of training. There is often a high expectation of the user to converse independently once he has received his communication aid, but it should be recognised that the child has had neither the relevant experiences nor developed the necessary conversational or social skills. He must be given time, training and support to enable him to become a confident aid user.

Some of these critical training issues are highlighted and discussed in *The jump from language boards to electronic/computerised communication devices* by Arlene Kraat (1985).

The communication device should incorporate adequate features for different functions and environments, e.g. communication, writing, note taking, lecturing or use of the telephone. It may also need to act as the user's interface to other systems, e.g. computer, environmental control system.

A clear visual display unit may be necessary where voice output would be inappropriate, e.g. conversations in the classroom, which would cause distraction, or private conversations in public areas (Fig. 26.5).

A device with good quality voice output and a less conspicuous visual display may be preferred by some users. The discreet visual display does not detract from the eye contact used in normal communication and will allow the impact of voice output to attract attention, talk to strangers or participate in group discussions.

The facility of an internal printer may be necessary for written messages or shopping lists with access to an external printer for essays and lectures, etc.

A flexible approach is essential and the user may require a variety of systems or aids to achieve total communication. In a familiar setting, facial expression, yes/no system and signing may be the most efficient method, whereas to a wider, uninformed audience the user may require a portable communication device with clear visual display and voice output (Fig. 26.6). In a school or college setting, however, the student will need access to a computer and printer.

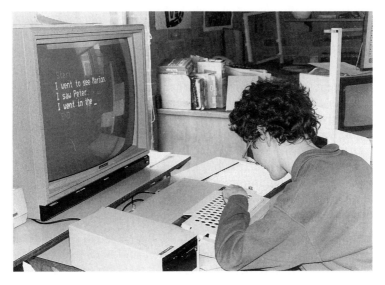

Fig. 26.5 A student with visual difficulties and poor hand function using a computer with a large visual display and keyguard.

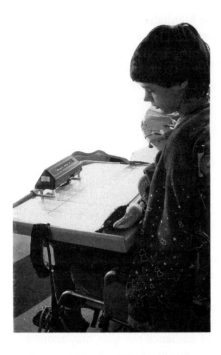

Fig. 26.6 A student with chin switches using linear scanning to communicate. The device is portable with a clear visual display and synthetic speech output.

Back-up systems are also essential to provide adequate cover, either in the event of a breakdown in a high technological device, or to enhance communication if a simpler system cannot provide sufficient information.

The user may also need copies or different presentations of his display for his various environments, e.g. a small chart for use in bed/hospital.

Combined communication and mobility

Developing control over one's environment and developing a sense of self as independent from the environment demand the skill to manipulate and interact with the environment in a locomotor (physical) as well as in a communicative sense (Baird 1989).

Developmentally, mobility and communication are interrelated skills and the acquisition of driving skills by multiply handicapped young people who are unable to speak, frequently brings benefits in many areas including an increased desire to communicate (Thornett & Moffat 1989). Technology should be used to help severely disabled people to overcome their motor disorder and enhance communication.

It is important that education should be extended for these young students, as often they not only mature later and have received less time in school than their able-bodied peers, but they are only just beginning to use their system or aids proficiently when education is due to finish. Training and support needs to continue, not only to monitor the augmented system or communication device, but also to keep pace with technological advances.

Further information and advice on computers, software and input and output devices for those with special needs may be obtained from The ACE Centre, Oxford, and The CALL Centre, Edinburgh (see list of addresses).

REFERENCES

Baird G 1989 Presentation at the First European Academy of Childhood Disability

Baker B 1982 Minspeak. Byte (Sept): 186–202

Bennett J 1987 Low technology. In: Enderby P (ed) Assistive communication aids for the speech impaired. Churchill Livingstone, Edinburgh.

Bliss C K 1949 Semantography. Semantography Publications, Sydney

Brown A 1987 Inputs and how to activate a communication aid. In: Enderby P (ed) Assistive communication aids for the speech impaired. Churchill Livingstone, Edinburgh

Carroll L 1985 Computers at Cheyne Centre for spastic children. The College of Speech Therapists Bulletin (Nov): 5

Charlebois-Marois C 1985 Everybody's technology. Carlcoms, Quebec

Fitzgerald E 1937 Straight language for the deaf: a system for instruction for deaf children, 2nd edn. Steck, Austin, Texas

Koke S, Neilson J 1987 The effect of auditory feedback on the spelling of nonspeaking physically disabled individuals. Hugh Macmillan Centre, Toronto

Kraat A 1985 The jump from language boards to electronic/computerised communication devices: some critical training issues. In: Conference report on communication through technology for the physically disabled, Dublin

Le Prevost P 1983 Using the Makaton vocabulary in early language training with a Down's baby. Mental Handicap 11: 28–29

McConkey R, Gallagher F 1984 Let's Play. Video course for parents of mentally handicapped children. St Michael's House Research, Dublin

MacDonald A 1984 Blissymbolics and manual signing—a combined approach. Communicating Together 2(4): 20–21

Masidlover M, Knowles W 1979 The Derbyshire Language Scheme, Educational Psychology Services, Ripley

Moffat V, Jolleff N 1987 Special needs of physically handicapped severely speech impaired children when considering a communication aid. In: Enderby P (ed) Assistive communication aids for the speech impaired. Churchill Livingstone, Edinburgh

Skelly M, Shinsky L 1979 Amer-Ind gestural code based on universal American hand talk, Elsevier, North Holland, New York

Southgate T 1990 Communication. (Edited by G M Cochrane) Mary Marlborough Lodge, Oxford

Thornett C, Moffat V 1989 Powered mobility and communication—a combined project. Isaac 'UK' Newsletter 8 (Dec 1989)

Walker M 1976 Language programme for use with the revised Makaton vocabulary. Makaton Vocabulary Development Project, Camberley

Walker M, Armfield A 1982 What is the Makaton vocabulary? Special Education Forward Trends 8(3): 19–20

Walker M, Grove N 1985 Communication before language. Makaton Development Project 152: 2–4

USEFUL ADDRESSES

The ACE Centre, Ormerod School, Waynflete Road, Headington, Oxford

Amer-Ind, 7 Chester Close, Lichfield WS13 7SX

Association For All Speech Impaired Children (AFASIC), 347 Central Market, Smithfield, London

Blissymbolics Communication Resource Centre (UK), Thomas House, South Glamorgan Institute of Higher Education, Cyncoed Centre, Cardiff CF2 6YD

The CALL Centre, University of Edinburgh, 24 Buccleuch Place, Edinburgh

Cambridge Adaptive Communication, 24 Fulbrooke Road, Cambridge CB3 9EE

Centre for Human Communication, DSA, Oak Tree Lane, Selly Oak, Birmingham B29 6JA, (Tel: 021 414 1661)

Concept Keyboard Company, Moorside Road, Winnall Industrial Estate, Winchester SO23 7RX

Dolphin Systems for the Disabled, Unit 96c, Blackpole Trading Estate, Worcester WR1 2RN

Easiaids, 5 Woodcote Park Ave, Purley, Surrey, CR8 3NH

Elfin Systems, Llanthony Road Trading Estate, Llanthony Road, Gloucester GL1 1SB

Foundation for Communication for the Disabled, 25 High Street, Woking, Surrey, GU21 1BW

International Society for Augmentative and Alternative Communication—ISAAC (UK), 198 City Road, London EC1 2PH

Learning Development Aids (LDA), Abbeygate House, East Road, Cambridge CB1 1DB

Learning with Rebuses, National Council for Special Education, 1 Wood Street, Stratford upon Avon CV37 6JE

Liberator, Whitegates, Swinstead, Lincs NG33 4PA

The Makaton Vocabulary Development Project, 31 Firwood Drive, Camberley, Surrey

National Centre for Cued Speech for the Deaf, 29–30 Watling Street, Canterbury, Kent CT1 2UD

Paget Gorman Society, 3 Gipsy Lane, Headington, Oxford, OX3 7PT

Pictogram Ideogram Communication, The George Reed Foundation, 1919 Scarth Street, Regine, Sasketchewan, Canada S4 P2 H1

The Picture Communication Symbols, Mayer Johnson, Dept K, PO Box 86, Stillwater, MN 55082, USA

Possum Controls, Middlegreen Road, Langley, Slough, Bucks. SL3 6DF

Rainbow Rehab, PO Box 546, Bournemouth BH8 8YD

Royal National Institute for the Deaf, 105 Gower Street, London WC1E 6AH

Toys for the Handicapped (TFH), 76 Barracks Road, Sandy Lane Industrial Estate, Stourport-on-Severn, Worcestershire DY13 9QB

Werth PC, Audiology House, 45 Nightingale Lane, London SW12 8SP

27. Education

H. Parrott   A.C. Bruce   C. Zergaeng

The aim of this section of the book is to look at how education is provided for young people with physical difficulties, and the various factors which affect choice. It will also examine the place of the national curriculum within the context of the young person with severe special needs and investigate particular areas of the curriculum which create significant difficulties for young people who have multiple disabilities.

Special education for pupils with physical disabilities has a short history in the British Isles, the first provision being made in 1851. Emphasis at that time was placed upon training for a trade; 'education' took second place. The Heritage Craft Schools—one for boys and one for girls—were founded at the turn of this century and provided a training in a very wide variety of skills, with which the scholars would be able to 'earn their place in the world as round pegs in round holes'. The founder, Dame Grace Kimmins, was strongly influenced by her husband, a psychologist with the London Education Board, to bring 'education' to the pupils. Government intervention was at first given in the form of support to the charitable organisations and individual enterprise. Later it provided a framework upon which the provision, which is now statutory, could be maintained. The present pattern can be clearly realised by briefly looking at the legislation over this century.

In 1921 the Education Act recognised four categories of handicap— blind, deaf, defective (comprising physical and mental disability) and epileptic. The parents of children within these categories were required to see that their children attended a suitable special school until the age of 16 and it was the responsibility of the local education authorities (LEAs) to provide the schools.

By the time of the 1944 Education Act, the education authorities were required to meet the needs of children with special needs within their general duty in both primary and secondary education. It also became the responsibility of the authorities to ascertain which children required special educational 'treatment'. Thus a new framework was formed, which categorised children according to handicap. This pattern remained until the Education Act of 1981, which, as a basis for much of the new legislation, accepted that categorisation acted as a barrier to providing appropriate education. Placing the child who had multiple disabilities was exceedingly difficult in the presence of definitions that were dependent upon, for example, an IQ score, or the decision of a general practitioner. In fact, the system was in danger of strangling itself, and special school placements rose between 1945 and 1977 by 100 000.

The 1944 Education Act described formal procedures for discovering handicapped children within the local education authorities. Parents could be fined for not complying with the request that their child should be seen by a medical officer who would advise as to whether the child suffered from 'any disability of mind or body' and to what degree. The LEA noted the report of the medical officer, teacher or 'other persons' and made the decision regarding special schooling. The LEA had then the two duties of notifying the parents and providing the 'treatment'. A certificate was produced and signed by the medical officer.

It can be readily seen that a medical model was the one used to satisfy the special educational needs of the child: the word 'treatment' was seen as fundamental to the process, assuming as it did that there was a cure to be found for a child with a special educational need; and placing the medical officer as the key professional. Although the system did become less formal over the years, there was an increasing awareness that much was left to be desired. The outcome of the arguments and discussions that took place was the Department of Education and Science (DES) circular 2/75 *The discovery of children requiring special education and the assessment of their needs*. This described the need for a multidisciplinary approach. This circular, the Warnock Report of 1978 and the ensuing Education Act of 1981 all had a major and lasting effect upon the education of children with special needs, particularly perhaps those young people who have physical and multiple disabilities.

The Education Act 1981 lays down that for every child for whom a form of special education is deemed necessary, a Statement is drawn up which describes the need and the proposals for meeting those needs. Many items of 'advice' can be added to the Statement and these can be drawn up by a wide variety of people, not least of whom are the parents, who have a strong and important part to play in the production or non-production of the Statement and the provision that is to be made. Others may be the community paediatrician, family doctor, health visitor, therapists, social worker, voluntary agencies, educational welfare officer, educational psychologist, inspectors and advisers in special education, school medical officers, medical consultants, teachers, and the members of child guidance clinics. Using the statement, it is the responsibility of the local education authority to identify for the child the special educational provision that is deemed to be the most appropriate.

PROVISION

The child with physical or multiple disabilities may be provided with special education in one or more of the following settings during his or her school life:

- An ordinary class with support
- As above, with a base to which to withdraw
- Part-time in special class
- Full-time in special class
- Part-time in day special school
- Full-time in day special school
- Residential special school
- Hospital school
- At home with tutor.

Local education authorities may not be able to provide this wide range of resources, but it is up to them to seek suitable provisions. If local provision is unsuitable, the authority must seek provision elsewhere. The advantages of working closely from the outset with the other statutory bodies of social services and health authorities can readily be seen: (1) the setting up of district handicap teams; (2) the greater liaison between LEAs and social services made necessary under the legislation of the 1986 Disabled Persons Act (information must be passed from one authority to the other regarding young people approaching 16 years of age who are the subject of a Statement); and (3) agreements that are being reached regarding the joint funding of some agency placements—non-maintained and independent schools for the multiply disabled have made it possible for there to be a greater understanding of the needs and the importance of ensuring the most appropriate provision is sought.

Since the passing of the Education Act of 1981 there have been great efforts made towards providing for special needs within an 'ordinary' mainstream setting. Many local education authorities are reviewing the place of their special schools with the basic principle as laid down by the Act, that there should be a concerted effort as never before to integrate the disabled within the limits of normal society rather than to segregate them because of their differences.

It is now well recognised that the majority of young people who have special educational needs may be able to receive a relevant education within a mainstream school, whether at junior or secondary age, and great steps have been taken by many local education authorities to ensure this is possible. For the young person who has physical disabilities it may be that an ancillary helper can be the solution to the problems of moving from class to class, and those of personal care during the school day. Many schools are taking also the introduction of the national curriculum as an appropriate time to ensure that young people with special educational needs can be catered for within the mainstream school.

At all times, however, the main factor must be to match the child's statemented needs with the provision. The Warnock Report of 1978 suggests that special educational needs require the following:

> The provision of special means of access to the curriculum through special equipment, facilities or resources, modification of the physical environment, or specialist teaching techniques; the provision of special or modified curricula; particular attention to the social structure and emotional climate in which education takes place.

It is accepted that for the majority of children who have both physical disabilities and special educational needs, the mainstream school should be able to satisfy the above points. However, there is no doubt that some children may not find the levels of expertise, the necessary level of adaptation of physical resources or the correct level of curricular modification outside the special school or unit. The Warnock Report defines special education thus:

> Effective access on a full or part time basis to teachers with appropriate qualifications or substantial experience or both; effective access on a full or part time basis to other professionals with appropriate training; and an educational and physical environment with necessary aids, equipment and resources appropriate to the child's needs.

If a special school, where these facilities and resources are available, is going to provide the most sensible solution to a child's education, then that school will be recommended, (taking into account the many questions that are bound to arise). The decision having been reached, it is the responsibility of the school chosen to provide the appropriate education for the child. The school will review the child's situation on an annual or more frequent basis, and decisions regarding continuing in that school will be made at the review.

As the child gets older, there may be a greater emphasis placed upon skills needed beyond school age. There is now general acceptance that a young person who has special educational needs will benefit and receive education until the age of 19. Significant strides have been made towards promoting appropriate further education for students with special needs. A number of special schools offer courses for students over the age of 16 and many colleges of further education now provide Link Courses, which can cater for the student with not only physical, but also intellectual disabilities. There are also a number of specialist residential colleges that cater for such students.

Of greatest importance must be the links, made at as early a stage as is feasible, with other agencies, which are going to have important roles to play in the lives of young disabled adults. There must be no reason for the good preparation work that the child and student has carried out to come to be of little use because of poor communication or lack of support and understanding.

THE NATIONAL CURRICULUM

The section of the 1988 Education Reform Act (ERA) which has had the most immediate effect on teachers and children is Section 10(2), which places a duty on the head teacher of every maintained school to implement a national curriculum within that school. The main principle of the national curriculum is that all registered pupils of compulsory school age, including those with a statement of special educational needs, share a right to a broad and balanced curriculum.

It is a disadvantage to be writing this at a time when professionals have had little opportunity to absorb and discuss the implications of the national curriculum for 'special needs' children. The concept of a nationally prescribed curriculum is in many ways at odds with the main philosophy of the 1981 Education Act, which emphasises the need for individual planning and close scrutiny of individual special needs. The dynamic of the national curriculum is for reference to normative attainment targets. There has always been a tension between the desire on the one hand to enable children with special educational needs to participate as fully as possible in activities in common with their peers and on the other hand to provide a detailed curriculum plan based on assessment of their individual needs. Nonetheless there is a responsibility to ensure that any potential for good in the 1988 Educational Reform Act is implemented.

As originally presented in 1987, the Education Reform Bill contained minimal reference to the application of the national curriculum to children with special educational needs. Clause 10 declared that 'a statement . . . of a pupil's special educational needs may direct that the provisions of the National Curriculum shall apply...with such modifications as may be specified in the statement'. By the time the Bill became the law in July 1988, section 19 had been added allowing for the 'disapplication' of the national curriculum to some pupils without statements for temporary periods. Section 18 of the Act is perhaps one of the most relevant to special schools:

> The special educational provision for any pupil specified in a statement under section 7 of the 1981 Act of his special educational needs may include provision:
> (a) excluding the application of the provisions of the National Curriculum; or
> (b) applying those provisions with such modifications as may be specified in the statement.

The Secretary of State has been empowered to make further orders and regulations that will affect children with special educational needs and these are, at the time of writing, eagerly awaited.

Advice was forthcoming in October 1989 from a Special Educational Needs Task Group contained in *A curriculum for all*, and this may form the basis for regulations to follow. It is encouraging to read in this publication that many of the recommendations are based on the excellent and appropriate work carried out in special schools. Its advice has allowed work to begin on assessing the best methods of using attainment targets in the core subjects of English, mathematics and science for children with physical and sensory impairment. Access to such normative objectives is certainly a challenge. As the document points out, the principle of entitlement to a broad and balanced curriculum 'does not automatically ensure access to it nor progress within it'.

The demand of the national curriculum to promote the development of what can be seen as 'the whole child' is not new to teachers in special schools. The emphasis here has long been on the fostering of mobility, communication, self-help and social skills. The very necessary emphasis on such 'non-academic' skills has led to criticisms of narrowness of curriculum and limited opportunities. The call in *A curriculum for all* is for special schools to extend their curricular breadth. This will take ingenuity and careful planning to ensure that the work of the special school is not diluted simply to show that it can offer the national curriculum.

The involvement of the various therapy professions has been fundamental to developing a sound scheme of work. There is a strong awareness in many special schools of the importance of planning for life after school. If the national curriculum aims to promote all such aspects of development it is likely to find broad acceptance in special schools.

At present there exists guidance for the three core subjects of English, mathematics and science. *A curriculum for all* also poses some questions for special schools to address, and exhorts them to shape their existing curriculum and the national curriculum into a single framework. Examples of how adaptations may be made to enable pupils with special needs to achieve attainment targets are given for each of the three core subjects. Advice at present is concerned mainly with Key Stage 1, i.e. 5–7-year-olds, and it is salutary to read in the Education Reform Act that 'some pupils with severe learning difficulties may be working towards statements of attainment in Level I throughout most or all of their school days'.

As the programmes of study are issued, careful reappraisal of a school's current curriculum and its relationship to the national curriculum will be needed. Many special schools already undertake almost constant review of their curriculum as changes in the nature of special school pupils have occurred, largely as a result of the 1981 Education Act. Work will need to be undertaken to see if a unified framework is possible. For those pupils that the National Curriculum Council see as forming 'the majority of pupils with special educational needs ... with difficulties of a mild, moderate or temporary nature' cohesion and access to the national curriculum should not prove too difficult. More problematic will be the provision of such a unified framework for children who have profound and multiple disabilities.

Concern is already being felt amongst teachers of children with profound physical and learning difficulties that they have been somewhat overlooked, representing, as they do, a very small percentage of the population of children who have special needs. The Special Educational Needs Task Group emphasised that the entitlement of a broad and balanced curriculum, the main principle of the national curriculum, applies to the whole range of disabilities. For example, it may be necessary for teachers of children with more severe physical disabilities to look beyond the guidance given regarding physical access to the curriculum in *A curriculum for all*:

> Some pupils with physical disabilities will need computers with adapted keyboards. Those with sensory or physical disabilities may require specific instruction in the use of sophisticated hearing, vision or other aids.

Such work is just the beginning and may well become a diverse pattern of exemption from, and modification to, the national curriculum.

Emphasis on the subject areas will be seen by many teachers to herald the return to subject specialists being appointed to special schools. Patterns of work have evolved away from this for some years, involving work drawn from a wide range of subjects. Whilst special school headteachers will need to demonstrate that they can offer a full national curriculum there should be no requirement to reintroduce the subject specialist. Rather it is a matter of utilising the skills available amongst the staff. Certainly, in the first levels and Key Stage 1 of the curriculum, for example, many subjects can be readily taught by good teachers without specialist qualifications. If they can become armed with carefully planned steps that allow special needs children who have more severe learning difficulties to work towards access to these first levels, then the marriage of the special and national curricula may not be such a stormy one as initially feared.

Anxiety may also be felt by parents. Encouraged perhaps with new expectations about their child's participation in a national curriculum, they may rightly want to see progress described in national curriculum terminology. As *A curriculum for all* points out, however, many pupils may spend their school career on Level One. How then to quantify a child's progress to parents faced with apparent stagnation?

It is at this point that special schools will have to display the courage of their convictions about the work they do. Such schools cannot afford to jettison the important work that has taken so long to establish with regards to mobility, communication and the acquisition of self-help skills. Such aims should be presented as programmes of study seen as prerequisite skills for entry to the national curriculum and will consequently be officially accepted as a positive alternative to disapplication. Much of what is special about special education can, with ingenuity, be matched to existing programmes of study. For example, analysis of the interaction and skills required in a specialist plinth-lying group will almost certainly reveal work relevant to attainment targets in each of the core areas.

It may be that many special schools find no positive alternative to disapplication. If the crude categorisation of children with handicapping conditions which preceded the 1981 Act were still in force, then such disapplication of certain subjects could readily be linked with certain categories. But since the Warnock Report there has been greater understanding of the wide diversity of patterns of disability and learning difficulty; categories included a wide range of special needs. It would be contrary to the spirit of Warnock and undermining of all the positive work in special education of the last decade to invoke disapplication by similar categorisation.

Section 16 of ERA allows schools to claim exemption from the national curriculum on the grounds of experimental or developmental work.

Once the initial fears about the incompatibility of approaches are reconciled, special schools will remain as places where new approaches to effective working with pupils with a wide range of difficulties can be fostered. Whether they feel that this should mean they can claim exemption from the national curriculum will depend not least upon the attention given to special schools by the legislative bodies.

LEARNING DISABILITY

Children who have severe physical disabilities generally have an associated learning disability resulting from central neurological damage and from the lack of opportunity for learning that a physical disability can cause. A child who cannot move himself cannot actively explore his environment, a child with limited or no hand function cannot play with objects and learn by trial and error how they fit together. The child with physical disabilities thus has less opportunity for incidental learning.

Young children are constantly asking questions and learning from the replies they get both about language itself and about the world. The child who has no speech is deprived of this opportunity for learning and indeed may be generally talked to less often than verbal children.

The physically disabled child is therefore very dependent on adults or older siblings to structure and facilitate his opportunity for learning. The more physically disabled the child, the more this is likely to be the case.

PRE-SCHOOL EDUCATION

There will be certain aspects of early learning that may need to be taught in a highly controlled way rather than naturally learned by the child. This is particularly the case with children whose mobility and hand function are affected. Parental involvement is vital at this early stage, and the Portage Early Education Programme reflects this and is now used widely by local authorities.

Portage is a home teaching programme that involves parents teaching their own children a range of skills with the aid of the home visitor, who assesses the child's skills by means of a checklist. Together parent and home teacher set appropriate teaching goals and achieve them through an individual programme of planned activities.

Many authorities also use peripatetic teachers of special needs to assist and advise parents. From the age of 2 years the local education authority may fund a child to attend a nursery school or unit which will cater for the child's educational needs. In practice, however, at this early stage it is often impossible to know exactly what the child's needs are going to be, and for this reason nursery units have an important role to play in assessment.

The general principles of remediating learning difficulties are outlined below:

- Diagnose and assess
- Define what the child is to learn
- Break down the task to be learned into small parts so that each part can be taught separately
- Decide how and when the child will be taught, and by whom
- Evaluate the effectiveness of the teaching by regular assessment of the child's progress.

The curriculum is usually set out in the form of a checklist in a wide range of skill areas such as fine motor skills, symbolic play, and language comprehension. This acts not only as an assessment of what the child's abilities are now, but also as a guide to the objectives for that child and as a measure of his progress. Within these structured activities there must be room for play. Many skills, such as sharing and imaginative play, are best taught in groups as fun activity.

A physically disabled child often has a wide variety of needs, which means that many therapists and other professionals may be involved. Communication between all involved with the child is of great importance and the value of a team approach cannot be overemphasised. There will be many areas in which professionals must work together; for example the speech therapist and teacher on language and speech difficulties, and the physiotherapist, teacher and occupational therapist on mobility and equipment. Group work has the advantage here in that a therapist and teacher can work together with the children in structured yet fun activity.

Early education for the child with disability must not be seen as taking place purely within the confines of the special school. Wherever possible efforts should be made to offer the child the opportunity of being in an ordinary playgroup, providing that the situation within the group is satisfactory in terms of attitude, staffing facilities and equipment.

If one is aiming to achieve a placement in the mainstream educational system for a particular child, then this aim—once realistically stated by all concerned—must be worked towards wholeheartedly. There may be particular necessities that must be looked at regarding, for example, toilet facilities and access within the proposed school. Therapists have an important role to play here and can act as the coordinators between the two establishments, special and mainstream. There must also be liaison between the teaching and ancillary staff throughout the preparation time. This liaison must not be lost once such a move has been made; a programme of therapy will need to be continued, as the physical problems that a child has to live with will not disappear when he is at an ordinary school.

THE SCHOOL-AGED CHILD

The first part of this chapter outlines the types of special educational provision in which a child with special educational needs may be placed. It also discusses the type of curriculum that will be required for different children depending on their learning and physical disabilities.

SPECIFIC LEARNING DIFFICULTIES

The largest group of physically disabled children suffer from central neurological damage, e.g. those with cerebral palsy. The following discussion will concentrate on this group of children and their basic educational attainments in reading, writing and numeracy. Possible remedial methods will be considered.

Concentration and distractibility

Children with neurological damage are likely to have problems of attention and concentration, and these difficulties will affect their attainment in all subjects. A quiet area of the classroom where there are fewer distractions, such as a corner that can be screened off, is required. A programme can be devised that will reward the child for completing a certain task within a particular time limit. This must be suited to the age and appropriate needs of the child, older children being encouraged to take responsibility for themselves.

Reading

Significant numbers of children with physical disabilities are retarded in reading (Rutter et al 1970). Furthermore, the rate of retardation appears twice as great in children with neurological damage. Cope & Anderson (1977) studied the reading attainments of children within units and special schools for children with physical disabilities and found that a high proportion of pupils in both types of provision were significantly backward in reading. Analysis of the results shows that the children of below average intelligence and poor visual perceptual skills are considerably at risk of being retarded in reading. This is a similar finding to that found in children with hydrocephalus (see Ch.13).

Children with neurological damage often have difficulties with skills such as figure–ground perception, sequencing, visual memory and visual discrimination (see Ch. 6, p. 100).

These are all skills that one would assume are necessary for learning to read, although research is inconclusive. Indeed, Bryant & Bradley (1985) argue that deficits in these skills may be a consequence of poor reading ability rather than a cause of it, as reading gives practice in those skill areas.

Whatever the cause, these children do have difficulty in learning to read and continuous assessment of a child's progress should be undertaken so that, if a child is failing, changes to the teaching method or material can be made.

A phonic approach to reading is likely to be more appropriate for a child who has visual perceptual difficulties, rather than a 'look and say approach', as the former would make best use of relatively good auditory skills. Many schools now operate paired reading, which involves the child reading books of his own choice together with his parent or teacher. The child gradually takes over the reading as he becomes more skilled and confident. This has been found a useful approach, as it can be very motivating for the child and helps him to learn to predict the language in books—an essential part of learning to read meaningfully. However, a child who has visual perceptual difficulties will probably need to have paired reading combined with a specific reading programme.

Many programmes are available that claim to remediate specific problems such as visual perceptual skills. However, the evidence of their effectiveness is inconclusive, particularly with regard to their effects on educational attainment. It appears that gains in specific areas, such as visual discrimination, do not necessarily generalise to other skills such as reading. The nearer the task is to reading the more likely it is to generalise; therefore, teaching visual memory skills is best done with words rather than with pictures or shapes.

Children with spina bifida and hydrocephalus sometimes learn to read fluently but with poor comprehension. It is therefore necessary to monitor these skills carefully and act accordingly.

Teaching the non-verbal child to read presents a challenge. Firstly it is necessary to establish that the child is able to retain a series of four to five words at a time, and has sufficient language comprehension to understand simple story books. The child can be taught using the usual methods, but the difficulty arises for the teacher in the way she checks which words the child can read.

This can be done in two main ways:

1. By teaching words which correspond to the symbols on the child's

communication chart. The child can then indicate the correct symbol for the word shown. (This will obviously be restrictive.)

2. By giving the child a multiple choice of words and asking him to select the word named. This may be done with flash cards, in a book with the teacher pointing to each word in turn, or on a computer with an array of words.

A relatively fluent reader (7–8 year level) can use a Cloze procedure, requiring completion of a missing word in a sentence, which will also test comprehension. Paired reading, although the child cannot read out loud, allows the child to work with real books and gain knowledge of sentence structures, which are needed in prediction skills. This is especially important in children with very poor hand control who are unable to pick up a book and read it for themselves. Page turners are not generally found to be satisfactory, and the child is therefore reliant on an able-bodied person to turn the pages for him. These children may become poor readers because of their lack of opportunity to read.

Writing

Many physically handicapped children have problems with handwriting due to gross motor difficulties or to other specific problems. These children may never write competently and will require alternative means of recording their work, such as a typewriter. Some children who write very slowly and form letters poorly may also benefit from learning to type in addition to writing.

Research findings indicate that neurologically damaged children are likely to have difficulties in learning to write. Wedell (1973) and Anderson & Spain (1977) have suggested that the problem of fine motor control is the main underlying cause of poor handwriting.

Anderson also states that poor perceptual and visuomotor difficulties probably hinder the child from making the correct spatial judgements that are necessary in writing. Those who are likely to have handwriting problems, such as children with spina bifida or hydrocephalus, will benefit from the teaching of pre-writing skills, which will develop fine motor control. Handwriting needs to be specifically taught, concentrating on the arm and hand movements accompanied by an auditory clue such as 'down, up and over' for the letter 'r'. Children should not be allowed to copy letters without learning to form them correctly as they will develop their own idiosyncratic ways of forming letters. Positioning of both pen and paper is important, and handwriting can often be improved with the aid of a triangular grip or even a different type of pen. An occupational therapist will advise on positioning and equipment available, such as a magnetic strip to hold the paper in place for the child who only has use of one arm.

Number work

It appears that a large proportion of physically handicapped children have difficulties with arithmetic. Indeed, Anderson (1973) found that 78% of neurologically damaged children were rated by their teachers as having significantly more difficulty in their number work than with their reading. More recently, research conducted with spina bifida children has found indications that these children—even when of average ability and only mildly handicapped—have definite problems with arithmetic compared to a non-handicapped control group (Halliwell et al 1980).

Gaddes (1980) has identified difficulties in language, reading and spatial imagery as leading to slow progress in acquiring numeracy. The problems of poor spatial imagery can be understood in term of the Piagetian model of child development. In the pre-operational stage, thinking is characterised by perceptual rather than by conceptual processes, so that a child at this stage will depend on his visual perception to a very large extent when making quantitative judgements. In the early stages, modern teaching of mathematics is largely concerned with teaching the child to make judgements of quantity independently of, for example, spatial arrangements. Activities to teach this concept include sorting, grading and counting objects, and visual, perceptual, perceptuomotor and fine motor skills are all required for the successful execution of such tasks. It is evident, therefore, that children with these problems may well experience difficulties in the early stages of learning mathematics. They may be helped by verbal descriptions of the tasks to aid their acquisition of number concepts.

As the child progresses, he will be required to record his work, and difficulties in sensory and motor organisation may cause further problems in setting out sums, arranging figures in the appropriate columns, and remembering the correct sequence in which to carry out the required computations. In addition to the problems of sensory and motor organisation, it must be remembered that many neurologically damaged children have attentional difficulties. Heskell (1972) has emphasised the significance of these factors in determining a child's level of attainment in arithmetic.

REFERENCES

Ainscow M, Tweddle D A 1979 Preventing classroom failure: an objective approach. John Wiley, Chichester
Anderson E M 1973 The disabled schoolchild. A study of integration in primary schools. Methuen, London
Anderson E M, Spain B 1977 The child with spina bifida. Methuen, London
Baker D, Bovair K (eds) 1989 Making the special schools ordinary? Vol 1, Falmer, London
Bowers T (ed) Managing special needs. Open University Press, Milton Keynes
Bryant P, Bradley L 1988 Children's reading problems. Blackwell, Oxford
Cope C, Anderson E M 1977 Special units in ordinary schools: an exploratory study of special provision for disabled children. Institute of Education, London

Department of Education and Science 1978 Special educational needs. Report of the Committee of Enquiry into the education of handicapped children and young people (The Warnock Report). HMSO, London

Department of Education and Science 1989 National Curriculum: from policy to practice. London

Gaddes W H 1980 Learning disabilities and brain function Springer–Verlag, New York

Halliwell M D, Carr J G, Pearson A M 1980 The intellectual and educational functioning of children with neural tube defects. Kinderchirurgie 31: 375-381

Heskell S H 1972 Arithmetical disabilities in programmed instruction: a remedial approach. C.C.Thomas, Illinois

National Association of Headteachers 1989 Guide to the Reform Act 1988. NAHT, Haywards Heath

National Curriculum Council 1989 Curriculum guidance: 2. A curriculum for all. Special needs in the national curriculum. NCC, York

Rutter M, Tizard J, Whitmore K (eds) 1970 Education, health and behaviour. Longman, London

Wedell K 1973 Learning and perceptuo-motor disabilities in children. John Wiley, Chichester

FURTHER READING

Cambridge J, Anderson E 1979 The handwriting of spina bifida children. Association for Spina Bifida and Hydrocephalus (ASBAH)

Cameron S, White M 1985 The Portage early education programme. A practical manual. NFER Nelson

Male J, Thomspon C 1985 The educational implications of disability. The Royal Association for Disability and Rehabilitation

Reason R, Boote R 1986 Learning difficulties in reading and writing. A Teachers Manual. NFER Nelson

28. The nursing care of the chronically sick or handicapped child

Mother Frances Dominica

INTRODUCTION

The physical care of a child who is handicapped or who has a life threatening, chronic illness is only a small part of what one would describe as nursing care. It is just as much a part of the role of the nurse to recognise and meet the child's emotional and spiritual needs, and indeed those of his family. Nursing care of such a child is about care for the whole child and his family, helping them to achieve the optimum quality of life throughout, even though the lifespan may be short, enabling the child to meet continuing handicap, diminishment of health, or death with dignity and helping the family to live on. The importance of being sensitive to the very different needs of each person and of being ready to respond in the way which is most appropriate to each individual cannot be stressed strongly enough.

THE CHILD AND HIS FAMILY

The changing social pattern

The position of a family with a chronically sick or handicapped child is dramatically different now as compared with previous generations. Due to developments in preventive and curative medicine, the occurrence of some forms of chronic sickness and severe handicap in children is much less frequent, but where such sickness or handicap do occur many who would once have died now survive with varying degrees of dependence. Although there are more extensive and improved facilities offering support to these families, the pattern of family life has changed and the involvement of the extended family is less common. The nuclear family, not infrequently a single parent family, can suffer feelings of isolation.

Learning from the family

Anyone involved in the nursing care of a child must see him in the context of his family. Care of the handicapped or chronically sick is different from care of the acutely ill; it is vital for the nurse to listen to and learn from the family, for it is the family that knows best the individual characteristics and needs of the sick child. This is especially important where the child has difficulty in communicating.

According to the severity of the child's disorder, the extent to which it involves and affects the family will vary. Although in some cases the practical problems are immense, they are seldom the worst of the difficulties facing the parents; very often the resulting problems are the most taxing.

Prolonged anxiety and grief of the family

However imaginative and understanding we are, as outsiders we can only begin to be aware of the strain and anguish which the family experiences physically and mentally. In the case of an acute illness or accident followed by death, the grieving process and mourning have the potential for being resolved over a period of time. Theoretically, at least, others accept this process. With chronic sickness or handicap the grief is cruelly prolonged and may often begin at the moment of diagnosis when it is recognised that there is no known cure, and there is not the same possibility of resolving or completing the mourning. Every stage of diminished ability or independence, every loss of function and each new sign of deterioration is a further cause of mourning to the family and needs the acknowledgement of those around, not least those professionally concerned. This grieving may bring with it the feelings of denial, anger, remorse and guilt as well as sorrow common to all bereavement. The need for the nurse to foster an honest and accepting relationship through all this is crucial.

Differing reactions of parents

It must be recognised that father and mother may react in very different ways to their distress, and their relationship may become strained because of the difficulty of one partner in understanding how or why the other is behaving in a certain way. Sheer physical exhaustion may affect communication and so things go from bad to worse. One or both partners may feel ashamed or guilty about their child's disorder and their own inadequacy in coping with it. It is generally easier and more acceptable for a woman to show her emotions than it is for a man to show his and it is particularly difficult for him in the social or work context. It is also traditional for the mother to fulfil the nurturing, caring role which reinforces the bond between her and her child, sometimes to the apparent exclusion of the father. Either parent may have periods of time when they distance themselves from the child as a form of self-protection. Arguments frequently occur as to the degree of protection the child needs, or as to the best treatment or the management of behaviour. The nurse needs to try to make both partners feel valued and to include them both in communications concerning their child, showing a sensitivity to the difficulties each faces and making positive suggestions about activities they and their child may be able to enjoy together.

We must be aware that the difficulties and frustrations may cause such stress that they lead even the most caring parents to abuse their child physically, and this needs to be seen as a symptom of the pain that they are suffering; it should be handled in a cautious but sensitive way. An isolated incident of physical abuse may occur, causing the parents enormous guilt, which, if talked over with someone who knows and understands the family, may be defused, so preventing further incidents. Whatever the circumstances, signs of physical abuse are a danger signal that cannot be ignored. The possibility of euthanasia goes through the minds of the parents of many chronically sick children, so terrible is the anguish of being helpless in the face of your child's suffering.

The effect on siblings

The disruption of family life inevitably affects other children in the family, who may feel neglected in favour of the sick child. In some cases this can lead to strong resentment, resulting in disturbed behaviour. They may also carry around a huge burden of sorrow, which may manifest itself in many ways and therefore may not be recognised for what it is. Irrational guilt, extreme anger and temper tantrums, or feigned sickness are examples of this. A sibling may have fears that he himself will suffer the same illness or even die, and he may well feel that he must protect his already over-burdened parents from this and other anxieties or strong emotions. Here the nurse may have an important role to fill, just as friend and confidante. Explanation and involvement appropriate to the age and temperament of the sibling may help to overcome some of the difficulties. Siblings who do in fact suffer from the same condition, for example inherited progressive disorders, have their own very special needs.

The effect on others

Grandparents, aunts, uncles, cousins, friends, neighbours and professional care-givers are all affected by the child's suffering. We need to be aware that as well as being a potential source of help, they are potential casualties in the unfolding of a particular tragedy.

The importance of continuing social contacts

Friendships and social contacts outside the immediate family circle are of immense value for all members of the family to provide relief, diversion and support during the child's life and, should it occur, after his death. It is dangerously optimistic to think that old friendships—which have been neglected during the child's life, often from simple lack of energy on the part of those caring for him or reluctance ever to be parted from him—can automatically be resumed later. Brothers and sisters should not be made to feel guilty about enjoying their own ordinary friendships, indeed these should be encouraged.

Dependence and independence of the child

Members of the family may sometimes be helped to adopt a slightly different approach from the instinctive one to protect at all costs, which sometimes lessens the quality of the child's life. Every child is dependent on his parents or parent substitutes during the early years of his life; gradually this dependence diminishes in a well child. Increasing independence is exciting and challenging for a young person, though some parents are reluctant to let go. How much more difficult it is for parents of a handicapped child to allow him to face the challenges of the outside world. Undoubtedly a society which is geared to the normal imposes restraints on those who are different, so we must do all we can to help the child and his parents to meet and overcome prejudices.

THE CHILD AND THE NURSE

Trust between child and nurse

There will be times when the nurse will be called upon to act as parent substitute. Trust and acceptance are essential to any satisfactory lasting relationship and this is certainly so between a nurse and a handicapped or sick child. Equally important to such a child is a feeling of self-worth and confidence which we must foster early on by an immediate readiness to accept him while acknowledging that it will take time for him to trust us. If this is to happen, our behaviour towards him must be consistent and our responses honest. If he trusts us enough, he may feel able to relax and perhaps to share some of his worst anxieties and his grief; it is remarkable how protective sick children feel towards their parents and they will often go to great lengths to spare them further pain, whereas someone they trust who is less closely related, but has some involvement and authority, may be taken into the child's confidence.

Flexibility in methods of treatment

Acute nursing care may often require textbook methods of treatment to ensure a satisfactory outcome. However, nursing a chronically sick child allows and indeed demands a greater degree of flexibility and creative use of imagination. The child's own knowledge of the best way of coping with the disorder will most often be the way we must adopt. It is clearly not appropriate to carry out a task in textbook fashion or even according to stated policy, if such action causes distress or unnecessary suffering, perhaps only through its unfamiliarity.

Commands and instructions issued by an apparently demanding or cheeky chronically handicapped child can be irksome to say the least, but we must remember that a child who lives with a condition usually knows what is best for him. He is not a textbook case; he is a unique individual with his own idiosyncracies and needs, which he understands better than anyone. The child's agreement must be sought if we wish to try a new procedure, showing him that we are anxious to do the best for him and not just determined 'to do our own thing'. All this assumes that his level of consciousness allows him to reason, relate and cooperate.

The need to be observant

In caring for the chronically sick there is a danger that we may not be sufficiently observant of changing needs, as these often come about very gradually. We need to be constantly assessing the child as he is and questioning whether our care remains appropriate. There is scope for imagination and resourcefulness, but always with consideration for the home situation if this is relevant. Change in treatment may sometimes provide the opportunity of helping the parents to accept further deterioration in their child's condition, which they may not have noticed or indeed may have chosen to ignore or deny.

Basic physical care

The nurse must give meticulous attention to the physical needs of the child. Her standard of care can make all the difference between constant discomfort and nagging reminders of his plight and freedom to focus his attention on positive and outgoing thoughts and behaviour. Care of skin and hair needs to extend to helping the child to feel attractive; well fitting, pretty or 'fun' clothes which he enjoys wearing are also a boost to the morale and these should be chosen or adapted with a view to ease of dressing and undressing. Dental care is as important, if not more so, for a sick or handicapped child as it is for a well child. Cleaning the teeth, despite the difficulties that handicap may present, a good diet and regular dental check-ups are all important. Diet needs to be imaginative and varied and it is not wise to give in to all his fads just because a child is handicapped. With loss of normal physical activity, bowel function is often impaired, if this is ignored, it will cause added discomfort and anxiety to the child. Before resorting to large doses of aperients it is good to try added fibre in the diet, if this is not contraindicated. Hydrotherapy, even just on the apparent level of play, can bring great relief to a child who has muscle contractures or paralysis, or who is emaciated. At its simplest, this can just take the form of the nurse allowing extended playtime in the bath. Indeed many forms of treatment or routine care can be transformed into fun-times if the nurse is prepared to adopt this approach.

The need for mental stimulus

Boredom and feelings of frustration may be overriding problems for the child whose activities are limited, and a good nurse will enable him to explore positive avenues of interest which will stretch him; she will not be shocked by displays of anger which may be a direct result of his frustration, but rather will help him to channel his energies. Education and mental stimulation are vital for the child who is capable of benefiting to however limited a degree. Ongoing relationships with peers can be a lifeline for the sick or handicapped child, and with a little wise encouragement the well child will be enthusiastic to include him in many ways to the benefit of both.

The danger of over-protection and over-indulgence

It is important to avoid overprotection and overindulgence, not to swamp the child with material goods (which, for many, is the instinctive response to a child's suffering, especially where it is acknowledged that the lifespan will be short) and to maintain discipline for the sake of the child. He needs to know that, as with other children, there are acceptable patterns of behaviour to which he is expected to conform. This structure is important to him for his own security in a world where many things already deviate from the norm. If he is over indulged or spoilt, his behaviour may cause further problems in an already overcharged family atmosphere and he may well become bewildered himself. His need is for physical and emotional love and strength, not material possessions.

THE CHILD WITH A LIFE-THREATENING DISORDER

Answering the child's questions

Most of what has been written applies to the child with a progressive, life-threatening disorder as much as to the child with a chronic condition which is not progressive. However, there are, of course, special things to consider for the former. If the child is aware of his deteriorating condition he may well ask questions. It is important to listen carefully to what he is actually asking; adults easily fall into the trap of assuming that he is asking a more complex question than he really is. The cardinal rule is never to lie to a child. This does not mean to say that he must be given the whole stark truth in one dose, but it is often possible to give truthful reassurance and allay the child's fears about the actual process of dying and death itself, always, of course, using terms which the child understands and being careful not to contradict beliefs held by his family.

The small child has a natural capacity to live for the present moment; recognising this can be used to advantage by those responsible for caring for him. If he is free of pain and discomfort and is surrounded by people he loves and trusts, he is less likely to be fearful for the future. The older child will have taken on more of the anxieties and complexities of an adult in facing dying and death. It must be categorically stated that there are no hard and fast ways of answering his questions or set methods of helping him to come to terms with the truth. So much depends on the nurse's own ability to absorb the impact of what is happening, emotionally and spiritually, and cope with them within herself. Platitudes and pat answers are less than helpful. At times when there seems to be nothing helpful to say, it is better not to use empty words, but rather to try to communicate reassurance through physical presence—just being there alongside through it all.

Symptom control

With great advances in the right use of drugs for symptom control, pain and other distressing symptoms associated with the terminal phase of illness need no longer be a feature. In spite of the development of these skills, it must be admitted that there is still room for research into pain control in paediatrics, for it is an acknowledged fact that the child's absorption of and response to drugs is different from that of adults. Optimum use of drugs depends not only on the doctor's skill in prescribing and titrating, but also on the nurse's awareness of her responsibility to be acutely observant of symptoms and changes, and to be prompt and accurate in reporting them. It should be remembered that optimum results in the use of drugs in pain control can only be achieved through regular and punctual administration.

The family can be spared some suffering by seeing their child relieved of distress and even where the child's level of consciousness renders him apparently unaware, it is important to continue to minimise the family's distress; for example the use of hyoscine can prevent the "death-rattle".

The family's involvement

The importance of the family's involvement throughout the child's illness cannot be stressed enough, but it is never more important than in the terminal phase. Communication between family and professional carers must be open and honest.

The family may well feel particularly inadequate at this time and will need constant reassurance and encouragement to be involved on every level as far as they are able. Many people are afraid of how death itself will actually occur and relatives should be helped to voice their fears, which may well be unfounded.

There are so many small, unobtrusive ways in which the sensitive nurse can help at this stage. The room can be kept fresh and comfortably tidy and the bed linen clean; the child can be cherished and tended lovingly. The family can be helped to talk to their child; they may not realise that hearing is one of the last faculties to be lost and that he may continue to hear long after he has ceased to be able to respond; it follows that they and others should be warned not to say things which may distress him. To hold him or just hold his hand or stroke him is natural and right.

Through all the strain of caring for a chronically sick or severely handicapped child, there will almost inevitably have been moments when parents have wished it would all end. With the actual death of the child, the family may need to be helped through the appalling confusion of the mixture of relief and grief.

Where it is at all possible, and that is surely more frequently than we sometimes assume, it is right for the closest relatives to be with their child when he dies. Brothers and sisters should usually be included, irrespective of their ages. Their bereavement will probably be more distressing if they have been excluded at any stage, especially at such a significant moment as the death of their sibling. The reality is usually gentler and less harrowing than the ordeal of experience by fantasy.

AFTER THE DEATH OF A CHILD

Another false assumption is that the best way to spare the feelings of the bereaved is to act with great haste after the child has died. We have all seen relatives walking away down the hospital drive with a plastic bag or a suitcase within an hour or so of death. How much more healing it is if we create an environment where there is no hurry, where parents and others are given as much time as they want to hold the body of their child, to cry, to talk, to be alone if they so choose. Can they not then be invited to wash and dress their child for the last time, in clothes they choose? It is not necessary to have the funeral on the first available day if this means that the bereaved feel rushed and are denied the time to say their goodbyes and to plan the service for their child. Many parents have never been face to face with death and may never have attended a funeral. They should be helped to understand that it need not be a take-it-or-leave-it handout from the priest or the minister, but something which they themselves can plan so that it is special for their child.

Through these early days we may be tempted to suggest that the relatives who are most distressed should have sedatives or hypnotics prescribed. This is rarely helpful as it merely delays the early stages of grief. It is far more healing to have people alongside who are not afraid to allow the members of the family to express their emotions openly, or indeed to show their own feelings. This applies throughout the months and years of grief following death.

Some relatives and friends will be responsive over the first weeks to the need that the bereaved have of support and friendship but after that such people will be few and far between. Then the general attitude begins to prevail—'best get back to normal and avoid all circumstances or conversations which serve as reminders of the one who has died'. It is at this point that grief, which is a natural response to loss, risks becoming suppressed and distorted to the extent that the natural response becomes a psychiatric disorder. I believe the reason that so many bereaved people end up needing professional counselling or psychiatric treatment is that the rest of us are afraid. Face to face with grief we feel inadequate or embarrassed, we make ourselves scarce and fervently hope that there is an 'expert' around to handle the situation. The nurse, especially one who has known both child and family, has an opportunity to play a vitally important part here, mostly by listening. It is not for nothing that we were given two ears but only one mouth! Let us never be tempted to say 'I know how you feel'. We do not. Even if we ourselves have lost a child, we cannot know how someone else at the centre of such a tragedy is feeling.

Forewarned is forearmed

I think it is helpful to warn parents or other newly bereaved people that the pious platitudes or unsought advice of others can be insensitive and hurtful; that however close the relationship between two people may be, they may grieve differently; and that the healing of grief is a very long, slow process. It is never complete. Parents will never 'get over' the death of their child. To suggest that they will is like saying, 'One day it will seem as if he never existed'. But given time, usually at least 2 years, and at least one person who hears them and seems to understand, life may begin to take on some meaning again. It will never be the same as it once was, but the pain becomes less acute and a new energy and enthusiasm are born. The capacity for enjoyment in life *is* restored.

CONCLUSION

It is humbling to be entrusted with the care of a sick child and most especially one whose life is drawing to a close. As nurses we may become deeply involved with members of the family and may see them at times when their defences are down and they are at their most vulnerable. We may be taken into the confidence of one or more members of the family and allowed an insight into problems and anxieties and patterns of family life which have not previously been shared. We are there not only as professional carers but as fellow human beings who must be able to be trusted implicitly and who are seen to be unafraid of the truth. There will often be times when we have nothing wise to say and when all we can do is to stand by, not trying to set ourselves up as having the answers. Simply by being willing to share the pain, however inadequately, we may help to dissipate it a little.

Staff support is extremely important in this emotionally charged work. It cannot be denied that it is draining and there must be regular opportunities for team members to share the joys and sorrows, perplexities and misunderstandings that inevitably occur. It should be added that a sense of humour in members of the team is invaluable!

There are chronically sick or handicapped children who will be cared for at home throughout; others may be in hospital or institutional care, and yet others will experience both types of environment. The nurse's involvement varies accordingly, but, however full or limited it may be, she does well to remember that the extent to which she brings comfort and support depends largely on how honestly she herself faces life and death. Pretence and evasion are rarely conducive to healing and wholeness in those for whom we care.

Being alongside children with chronic sickness or handicap and their families, we absorb some of their grief. But we also share some of the good things: learning to think of time in terms of depth rather than length; enjoying the swift growth of real friendship; bypassing the usual obstacles of class, creed, colour, age, education; having 'all one's sensitivities heightened' as one father put it. And we begin to recognise and revere the nobility and beauty in every man, woman, and child because tragedy lifts the mask of pretence and truth is revealed. There can be few kinds of nursing more demanding or more fulfilling.

FURTHER READING

Dominica F 1987 Reflections on death in childhood. British Medical Journal vol 294 (10.1.87)

29. Caring for children with special needs

R. Marchant

To care for—to look after, to take thought for, to provide for, to protect, to watch over, to guide, to attend to, to take trouble over, to have regard for, to feel concern for, to be responsible for . . .

Oxford English Dictionary

A great many people are concerned with the care of children with special needs: families and friends; substitute families; many professionals in medicine, nursing, therapy and education; and a whole range of direct care workers. This chapter is about caring for groups of children in settings other than families. The key issue addressed throughout is that of service quality in child care—What matters most for children and their families?

Services for children with special needs are changing rapidly, in a context of both creativity and controversy about the best way forward. Within child care services 'group care' is rapidly emerging as a field of theory and practice that cuts across traditional disciplines (Ainsworth & Fulcher 1981, 1985).

Throughout this chapter 'group care' or 'residential care' refers to care of the child in a setting other than a family. This is deliberately broad-based, and includes any service setting which has 'care' as one of its functions and which provides for children in groups; for example, residential schools, children's homes, group homes, hospitals and respite care units.

The care provided by these services may be temporary or permanent, and on a part-time or full-time or flexible basis. This chapter focuses on the needs and experiences that all children have *in common* in their use of care services. The key question throughout is: *In all of the above settings, with all children, what matters most?* It is this questions of quality which provides our central focus, and an assumption is made throughout that all human services are ultimately accountable to the people they serve: in this instance, children with special needs and their families.

The starting point for looking at service quality is therefore with the person or people relying on the service. How might a good service look from the child's point of view?

The following ideas are based on discussions with children and families and on experience within residential services, and together give the basic structure for the rest of this chapter. They are presented as a child might present them to encourage us to take the child's perspective as much as is possible.

A good service for me would:

- Value me as a unique individual—let me be me
- Let me build genuine relationships—really care about me
- Meet my needs—both ordinary and special
- Involve my family in my care and in any decisions about me
- Recognise me as a child first with a handicap second
- Let me influence the way I live—give me real choices
- Enable me to learn and change and grow
- Be flexible and responsive and accessible—adapt to me.

This chapter looks at ways of building these values into services and translating them into practical realities. We begin with a brief look at definitions and images of residential care, then work through the above eight sets of issues, and end with a broader look at the organisational factors that affect service quality.

DEFINITIONS AND IMAGES

Residential child care has an unfortunate history and a mixed reputation. It is frequently regarded within human services as 'the poor relation' (Potter 1986) and, as Atherton (1986) notes, residential care is definitely the unglamorous end of social work practice. Outside the world of professionals there are also surprisingly high levels of agreement about residential child care—in it's traditional and legal sense of provision for children 'in care' it is 'a feature of society that is almost universally condemned across class, age, interest and political outlook' (Lee & Pithers 1980). Those perhaps in the best position to comment—the children, parents and careworkers directly involved in residential care—tend to hold similarly negative views and images (Whittaker 1984).

Some of these negative perspectives are firmly grounded in the known damaging effects of 'traditional' forms of residential care: the rigidity, block treatment, depersonalisation and social distancing described by Goffman (1961) as features of large institutions, and the more recent documentation of the damaging effects and deprivation experienced by disabled children in hospitals and residential services (Oswin 1971, 1985). In more general terms the disabling influence of institutional care has been well documented in research demonstrating that residential institutions can actually *require* their residents to remain dependent (Miller & Gwynne 1982).

These powerfully negative views and images of residential care are reflected in and compounded by the generally low status of direct care workers. Whether employed as nursing auxiliaries, house parents, care assistants or support workers, staff caring for children with special needs are usually poorly paid, offered minimal training and little support, and are rarely involved in decision making. They are likely to be seen by other professionals as having strong relationships with 'their' children, a good heart but few skills (Knoll & Ford 1987).

The staff themselves may adopt this devaluing of what they do, and create for themselves a limited and limiting definition of their role as 'just' caring: doing the things that no-one else wants to do—feeding and toileting and bathing and changing. Yet although there can be 'good' caring and 'bad' caring, there is no such thing as 'just' caring: some intrinsic features of residential child care make this a service with a central place in family support and child development.

One of these is *time*: residential care is by far the most significant service in a child and family's life in terms of time. Even children who stay at a residential school just on a weekly basis will spend *at least 75% of their time in the residential part of the service*. No other service offers anything like this amount of involvement in a child's life.

Secondly, *the nature of the task*: care work is concerned with the details of life and in this lies both its strengths and its risks. Direct care staff are in a unique position to get to know children, to build strong relationships with them and to teach, support and enable their growth. They are also, because of the very intimacy of their involvement, in an unusually powerful position to have a negative as well as a positive impact in the child's life. Residential work has been described as 'total immersion in the minutiae of day to day life' (Potter 1986) and Atherton (1986) speaks of 'doing good in minute particulars'. Ordinary everyday events are a powerful medium for influence and this is particularly so for children. Children without doubt view their carers as central figures in their lives, and often form strong lasting attachments with direct care staff.

Working with children in groups and working with the 'shared life space' of children is both a challenging and demanding role, and residential care can be a creative and liberating force (Lee & Pithers 1980). Seeing residential care in this way requires a real redefinition of the function of these services and a radical rethink of the role of direct careworkers. Knoll & Ford (1987) argue for 'the definition of a new type of role that really has no parallel in our culture . . . direct service workers . . . as aides, educators and facilitators'.

Summary. Services are changing fast and residential care increasingly means providing care for a child for some of the time rather than for all of their lives. Davis (1981) defines three main models of residential child care: *family substitute*, which replaces care by the family; *family supplement*, which aims to enable the family to continue to care; and *family alternative*, which aims to provide another option altogether—something different to family care. Many residential services may of course fulfil all three of these roles for different children. However, there is increasing recognition that the first choice for family substitute care is another family rather than a 'care' setting. Given this welcome trend towards finding alternative families for children who need them (including in recent years those children with very special needs—see Argent 1986), and given our focus on the care of children in groups in settings *other than* families, we will work on the basis that the majority of children receiving group care will have involvement with their families, whether substitute or natural.

With these basic thoughts on residential care we move on to look in more detail at the eight issues of service quality outlined earlier. For each one we will look at its relevance in terms of service quality and then work through some practical suggestions for building these values into services.

1. Design around individuals: 'Value me as a unique individual— let me be me'

One of the key criticisms levelled at institutions is their treatment of everyone as the same: the depersonalisation and deindividualisation of people.

How can a service ensure that children and families are always recognised as individuals?

Build the service around the needs of individual children and families: start from scratch by asking what does this particular child and family *need* rather than what do we offer. Make individual planning systems genuinely individual: careplans or individual plans are more likely to be relevant and individually meaningful if they are put together by the child, their family and those very closely involved with the child rather than by a panel of distant experts. They are also much more likely to be put into action if they have the commitment of front-line staff.

Support individual keyworkers in taking responsibility for coordinating the care of each child. Make it their task to become acutely aware of the child as an individual: who they are, how they feel, what is important to them, etc.

Avoid speaking of and thinking of the children as one (them, that lot, the kids, the group) or, worse, subdividing the children by some shared characteristic (the feeders, the walkers). Actively fight assumptions such as 'they're all the same' and the discussion of children as 'types' by their handicap. Insist that children are spoken to and about at all times using the names by which they or their family wish them to be known. Make the children's bedrooms or living spaces as different as possible: details matter—even down to one's own flannel and towel and duvet cover as well as personal possessions (and of course clothes).

Work with staff to emphasise the differences between individual children; introduce new staff or new children carefully and on a one to one basis, and make the introductions two-way. Encourage individual routines that replicate the child's lifestyle at home as far as possible and, unless there is good reason not to, do things the way the child is used to doing them rather than the way they 'have always been done' within the service.

2. Enable strong relationships: 'Let me build genuine relationships—really care about me'

One of the often heard assumptions among residential care staff is that getting 'involved' with the children (or getting too involved) is dangerous. Yet research among children receiving residential care has found again and again that the quality of the relationships between staff and children is considered by children as *the* single most important feature of care (Whittaker 1984, Potter 1986). Families also are clear about wanting to build relationships with familiar and trusted staff who are honest and open. The personal touch or commitment is what brings alive the process of caring (Atherton 1986).

How can a service facilitate good relationships between staff and children?

Minimise the number of staff involved with each child: have small teams of staff working with small groups of children. Allocate work by child and not by task, i.e. plan routines such that each staff member carries out all the care for a small number of children rather than planning routines around tasks. Actively support the making of individual relationships: recognise the dangers or risks involved in this—favouritism/over-identification and work to prevent them through staff support and supervision.

Build the expectation of strong relationships into job descriptions, into induction and ongoing training, into staff appraisal and development. Do everything possible to enable staff to retain their emotional openness. Work on the basis that the main resource one has as a carer is oneself and use supervision, group work and teaching to support staff as real people with real feelings that are central to their work.

Value staff as important and worth investing in; aim for high staff continuity over time. Look at the broader organisational supports that encourage staff to stay. Create a culture that actively values the making of two-way relationships between staff and children. Use measures of engagement as indicators of quality—how much time do children spend interacting with staff or with each other?

Teach listening skills to all front-line staff. One of the major unmet needs identified by children with disabilities is the chance to talk about difficulties or concerns (Madge & Fassam 1982). This does not mean that every child with a disability needs professional counselling, simply that they need someone who will spend time with them actively listening and helping to explore problems.

Value relationships between children and staff. As Bettelheim (1950) pointed out, 'Love is not enough'—relationships between children and their paid carers cannot be left to chance. A helpful relationship for a child is an enabling one. Caring means conducting, guiding, supporting and facilitating rather than doing things for or to the child. The relationships between children and their carers are highly personal and intimate, and   very important to both parties. They need to be recognised as such.

3. Meet individual needs: 'Meet my needs—both ordinary and special'

The basic assumption that services should be designed to meet the child's needs seems too obvious to need stating. Yet creating services that are genuinely needs-oriented is an extremely challenging process.

How can a service meet the very different needs of the individual children served?

Be clear about service aims. No single service can or should even attempt to meet all of a child's needs: services work best if they are clear and coherent about their function(s). Involve front-line staff in defining service aims. There are a number of new ways of working with staff which are extremely helpful in working towards this goal; for example, the programme design session (Yates 1980), which focuses on three basic questions:

Who are the people?	What are their needs?	What would it take to meet those needs?

This approach encourages staff to look creatively at what their service is for. Within child care services this process quickly identifies the potential tension between the needs of the child and the needs of their family—most obvious in the provision of respite care—and can prove a very useful way of enabling staff to think more deeply and more freely about the children and families whom they serve.

Address the possible tension between creating 'ordinary lives' and meeting special needs. Many children who receive residential care have very special needs and are likely to need skilled help in order to live ordinary lives. In order to meet the diversity of needs of children, staff must be equipped with some real skills in addition to the basics of good physical care.

Teach staff about the ordinary needs of all children—love and security, new experiences, praise and recognition and responsibility (see Kellmer Pringle 1975 for a full discussion). Teach staff about the special needs of the children whom they care for. This kind of teaching is far more likely to be effective if based around the needs of the actual children with whom the staff are involved.

Equip staff with skills and support in the setting of limits and handling of behaviour that challenges those limits; both are necessary skills in any group work with children with or without special needs. Involve front-line staff and families fully in the planning of care for each child, again making this a process led by need as much as is possible.

4. Work in partnership with families: 'Involve my family in my care and in any decisions about me'

Recent research has found that in many residential services families are not included and sometimes they are specifically excluded (Burford & Casson 1989). The inclusion of families in child care planning is an essential that needs to be actively encouraged: parents love the deepest, know the child the best and are around the longest. Even those parents who are unable to care for their child at home often provide the most permanence and continuity in a child's life over the years.

How can a service involve families in the care of and planning for their child?

Work hard with staff to define their role as clearly distinct from parenting (*unless* the care being provided is family substitute care). Include parents in all planning for their child. Create both formal and informal mechanisms for ensuring this happens; for example, a central role for parents in assessment and individual planning; clear lines of communication via named keyworkers for each child; active inclusion in all decisions however 'small', like haircuts and choosing clothes.

Work with parents in ways that suit them—adapt to their style. See McConkey (1985) for a number of useful suggestions for ways of doing this. Encourage close links between the service and the family. Communicate clearly and honestly and encourage regular visits by the family members to the service and by staff to the family home if parents are happy with this.

Teach staff about family systems and relationships in ways that enable them to understand more easily and relate more sensitively: the concept of no-fault communication is very helpful here (Burford & Casson 1989). Create forums for parental involvement in the planning of the whole service, through parent/staff meetings or quality circles.

5. Be child-centred: 'Recognise me as a child first—let me live life like other children do'

Another common and damaging experience of many children with special needs is that of living life very differently from other children and being separate and segregated from the ordinary world. Services for children need to be primarily child orientated. As noted in the conclusions of *Ask the children*, a research project that involved interviewing a number of disabled and able-bodied children: 'the disabled and the non-disabled are not really all that different' (Madge & Fassam 1982). Yet services often reinforce the differentness of the people they care for, whether through their physical location or style of building, mix of disabilities, routines and rhythms, lifestyles, etc. (Wolfensberger 1978).

How can a service minimise a child's disability and recognise him as a child first, while still meeting his special needs?

Base the rhythms of residential child care as far as possible on those of ordinary family life. Take part in community activities on an individual basis. Actively support home-based friendships and links with local groups; use local facilities (shops/clubs/sports) and local services (social/educational/medical) wherever possible.

Make the patterns of daily living as 'ordinary' as possible: the fragmentation of tasks in institutions can have a number of detrimental effects on children's lifestyles. This is a list of the people regularly involved in the life of one child in one residential school/hospital: care staff, night staff, drivers, porters, nurses, teachers, classroom helpers, physiotherapist, occupational therapist, speech therapist, social worker, psychologist, doctor. This array of people with direct contact is then backed up with a less visible and even larger team; for example, laundry workers, cooks, dieticians, administrators, secretaries, etc. This fragmentation of tasks can add to the discontinuity of the child's care, by making apparently simple activities complex (e.g. going out), and by limiting the child's experience (e.g. of food buying and preparation and of looking after clothes) and often by slowing down the process of decision-making and making communication very difficult. While there is a real need for multidisciplinary work with disabled children there are also strong arguments for taking skills and expertise in through front-line workers wherever possible, and for having the tasks of daily living take place close to the children.

Design the service such that it is child orientated. This means ensuring that the ordinary needs of children are central. One of the main needs of all children is to play. Play is the business of childhood: 'Play is, for the child, his most important and serious activity' (Stallibrass 1976). Children with disabilities may need skilled support and help in order to be able to play. All staff need to understand the value of and development of play, and to have the practical equipment and knowhow to enable even the most severely disabled child to participate in play activities. The service as a whole must recognise the value of play, which means allowing or even encouraging noise and mess and occasional chaos!

Another essential lesson of childhood is learning to be with other people, and residential services need to help develop in children the 'social skills' that are necessary for all of life. All children gain from time with peers free from adult influence, and this is something that many children with special needs miss out on. Interaction between children with severe communication difficulties may need to be creatively encouraged. Sometimes the most basic things like seating arrangements can help. There has been little recognition of the power of the group in residential care, but research is now showing what many staff have known for a long time: that the group can be a powerful tool for influencing and changing behaviour, for stimulating creativity, for increasing social learning and for achieving tasks (see Ch. 11; see also Ross & Thorpe 1987).

6. Empower the child and his family: 'Let me influence the way I live my life—give me real choices about things that matter to me'

Institutions, by their size and nature, often take power away from people, whether through loss of identity or loss of autonomy. Institutional living can encourage passivity and the fragmentation of roles and tasks can make it very difficult for an individual to assert any real control over their own life. It is sometimes suggested that children with disabilities need to *learn* to come to terms with lack of control over their own lives to prepare them for the hard reality of life with a handicap. However, if services are to change, then equipping young disabled children with the confidence and ability to take maximum control of their own destiny is an essential foundation stone for this change.

How can services empower children and their families?

Set out a charter of rights with the children in simple straightforward language: this a useful exercise for direct care staff with the group of children they work with. Such a charter might include items such as 'I can choose what I wear and what to drink and what time I go to bed up till 9.30 pm and 11 pm at weekends.' This process serves to enable the child to take control but also to recognise that there have to be limits to this control when living as part of a group. Such an approach is particularly useful with older children and teenagers; children need boundaries and are happy with limits and sanctions as long as these make sense and are seen to be fair and reasonable (Whittaker 1984).

Enable children to take control. Participating and making choices is as important for the most severely handicapped child as it is for the more able children. Giving control to very disabled children might be a more challenging process, but every child who is able to indicate yes or no (do you want to or not?) can usually also make choices (this one or that one?) through eye-pointing or gestures. Enabling children to take control is time consuming and can be surprisingly exhausting. Staff need to be actively supported in working to involved children in decision-making.

Another powerful reason for actively encouraging assertiveness among children with disabilities is the prevention of ill-treatment and abuse. Recent research suggests that a child's susceptibility to abuse increases with the severity of their handicap and that the likelihood of detection decreases (Morgan 1987, White et al 1987). It appears that compliance among children with special needs may be a factor increasing their vulnerability (Blyth & Milner 1989, Daar-Watson 1984).

Most children in mainstream schools are now likely to be taught some version of 'good sense defence' (e.g. the Kidscape teaching materials), and preventative teaching is just beginning in special schools. The teaching needs careful adaptation, particularly for children who receive intimate physical care, and the involvement of parents and all who work closely with the child is essential to the success of any preventative programme. A second major factor in the prevention of abuse is the awareness of child care staff about child protection issues in general and the importance of assertiveness in particular. Respecting the child's right to make choices and say no can be a foundation stone for effective 'good sense defence' teaching.

7. Develop competence: 'Enable me to learn and change and grow'

Caring in the traditional sense has often meant doing things *for* children. To enable children with disabilities to develop skills and to grow personally requires staff who define their role much more in terms of doing *with* children. This is quite a shift in emphasis and needs actively supporting. Doing with often takes more time and effort than doing for, and this needs to be explicitly recognised in staff training and staff supervision.

Services can also further disable children by limiting their experiences of and access to the 'outside' world. Goffman (1961) pointed out a major irony inherent in the idea of institutionally based 'rehabilitation', where everything that goes on within the institution is the opposite of that which goes on without, which means that the better one becomes adjusted to the inside the worse one is adjusted to the outside by definition.

How can a service enable children to develop real and useful skills?

Plan a child's daily routine around the things she *can* do rather than the things she can't. For example, if a child is able to help hold a toothbrush and to choose breakfast with help, the morning should be planned to give sufficient time for full involvement in these activities. Ensure that all child care staff understand the value of participatory and incidental learning. A useful parallel for staff is the similarity in the ways in which they learn their jobs: learning by doing is the most common (some would say the *only*) way of learning to care, and learning by doing is something often denied to children with disabilities because of the creativity needed to involve them in day to day life. Teach staff to teach: use effective systems of positive learning and build in regular opportunities for children to practise the skills learnt.

8. Be user friendly: 'Be flexible and responsive and accessible— adapt to me'

Since children with special needs are all so individual and so different, our services and approaches to them should be similarly varied. Adapting to the child, rather than expecting the child to adapt to the service, again takes planning and thinking.

How can services be more flexible and friendly for the people using them?

Replicate the child's home routines as far as is possible. Whether this is bedtime or the order of events on getting up, make it the business of the keyworker or main carer drawing up the initial care plan to find out how things happen at home. This flexibility needs to extend beyond the basics of routine to include specific requests of parents; particularly important for children receiving respite or shared care. The question of 'who knows best' will often rear its head through this process and this is where the concept of partnership with parents is truly essential.

Make the services available at short notice as and when the parents need it. Developing a truly flexible residential service is extremely diffi-cult and requires very creative use of resources. Employing part-time and relief (sessional) staff to work as required dramatically increases flexi-bility but has costs in terms of discontinuity, by increasing the number of staff. Another approach is to build in the expectation that staff roles will include a number of tasks other than direct care, for example keyworking; supporting children in schools and outside activities; training and private study and secondary care tasks—housework and care of clothes, etc.: roles that can be 'fitted in' around the demands of child care.

Increase flexibility on a day to day basis by giving individual staff greater control over their own working pattern. Build in 'float' hours or unallo-cated hours onto the rota to be used for specific activities with the child, for additional cover when needed, for supporting the child at home or for keyworking tasks.

The responsiveness of the service is directly linked to its internal flexibility and ability to adapt to each child's particular needs. But responsiveness is also a function of staff attitudes. For example, the suggestion of providing a respite service 'on demand' to parents often meets with cynicism and mistrust from care staff and other professionals, who feel that parents will abuse and misuse this control over the service. Yet it seems likely that the opposite may be true: provision of truly flexible responsive respite care available on demand might actually decrease the rate at which parents use the service (see Ch. 30, p. 510).

Fight anonymity: have one named person within the care service whom the family and child know is 'theirs'. Whether this is a keyworker or frontline manager, ensure that they have sufficient autonomy and authority to be able to make day to day decisions, and adequate training and support to be able to make them well.

Summary. We have considered eight features of service quality in child care from the child's point of view. These can be listed as follows: *let me be me; really care about me; meet my needs; involve my family; let me be a child first with a handicap second; let me influence the way I live; help me learn and be flexible and friendly.* We conclude by looking at the broader issues that enable services to build in these values.

ORGANISATIONAL FACTORS THAT AFFECT SERVICE QUALITY

The two key features of effective organisations in terms of the above criteria are: (1) the value base of the service; and (2) issues relating to staff support.

The *value base of the service* needs to be, above all, explicit. Clarity of aims and accessibility of values are critical ingredients of successful services. It is the role of leaders in human services to be 'expert in the promotion and protection of values and principles' (Burford & Casson 1989) and this is particularly true when services are undergoing rapid change and development, as is currently the case in residential services for children with special needs.

These values need to be built into the very foundations of the service, written into operational policies and explicitly referred to in job descriptions. They must form a central part of all staff induction and training, and the recruitment of staff needs to take into account likely personal commitment to such values. Front-line staff in child care need to know not only what to do and how to do it but *why* it is important. 'All good residential care is based on commitment, enthusiasm and a sense of purpose' (Potter 1986). Commitment is something that can be actively cultured (Provencal 1987), and a key mechanism for the culturing of commitment is *staff support*, which is our second feature of good organisations.

How might good staff support appear to the front-line staff working in child care? As with the children, staff do not come neatly packaged and therefore neither should our approaches to them. But there are some features of good staff support that are reasonably universal. From the point of view of a direct care worker, good staff support would:

- Value me
- Enable me to work well and notice when I do
- Stretch me: teach me things I will find useful
- Make sure I have the resources and back-up that I need
- Encourage me to develop new skills and better practices
- Support me in exploring the values on which the work is based
- Encourage me to stay and to keep going.

Supervision is one approach to staff support that has been well tried and tested, and acts to provide individual support through regular, structured sessions with someone specifically trained in listening or counselling and problem-solving skills. Supervision has been described as 'the process of talking to someone else involved in the same system about what one is doing in order to be able to do it better' (Atherton 1986). Supervision aims to improve the quality of life within a service by enhancing staff performance.

Whether or not formal supervision is used as a model for staff support, there are some basics of good management of particular relevance to child care staff. Firth (1983) gives the following as features of effective support in residential services: someone with time to listen, who holds similar values, helps clarify issues and keep things in perspective; someone who cares about what's happening to *me* and who notices when there's something wrong without me approaching them; someone who makes us feel we're doing a good job, who recognises our successes; someone with clarity of vision, who is confident and gives us confidence.

A service that cares for and values its staff is far more likely to enable them to be able to really care for and value the children they serve. It is this culturing of commitment, this supporting of involvement which enables staff to care in the positive sense of the word. Interestingly, the origin of the word 'care' has links with grief and trouble, hence 'to care' is also defined as:

... to sorrow, to grieve, to be troubled; an object or matter of concern; a burden, a state of anxiety; a serious or grave mental attitude ...

It is not possible to care well and to be indifferent. Caring is an emotional business, and the only way to do it well is to really care. To do this and to keep on doing it takes both personal resources and commitment and also the support and back-up of an organisation designed to enable and encourage caring as a process of value in its own right.

REFERENCES

Ainsworth F, Fulcher L (eds) 1981 Group care for children: concepts and issues. Tavistock, London

Argent H 1986 Find me a family. Pergamon, London

Atherton J S 1986 Professional supervision in group care. Tavistock, London

Bettleheim B 1950 Love is not enough. Tavistock, London

Blyth E, Milner J 1989 Compliance and abuse. Special Children 1989 (October): 8–9

Burford G, Casson S F 1989 Including families in residential work: educational and agency tasks. British Journal of Social Work 19: 17–37

Daar-Watson J 1984 Talking about the best kept secret: sexual abuse and children with disabilities. The Exceptional Parent 1984 (September): 15–20

Davis A 1981 The residential solution. Tavistock, London

Firth H 1983 Training support staff. In: An ordinary life. Kings Fund Centre, London

Fulcher L C, Ainsworth F (eds) 1985 Group care practice with children. Tavistock, London

Goffman I 1961 Asylums. Anchor, New York

Kellmer Pringle M 1987 The needs of children. Hutchinson, London

Knoll J, Ford A 1987 Beyond caregiving: a reconceptualisation of the role of the residential service provider. In: Taylor et al (below)

Lee P, Pithers D 1980 Radical residential child care: Trojan horse or non-runner? In: M Brake, R Bailey (eds) Radical social work practice. Edward Arnold, London

McConkey R 1985 Working with parents: a practical guide for teachers and therapists. Brookline, Cambridge, MA

Madge N, Fassam M 1982 Ask the children: experiences of physical disability in the school years. Batsford, London

Miller E J, Gwynne G V 1972 A life apart. Tavistock, London

Morgan S R 1987 Abuse and neglect of handicapped children. College Hill, Boston

Myers D, Cochrane C 1980 Children in crisis: a time for caring, a time for change. Sage, London

Oswin M 1971 The empty hours. Penguin, London

Oswin M 1985 They keep going away. Blackwell, London

Potter P 1986 Long-term residential child care: the positive approach. Social Work Monographs, Univ. of East Anglia

Provencal G 1987 Culturing commitment. In: Taylor (below)

Ross S, Thorpe A 1987 Groupwork with children. In: Lishman J Working with children. Kingsley, London

Stallibrass A 1977 The self respecting child. Penguin, London

Taylor F, Bicklen D, Knoll J 1987 Community integration for people with severe disabilities. Teachers College Press, Colombia

Watson G 1989 The abuse of disabled children and young people. In: Child abuse and neglect—an introduction. Open University Press

White R et al 1987 Physical disabilities as risk factors in child maltreatment: a selected review. American Journal of Orthopsychiatry 57(1): 93–101

Whittaker D et al 1984 The experience of residential care from the perspective of children, parents and caregivers. Univ. of York

Wolfensberger W 1978 The ideal human service for a societally devalued group. Rehabilitation Literature 39(1):15–17

Yates J 1983 Operational procedure for programme design sessions. In: Normalisation training through PASS 3: Teamleaders' manual. Atlanta, Georgia

USEFUL ADDRESSES

Keep Deaf Children Safe Child Abuse Project, c/o Nuffield Hearing and Speech Centre, 325 Grays Inn Road, London WC1X 0DA

Kidscape, World Trade Centre, Europe House, London E1 9AA (Tel: 071-488 0488)

30. Caring for children living away from home: policy and legal framework

P. Russell

The Office of Population and Census Survey Reports (1989) indicate that there are 360 000 disabled children living in the United Kingdom. Of these, 355 000 live at home. But if 5000 children cannot live with their natural families (for a number of reasons), and an unspecified number of the 360 000 children spend time away on respite or short-term care, we need to understand why and where good quality alternative care can be provided. The OPCS Reports give some worrying reasons about *why* disabled children cannot continue to live at home. 8% of a sample of 1000 children living away from home had suffered sexual abuse. A further 7% had been physically abused. 33% of the children had unsuitable family homes. Unsuitability might include parents in prison or who had a history of drug misuse. 25% had 'problems' at home (which could be linked to lack of family support). 33% of the children were found by natural *and* foster families to have such significant health or behaviour problems that they could not be managed in an ordinary home. The Reports do not specify the nature of these behaviour and health problems. But it is reasonable to assume that some family breakdowns could have been prevented if the families concerned had received better help and counselling earlier.

In terms of planning for suitable residential or foster care, the OPCS Reports show that only 12% of families with children at home had a social worker. Only 72% of the *foster* families regularly saw a social worker, although they were caring for disabled children. The most frequent source of information and help was likely to be a *doctor* (GP or hospital specialist) and the lack of routine referral to social services suggests that everybody working in child health services must take a positive role in terms of telling parents about sources of help, in sharing information and in identifying special difficulties such as behaviour problems early enough for intervention to be effective. It is important to remember that 94% of all the disabled children in the OPCS study were regarded as having significant behaviour disorders for some of the time. As behaviour difficulties are the most likely to impede integration in education (and leisure or respite services) it is obvious that many families are coping with unmet needs.

The evaluation of Honeylands (Brimblecombe & Russell 1987) found that parents of children with the most difficult behaviour problems were often the least likely to use respite care (although they needed it the most). One parent described herself as 'too tired' to negotiate for a break. Other parents felt that no-one would want to care for their child because of the behaviour problems, and were frightened of being rebuffed if they wanted help. Children with severe behaviour disorders do, of course, pose enormous problems in any form of group care. At Honeylands it was acknowledged that one child with very severe behaviour problems did pose a risk to other fragile and less mobile children unless intensive and additional help was available. However, without the opportunity for a break, the risk of family breakdown is multiplied and the children's difficulties escalate instead of being resolved. Working with young children with behaviour problems right from the start is therefore a crucial measure in prevention of family breakdown and avoidance of the need to find substitute care.

Family (and residential) placements may not only break down because a child is seen as difficult and because behaviour has become a major problem. Behaviour itself may be a response to major changes in a child's life. Berridge (1987), looking at foster placement breakdowns, found that breakdown was most likely for *any* child if 'profound social, emotional, geographical, educational and economic changes' occurred simultaneously. Where a child has a disability, such major changes (which could include the significant and often negative consequences of divorce or redundancy) would create a double jeopardy and family systems could break down.

Berridge's study also highlights the consequences of 'significant personal relationships and the importance of permanence' in children's lives. Children living away from home who were able to retain contact with friends and schools, or be placed with siblings, seemed to fare much better than those who had to face new relationships on all fronts. Education may in fact be the stable factor in disabled children's lives and the procedures of the 1981 Education Act (whilst not designed to provide planning for day-to-day living) still offer a unique opportunity to involve all relevant professionals in planning for children's future development. The conclusions of the Berridge study are also timely reminders of the need to provide continuity for parents as well as children and to acknowledge the problems for many families in constantly working with new and changing professional advisers. Indeed discontinuity may be a significant factor in avoiding family breakdown in the first place and keeping a child within the family home.

DEVELOPMENTS IN FOSTER CARE AND ADOPTION

When children cannot live with their natural parents, there have been encouraging developments in substitute family care. Many local authorities now run foster schemes for disabled children, some using the specialist fostering schemes of Barnardo's, the British Adoption and Fostering

Agencies, or Parents for Children. The past 5 years have seen major advances in successful fostering for even the most severely disabled children, with enhanced allowances and a range of support services from loan of equipment to home helps and respite care.

The majority of placements for disabled children will be with families who have been specially recruited and trained. Many families have some existing interest in or knowledge of disability and it is clear that some 'atypical' fostering (and adoption) placements work very well. Examples of such atypical fostering arrangements include one family with three disabled children; a single man who has adopted a teenage boy with spina bifida; an older couple who befriended and subsequently fostered a girl with Down syndrome and a serious cardiac condition, and her two brothers. However, goodwill alone is insufficient, and careful assessment is necessary of any prospective caring families. An evaluation of placements by Parents for Children found that the substitute families were remarkably like natural families. A predisposing favourable factor was the foster family's own social and family networks, as well as their interest and willingness to learn. In effect, families who were isolated were likely to experience difficulties like any ordinary family in the community. Even if the family did not have social or personal problems, there would still be a need for respite care, and for opportunities to 'have a break'.

Many foster parents with disabled children also have a special role in maintaining links and helping natural parents and siblings to keep in touch. Many parents of disabled children still feel ambivalent about the use of foster placements (which are often seen as indicating an incompetent parent). Advocates of foster placements should emphasise the positive contribution of shared care for the child concerned and create time and space for natural and substitute families to get to know each other. If children are moving out of residential care (particularly residential care in a hospital or NHS setting), there may be major anxieties about not only the quality of care but also the security of the placement being offered. Parents whose children live in NHS provision are not required to contribute to the residential costs. Although local authorities may (and many do) waive charges, they may legally require parents to contribute on a means-tested scale to their child's placement costs. Some parents have been particularly indignant when they had not accepted the need for a move and, again, social services and child health personnel need to collaborate in helping parents accept that a move is the best possible decision.

The decision to agree that a child with a disability should be adopted will also be very problematic and, wherever possible, parents should be helped to come to a voluntary agreement. Local authorities can, subject to certain conditions, seek a court order for the relinquishment of parental rights. But agreement, if at all possible, is likely to be the happier solution for all concerned and will enable an older child to possibly retain contact with grandparents and other friends and families. Adoption Allowances are now available to encourage the adoption of children by families who would not otherwise have been able to offer a child a permanent home; they are often little known or discussed by prospective adoptive parents, but they offer an invaluable additional income in caring for a child with special needs. Foster and adoptive parents are of course eligible for the Attendance Allowance and other Department of Health allowances relating to disability.

RESPITE OR SHORT-TERM CARE

The large majority of disabled children live at home. However, the development of respite care over the past decade (with some 300 schemes now in operation) has shown the importance that parents place upon 'having a break' and the value for children of opportunities to sample another family's lifestyle and leisure activities. Historically, respite care developed as an emergency service, usually providing short-term care within a long-stay hospital or other institution in order to meet a family crisis. Such respite care was often offered in 'block bookings' for summer holidays or other periods and was often distant from families and friends. However, there has been growing concern to develop flexible and local family support services which include respite care as one of a range of options for individual families and children. This shift in thinking sees respite care as part of an *integrated* service and not a special one-off intervention. In Oswin's words (1985), 'short term care should be regarded as a very specialist service needing clearly defined aims based on principles of child care practice and requiring continuous monitoring of standards with an emphasis on how it might be affecting individual children'. Oswin was stressing the need to think of children first, because she had identified a potential tension in respite care, which is frequently directed at supposed parent relief and not necessarily regarded as one part of an individual family support plan. Taking a child away may not solve the problems in a family where there are other factors (such as not coping with difficult behaviour) that await the child on his or her return home.

A number of studies on respite care have suggested that there are certain key principles to be followed:

1. That it should be a *local* service, where children can continue to attend school as if living at home.

2. That the service offers good quality *child care*. Although 11 000 individual respite care placements took place in mental handicap hospitals in 1988/9, hospitals are not good places for giving families 'breaks' and every effort should be made to find community support.

3. Availability on *demand*. Many parents want very short periods of respite care (often on a babysitting rather than residential basis). But they need it to be available at short notice. A number of schemes operating

respite on demand (such as the Somerset and Leeds respite family schemes) have proved that families do not abuse the service and welcome the 'ordinariness' of being able to leave their children as if he or she did not have a disability.

There is also awareness of the need to protect children and carers. The legal basis of respite care has always been poorly defined, but local authorities will now be required to use procedures adopted for the registration of foster parents and a number are introducing agreements or contracts (together with insurance schemes).

A particular problem in some respite care schemes has been apparent underuse, despite parental appreciation of the availability of such a service. The Honeylands evaluation (1987) and the DOH Social Work Inspectorate study of respite fostering in Norfolk and Oxfordshire (Banks & Grizzell 1984) both identified a number of families who emphasised the importance of guaranteed availability of respite care in enabling them to maintain severely handicapped children at home. Two families in the Honeylands study (Brimblecombe & Russell 1987) actually claimed they had used emergency short-term care when in fact they had never done so. But so real was their perception of the service offered that they felt secure enough to feel that they had used it and found it a critical factor in continuing family care.

Evidence about the ability of short-term respite care to alleviate family stress is inevitably subjective. The Avon research (1987) emphasises the fallacy of assuming that respite care is a universal panacea for all family problems. This study found that 'many of the *user* families had unmet needs as did many of the non-user families' . . . in both groups! The Honeylands evaluation suggests that many families may in fact need relief, but will still only use respite services on an incremental basis. Hence family relief may not be instantaneous and, indeed, measurements of stress levels in families in the Honeylands studies suggested that some families were actually *more* stressed at the start of using a service than before they did so. Overall stress levels were clearly significantly reduced after a period of time. But the stresses associated with letting a child go to another family or unit for the first time are frequently underestimated. The DOH Inspectorate Report (1984) in Oxfordshire made a similar point, noting the stages through which parents needed to go in becoming positive utilisers of respite services. This study identified three hurdles for potential users to overcome, namely using the service chosen for the first time; leaving the child overnight; and placing a child for a longer period while the parents went away on their own.

Although there has been no comparative research into parental satisfaction with different models of respite care, it seems that parents are more likely to be satisfied if a service is clearly linked to a voluntary organisation, school or a wider service like Honeylands or Preston Skreens in order to put the service in context and to ensure that respite care is a rewarding experience for the child. Respite care should also be seen in the context of the child's overall needs. Families who are using respite care (perhaps in different settings) to the extent that the child spends little time at home may need counselling about whether permanent fostering arrangements are needed.

RESIDENTIAL SCHOOLS

There are 2500 independent residential schools in the United Kingdom. Not all are special schools, but children with disabilities and special needs are increasingly attending ordinary residential schools. Falling demand for residential education has meant that many schools are changing to meet new demands. As the schools are developing greater capacity, many local authorities have been closing residential homes and looking to fostering and adoption to provide care for separated children. Although there are no official statistics on the number of children with disabilities and special needs who are living at residential schools for 52 weeks a year, there is concern that the number is rapidly growing. The passage of the Children Bill through Parliament led to considerable debate about the quality of some of this provision and about the problems of *inspecting* independent schools. Although HMIs have general duties to inspect schools, many of the newer independent schools are residential homes with education on the premises. They may be awaiting recognition by the Department of Education and Science as efficient. Pending that approval, they are registered as residential homes by the local authority in which they are situated. But registration officers do not usually have much experience of children's provision and their powers and duties are in any event circumscribed. As a result of concerns raised in the context of the Children Bill, amendments were laid for the first time that:

It shall be the duty of—(a) the proprietor of any independent school which provides accommodation for any child, and (b) any person who is not the proprietor of such a school but who is responsible for conducting it—to safeguard and promote the child's welfare.

To implement this duty, 'any person authorised by the local authority' may enter the school 'at any reasonable time' to carry out an inspection of premises, children and records in the manner as is laid down in regulations. This duty is an important one because it emphasises the principle of the Children Act that the *child's* welfare is paramount and the local authority is the child's agent in ensuring that any needs are met. The funding of the new inspection arrangements has also yet to be resolved. The Association of Metropolitan Authorities has estimated that it could cost £4 million a year to properly inspect all residential schools and has suggested that proprietors might be expected to contribute to this cost as do proprietors of private residential homes through the payment of an annual registration and inspection fee. Whatever arrangements are finally agreed, it is important that any professional visiting a school should be aware of the importance of looking at the overall quality of *personal care* in addition to any education offered and should notify the social services department if there is cause for concern. Children with disabilities are the most likely to attend residential schools very distant from their place of origin and to be unable to communicate with family or friends without help. In view of the growth of residential education as a means of providing *social care*, vigilance is important—whilst acknowledging the major contribution that many residential special schools offer to children with special needs.

THE CHILDREN ACT 1989: THE LEGAL FRAMEWORK FOR CARING FOR CHILDREN

The *Children Act 1989*, which received Royal Assent on 16 November 1989, is the most comprehensive piece of legislation that Parliament has ever enacted about children. It draws together and simplifies existing legislation to produce a more practical and consistent legal code. The Act strikes a new balance between family autonomy and the protection of children, and in order to achieve these goals it lays specific duties upon social services departments, education and health authorities to work together more effectively in the best interests of children.

I Parental rights—and responsibilities

The Act introduces a new concept of *parental responsibility* as opposed to parental rights. Clause 3 notes this as 'all the rights, duties, powers, responsibilities and authority which by law a parent of a child has in relation to the child and his property'. A feature of the Act is that it acknowledges the extended family as well as the parents. If, for example, the court considers that it is better for the child to make a residence order to a grandparent or other suitable person, rather than a care order, they may do so. There is much greater flexibility available in determining where and with whom a child should live. This should be particularly helpful when a child has a disability.

Parents not only acquire responsibilities with the new legislation. The transfer to the local authority of parents' legal powers and status can now only be achieved through a court hearing. Otherwise services to the family must be arranged on the basis of a *voluntary partnership*. The concept of partnership is linked to prevention of family breakdown and the removal of the stigma that often associates itself with social services involvement. This is particularly important in relation to children *not* subject to care orders but who may have been accommodated by the local authority (or health authority) for some time. The local authority will have as its first responsibility a *welfare duty* that takes into account the wishes of the child and his parents, as well as the child's ethnic origin and cultural and religious background. Subject to this principle, regulations will provide *voluntary agreements* between the local authority, the parents and the child (if appropriate). These new agreements will include a number of provisions but they are not legally binding on parents.

The local authority is placed under a duty to do all that is reasonable in all circumstances to safeguard and promote the child's welfare. If, in the longer term, an agreement does not work, the local authority may seek a Court order. If, by the time the Court hears the case, the parents' own circumstances have changed for the better, there may be debate about the degree of harm to which the child is now being exposed. The definition of *harm* can include the child's mental and physical development, and advice on the nature of disability will be essential.

If a Court order is sought, the child will have 'party status' and a guardian ad litem report will be obtained. The Court must take account of all factors in a checklist but also must consider whether it is better for the child to make no order at all. If, however, a care order is made, parental rights of contact are safeguarded or possibly decided by the court, and every effort will be made to maintain family links if at all possible.

II Assessment: a new partnership between parents, professionals and the child

The duty to identify children in need (see III below) will require local authorities to develop assessment arrangements within agreed criteria that take account of the child and family's preferences, ethnic origins and any special needs relating to the circumstances of individual families. These assessment procedures are expected to complement existing statutory procedures of assessment, such as those already operational under the 1981 Education Act. Formal assessment under the 1981 Education Act already involves collaboration between health, education and social services and a child's Statement of Special Educational Needs is likely to provide an important component in any social services assessment processes. As with the 1981 Act, social services departments will be expected to involve both parents and children in any assessment and decision-making processes.

In some circumstances, more formal procedures may be necessary. In cases that go to court, the court will have to be advised (amongst other things) of the likely effect on the child of a change in circumstances and the ability of the child's parent to meet his or her needs. The court will further be guided by the assessment of the report writer as to whether the making of an order will be better for the child than making no order at all. A high level of skill will be required to determine whether a child is suffering or likely to suffer significant harm. 'Harm' will be construed not only as actual physical or sexual abuse but also factors arising from the state of the child's health or development.

A court may require that an Assessment Order is made. This order will specify the nature of the assessment, the people to carry it out and any arrangements required for the child to live away from home during an assessment. The *Child Assessment Order* is a new order which provides for cases where (a) there is reasonable concern about the child, (b) his or her carers are uncooperative, but (c) there are no grounds for an emergency protection or care or supervision order. The main purpose is to help the local authority in carrying out investigative duties (which would probably not require an order if the parents concurred with the assessment) or to enable an authorised person (who could be a doctor, psychologist or any person appointed by the court) to carry out an expert assessment of the child's circumstances.

Child Assessment Orders are only available to local authorities and authorised persons and can only be given when due notice has been given to those affected (e.g. parents). They do not involve a child being removed from home, unless the court so directs. They can be appealed against and can only last for up to 7 days. In contrast, *Emergency Protection Orders* can be sought by anyone and are usually made without notice. There is no right of appeal and the right of *challenge* is restricted to 72 hours. The applicant gains parental responsibility for the child. In the case of Assessment Orders, the applicant gets only the right to carry out activities relating to assessment.

The two orders are intended to complement each other, but there has been widespread concern that the Child Assessment Order may be used sometimes inappropriately in borderline cases, because it is less invasive of family life and rights. Courts can use their judgement and powers to treat an Assessment Order as an Emergency Protection Order if they feel this is more appropriate. *Interim Care* or *Supervision Orders* will also sometimes overlap with Assessment Orders, the use of a particular order being dictated by the court's assessment of the degree of harm that a child is likely to suffer or to be at risk of suffering.

It is important to remember that a Child Assessment Order does *not* authorise an assessment or examination which the *child* refuses to undergo, if the child is regarded as having sufficient understanding to make an informed decision about this question (Section 43(8)). Discussion around 'sufficient understanding' and the Data Protection Act suggest that children and young people with learning difficulties are not exempt from this right. In cases where there is concern about the child's ability to give an informed decision, a guardian ad litem may be appointed to act on behalf of the child and to provide an independent voice.

Throughout the new legislation, the theme of listening to children is given major emphasis. The Act contains a checklist of matters to be considered in most court hearings with regard to the child's best interests.

As *An introduction to the Children Act* (1989) notes, 'The checklist of particular matters to which the Court is to have regard in reaching decisions about the child is headed by the child's wishes and feelings and highlights the great importance attached to them'. The guide goes on to say that 'the Act in the area of private law seeks to strike a balance between the need to recognise the child as an independent person, to ensure that his views are fully taken into account and the risk of casting on him the burden of resolving problems caused by his parents or requiring him to choose between them'. *As well as incorporating his or her views in the checklist, the court may permit a child to request an order about his or her own future.* If the Court commissions a welfare report, it must ensure that the child's views are included within it.

Because the Courts have new and much wider powers to intervene, it is hoped that they will be able to use these powers to protect children from risk or harm wherever they live, but also to avoid 'unwarranted intervention in their family life' (op. cit.). For children and young people with disabilities and special needs (in particular those with severe learning difficulties or communication problems), involvement and support during such assessment will require new strategies in training and support and also in avoiding premature assumptions about the inability of such children to contribute to discussions on their own future. The growth of the self-advocacy movement for adults will need parallels for work with children and young people if assessment is to become the participative process envisaged in the Act.

III Local authority support for children and families

The Act introduces a new concept of *children in need*. This is defined as meaning that a child will be regarded as being in need if:

a. He is unlikely to achieve or maintain, or to have the opportunity of achieving or maintaining, a reasonable standard of health or development without the provision for him of services by a local authority under this Part [of the Act];
b. His health or development is likely to be significantly impaired, or further impaired, without the provision for him of such services; or
c. He is disabled, and 'family', in relation to such a child, includes any person who has parental responsibility for the child and any other person with whom he has been living.

For the purposes of this Part, a child is disabled if he is blind, deaf or dumb or suffers from mental disorder of any kind or is substantially and permanently handicapped by illness, injury or congenital deformity or such other disability as may be prescribed, and in this Part of the Act—'development' means physical, intellectual, emotional, social or behavioural developments; and 'health' means 'physical or mental health'.

The new definition of need provides the basis of a general duty now imposed on local authorities to provide services for children in need *'so far as is consistent with that duty to promote upbringing of such children by their families*'. This general duty is supported by other specific duties such as facilitation of 'the provision by others (including in particular voluntary organisations) of services' and by schedules which will spell out the nature of these services. It is generally anticipated that these provisions should encourage local authorities to provide respite care and other support services as a means of supporting disabled children with their natural families.

For the first time local authorities have a general duty to provide day care services and supervised activities for *children in need* aged 5 years and under, and not at school; and for school age children outside school hours and in school holidays. It is hoped that these general duties may improve the range of holiday, respite and other services for disabled children living at home or with foster families. As Schedule 2 of the Act requires local authorities to identify children in need and to publish and advertise the services provided—*in addition to maintaining a register of disabled children*—the Act may result in a wider range of out-of-school activities for children with special needs, with correspondingly better information on their whereabouts for both parents and professionals.

IV Charging for services

As noted above, social services departments have new duties to provide services for 'children in need'. Services provided 'as the authority considers appropriate' can include family centres, day care, provision for the under-5s, respite care and any other provision which will support child and family. The availability of such services has to be publicised. For disabled children, the Act (Schedule 2, Part 1) requires that:

Every local authority shall provide services designed:

a. To minimise the effect on disabled children . . . of their disabilities; and
b. To give such children the opportunity to lead lives which are as normal as possible.

One major concern which has arisen with regard to support services such as respite care is the potential deterrent to families if charges are introduced. At present, charging for respite or support services in social services or health authorities is almost unheard of. Under the Children Act (Schedule 2, Part III, Para 21), local authorities acquire a new duty to consider whether they should charge parents. But they 'may only recover contributions . . . if they consider it reasonable to do so'. The definition of 'reasonable' will vary between authorities and has parallels with the NHS and Community Care Act, which makes similar provisions for charging for certain services. Both the Children Act and the NHS and Community Care Act distinguish assessment, advice and counselling (which will be free) from practical services such as respite care, laundry or day care which could be charged for. However, the OPCS Reports

(1989) have clearly indicated (a) the lower level of income in families with a disabled member as compared to their counterparts in the wider community; and (b) the existing additional costs of caring for a disabled child.

Historically many local authorities have deliberately chosen *not* to charge for services such as respite care on the grounds that they were therapeutic and also preventive (possibly saving the considerable costs of a family breakdown and permanent residential care). The Children Act and the NHS and Community Care Act emphasise the importance of keeping families together. 23% of families interviewed in the OPCS wanted domiciliary family support services to ensure that this happened. There will clearly need to be careful evaluation of policies with regard to charging for services—and the negative consequences of so doing. Additionally, at present parents are not asked to pay for services provided in a health or education setting and there could be a shift back to outdated models of respite care if families felt unable to pay for respite and other care provided through social services.

V Children in a multicultural society

The Children Act—for the first time in any UK legislation—acknowledges the need to be sensitive to cultural and ethnic issues when providing services. Section 22(5) requires that 'local authorities must also give due consideration to the child's religious persuasion, racial origin and cultural and linguistic background'. This means, for example, that when a local authority social services department exercises its new powers under the Act to provide day care for children and other supervised activities in holidays or outside school hours, the authority must take into account 'the different racial groups to children in their area who are in need belong' (Schedule 2). As the Act also requires social services departments to review such day care or out-of-school provision with the appropriate education authority, there will be new opportunities to ensure that cultural and ethnic differences are acknowledged and that services are acceptable to the families concerned.

VI Consultation with education authorities

If a social services department that looks after a child proposes to place the child in an establishment at which education is provided for the children who live there, they *must* consult the local education authority first. If the child has a statement of special educational needs, then the education authority who made the statement should be consulted. The education authority should also be informed 'as soon as it is reasonably practicable' if a child goes to live in such an establishment. Section 28(4) is intended to help prevent the growing number of social services placements of children with special needs in independent or non-maintained residential schools (frequently on a 52 weeks a year basis) for primarily social care reasons. There is also growing concern about the lack of attention given to continuity and quality of education during assessment of children living away from home, and the negative consequences of inappropriate or frequently disrupted placements.

VII Education supervision orders

The Children Act creates a new kind of supervision order, which may be made on the application of an education authority. *Education Supervision Orders* are administered by the education authority and last for up to 1 year in the first instance. Education authorities must consult their social services counterparts before making such orders. They can only be made if the child is of compulsory school age and is not being properly educated (i.e. 'is not receiving efficient full-time education suitable to the child's age, ability, aptitude and any special educational needs he or she may have' (Section 36(4)).

The Children Act abolishes the old Truancy Orders. Debating the Children Bill in the House of Lords, the Lord Chancellor noted that truancy should no longer be a primary reason for removing a child from home, because the cause of truancy might be *school* based rather than home based. Failure to educate a child properly (including sending him to school) is not a sufficient reason to issue a care order under the new legislation. But the court may make such an order if it finds that the child is suffering significant harm, since 'harm' may be defined as the impairment of development (whether physical, intellectual, emotional, social or behavioural development). Hence Education Supervision Orders can be applied to children with disabilities when there is concern about the quality or quantity of education being provided.

Education Supervision Orders will involve the appointment of a supervisor, who will have the primary duty to advise, assist and befriend child and parents and as far as is practicable to ascertain their wishes. He or she will endeavour to 'secure the child's proper education'. Smith & Grimshaw (1989) point out a potential tension between the new support and advisory role of a supervisor and the punitive powers that still remain to bring parents of non-attenders before a magistrate and impose fines.

VIII Notification of children accommodated in certain establishments

Local authorities *must* be informed by health and education authorities, residential care, nursing or mental nursing homes of any child who spends *at least 3 months* in their provision. Social Services Departments now have new duties to ensure the welfare of children in such establishments and have the right to inspect as required.

The social services department within whose catchment area the child lives must 'take all reasonably practicable steps to enable them to decide whether the child's welfare is adequately safeguarded and promoted while he stays in the accommodation' (Section 85(4)). During the discussions of the Child Care Law Review Working Party, the primary concern about children living in such accommodation was the confusion which often existed between the theoretical purpose for the placement (for example, respite care, medical treatment or education) and the real purpose which was to provide a residential service. Such children, who frequently were not in the care of a local authority, were often 'forgotten' in terms of child care policy, and their future was inadequately planned as a consequence. In practice, in the 1990s—with the gradual closure of long-stay hospitals—such children are more likely to be living in independent educational establishments. But a significant number will be in small NHS units, sometimes for extended periods of respite care because of family problems and lack of alternative provision. Now social services must have a general overview of all children's care and general welfare.

As part of this new provision, health and education authorities must also inform the social services department for the area in which a child or young person proposes to live, if a child has reached the age of 16 and leaves accommodation that has been provided for at least 3 months. In theory this should encourage more effective implementation of procedures under the 1986 Disabled Persons Act and the forthcoming NHS and Community Care Act, which will require social services departments to make new arrangements for the care and support of people with special needs in the community.

IX Child protection and independent schools

Because of significant concern about child protection in independent schools, the Act gives new duties with regard to all children so accommodated. An independent school is defined as 'any school at which full-time education is provided for five or more pupils of compulsory school age, not being a school maintained by the local education authority, a grant maintained school or a special school maintained by the education authority'. The 'five pupils' includes schools that are primarily nursery schools but which happen to have any group of five children of school age. Hence private nursery schools or post-school provision that includes five or more children or young people of school age will come under the provisions of Section 91(1).

The social services department must take all reasonably practicable steps to enable them to decide whether the child's welfare is adequately safeguarded and promoted in the school (section 87(3)). If they consider that the child's welfare is not being adequately safeguarded, the social services department must notify the Secretary of State. Social services may authorise people to enter the school in order to exercise their welfare duty and may (subject to regulations and guidance) inspect the school premises, records and the children. The right to inspect the *children* is of particular significance with regard to children with special educational needs. They are the most likely to have communication difficulties and to be placed at some distance from their family home. Vigilance from social services departments will offer significant new protection. HMI duties are unaffected by these new powers for social services.

Additional controls are provided when an independent school accommodates a pupil who is under 16 *for more than 2 weeks in the school holidays*. A person who proposes to care for and accommodate a child in these circumstances *must* give written notice to the social services department (unless already exempted by them). The child is then regarded as a privately fostered child and is protected by regulations relating to such fostering arrangements. Residential *holidays* are not so covered and there has been concern about the quality of care and protection on some of the wide range of group holiday activities now available.

Anderson & Morgan (1987) have identified 923 independent schools in the United Kingdom, with 127 250 boarder pupils. They estimate that there are approximately 5320 pupils (i.e. 4%) with special educational needs. Inspecting these schools will have major resource implications for both social services departments and education authorities. It should also be emphasised that the new arrangements apply to *all* independent schools and not only to those providing for special educational needs. Although the idea of inspecting Harrow or Eton would seem quite alien to many authorities, *all* residential establishments caring for children need careful monitoring. Hopefully the Children Act will refocus attention not only on the quality of education offered in residential schools, but also on the wider needs of children living in them.

X Children living in NHS provision

As noted above, there is a new duty imposed on health and education authorities to notify social services of any child placed with them for 3 months or more. The social services department concerned would usually be that which serves the area in which the child *usually* lives. If there is no such local contact, then the department in whose area the accommodation is located will take responsibility.

Once notified, social services departments must take all reasonable practicable steps to enable them to decide if the child's welfare is 'adequately safeguarded and promoted' (Section 85(4)).

Social Services must also decide if they should exercise any other powers under the Act. The Department of Health's Child Care Law Review Working Party (1988) gave serious consideration to fears about abandonment of children with disabilities in NHS provision because of lack of earlier intervention to encourage and support parental involvement. The 1989 Children Act empowers local authorities to provide a range of services (Part III) which can, for example, promote contact between a child and family or provide day services such as holiday and after-school play schemes.

Where a residential care, mental nursing or nursing home is registered and regulated under the Registered Homes Act 1984, social services have a power to enter the establishment in question in order to discuss whether the child's welfare is adequately safeguarded and promoted while he stays in the accommodation.

XI Local authority funding of provision outside the United Kingdom

The Children Act sets out a number of principles that should guide the local authority's choice of placements for a child. The welfare duty on social services departments includes generally providing accommodation 'which is near to the child's home' and friends and family.

However, social services departments may now arrange or assist in arranging for a child to live outside England and Wales with the approval of every person who has parental responsibility for a child, or the court, if the child is in care. The child is required to consent if he or she has sufficient understanding. This means that children can be funded to attend the Petö Institute in Budapest or other special treatment centres, providing that the decision is being seen as in the best interests of the child. There are of course, no additional resources for such provision. However, local authorities now have the legal right to make such placements if they wish.

XII Child protection

The OPCS Reports on the lives of disabled people in the UK (1989) indicated that 15% of children with disabilities living away from home did so because of physical or sexual abuse. A further 33% had 'unsuitable family homes'. Children with disabilities are, therefore, not immune to the risks from adverse family circumstances that affect their able-bodied peers. Although the spirit of the Children Act is one of partnership with parents and voluntary agreements, the histories of Jasmine Beckford, Kimberley Carlile, Tyra Henry and many others show the need to have clear procedures to protect vulnerable children.

Courts may now make an *Emergency Protection Order* 'if, but only if, it is satisfied that there is reasonable cause to believe that the child is likely to suffer significant harm'. The court may also make an order if the local authority shows reasons to suspect that a child may be suffering harm or if parents refuse access to the child 'unreasonably'. These orders can, however, only last for 8 days and can only be extended once for 7 days. After 72 hours, parents or the *child* can apply to challenge the order. The order may have a direction regarding a medical examination of the child attached. However, despite considerable debate, a medical examination *cannot be enforced against the wishes of a mature child.* Courts may impose *Child Assessment Orders* to enable a Court to order such an examination and to take advice from a range of professionals and agencies about the wellbeing of the child. Local authorities have an active duty to investigate where there is 'reasonable cause' to suspect that a child is suffering or likely to suffer significant harm and can apply for Emergency Protection Orders where they encounter difficulty in gaining access to a child or where there is considerable concern about the child's safety.

CONCLUSION

The Children Act presents major challenges to health and education authorities as well as social services departments and their professional staff at a time of other significant changes. However, the 1981 Education Act laid down statutory duties (and associated guidance such as Circular 2/89 on Assessment and Statements) which have clearly demonstrated that multi-professional assessment and collaboration can work. The new assessment procedures of the Children Act are likely to draw upon good practice in the special educational needs field. The Child Care Law Review Working Party seriously considered (albeit ultimately rejecting) the feasibility of utilising the 1981 Act model of assessment and statementing within their own child care strategy. The NHS and Community Care Act 1990, looking at assessment for services in adult life, commends the seamless service principle within children's services of compatible and complementary legislation. The Children Act, 1981 Education Act and the NHS and Community Care Act 1990, whilst daunting in their new duties, also clarify the contribution of education and give teachers and administrators new powers as well as duties to work with children and parents and to ensure that children with special needs are not seen as part of a separate service but included within mainstream legislation and strategic thinking for the 1990s.

REFERENCES

Anderson, Morgan A 1987 Provision for children in need of boarding/residential education. The Boarding Schools Association
Banks S, Grizzell R 1984 A study of family placements schemes for the shared care of handicapped children in Norfolk and Oxfordshire. Social Services Inspectorate, Department of Health
Berridge D, Cleaver H 1988 Foster home breakdown. National Children's Bureau
Brimblecombe F, Russell P 1987 Honeylands: developing a service for families with handicapped children. National Children's Bureau
Department of Health 1991 Patterns and outcomes in child placement. Messages from recent research and their implications. HMSO, London

Department of Health 1991 The Children Act 1989 Guidance and regulations. Volume 1, Court orders. HMSO, London

Department of Health 1991 The Children Act 1989 Guidance and regulations. Volume 2, Family support, day care and educational provision for young children. HMSO, London

Department of Health 1991 The Children Act 1989 Guidance and regulations. Volume 4, Residential care. HMSO, London

Department of Health 1991 The Children Act 1989 Guidance and regulations. Volume 5, Independent schools. HMSO, London

Department of Health 1991 The Children Act: guidance on children with disabilities. HMSO, London

OPCS (Office of Population and Census Surveys) 1989 Report 6, Disabled children: services, transport and education. HMSO, London

Oswin M 1985 They keep going away. Basil, Blackwell

Pahl J 1984 Families with handicapped children: a study of stress and a service response. Health Services Research Unit, University of Kent

Robinson C 1986 Avon short term respite care scheme: evaluation study. Department of Mental Health, University of Bristol

Russell P 1989 The Children Act: caring for children living away from home—the policy and legal framework. Voluntary Council for Handicapped Children, National Children's Bureau

Russell P 1990 The Children Act: challenges and opportunities for children with disabilities and special needs. British Journal of Special Education, March 1990

Russell P 1991 Children with disabilities—The Children Act. In: Oliver M (ed) Social work and disability. Butterworth–Heinemann, Oxford

The Children Act 1989 HMSO, London

The Children Act 1989 Highlight. National Children's Bureau

The Children Act 1989 An introduction to the Act. Department of Health

31. Social integration, sexuality and sex education

S. Dorner

INTRODUCTION

The last 20 years have seen some helpful changes in the prominence given in Britain to problems of social integration of children and young people who are disabled. Even though much of what emerges in the professional literature is descriptive and inclined to be broadly exhortatory, the present decade has fairly clearly been a more encouraging period when systematic proposals have been made to put into action some of the principles of normalisation and integration (e.g. in education policies) to which young-sters with disability are entitled. It is also relatively recently that some of the attitudes implied in the pejorative use of terms like 'overprotective' have come to be questioned; there is evolving a less judgmental recognition of the dynamics in families and the limited opportunities in social contacts that make it hard for those with disability to take their full place in society. Finally there are encouraging signs of an increased willingness to listen to disabled children and young people themselves and to ensure that their voices will be heard (Madge & Fassam 1982, Brimblecombe 1987).

This is not to say that the problems of social integration are close to being resolved. General social attitudes, financial constraints, limited facilities and other factors still mean that as far as true integration is concerned, we are still in the foothills of a landscape that contains Mount Everest as the final peak to conquer. One of the most ironic of paradoxes is that the problem of integration is seen, in the way we use language, as a problem 'of the disabled' rather than as a problem of people and their social relation-ships, whether disabled or able-bodied.

FRIENDSHIPS AT SCHOOL

Not surprisingly, the question of friendships is vitally important to the sense of well being and self-esteem of disabled children and young people, just as it is to anyone else of their age. Within the setting of school the picture is fairly encouraging in that the great majority of young people report friendships, occasionally with one friend only, but usually with more. However, studies indicate differences between the physically dis-abled and the able-bodied.

Firstly, roughly 10% of disabled children do appear to be almost entirely without friends, even at school, and secondly it is much more likely, as one would expect, that the able-bodied group will have friends, not just at their own school but at other schools as well (Madge & Fassam 1982). Thus there appear to be limits set on both numbers and choice for disabled children at school.

Further, where self-reporting forms the basis for the relatively positive picture at school, a note of caution is necessary since it has been shown that teachers at both special and mainstream schools quite often tend to see disabled pupils as being rather solitary and more often to be described as 'not much liked' (Anderson & Clarke 1982). However, in a more recent study of children with spina bifida (Lonton et al 1986) around 80% of teachers felt that the physically handicapped were fully accepted by their peers.

Teasing is occasionally reported and bullying can also occur, but studies agree that this is not common.

FRIENDSHIPS OUTSIDE SCHOOL

The fact that handicapped youngsters usually have friends at school, however encouraging this may be, does not resolve the issue of social integration; studies that have investigated friendships outside school reveal a disturbing problem. The overwhelming majority of able-bodied children see their friends outside school. The figures are of the order of 80–90%. In contrast, Anderson & Clarke found that the figures for disabled adolescents having no friends outside school range from 30–60% depending on the type of school attended. Madge & Fassam (1982), studying a wider range of age and disabling conditions found rather similar percentages of friendless children as far as their contacts outside school were concerned. Dorner's study (1976) indicated that 40% of spina bifida teenagers had no friends outside school or college.

SOCIAL AND LEISURE ACTIVITIES

Not only are the opportunities for contact with friends limited for disabled children, but problems also arise in what is available to them to further their leisure time interests. PHAB clubs or similar organisations are clearly exceedingly helpful and most older disabled youngsters belong. However, attendance is often restricted to one single club rather than access to a range of activities and organised groups for the able-bodied, and interests that are very common, e.g. sport, are often very difficult to develop because of lack of facilities. Thomas et al (1989) describe a progressively worsening situation where disabled young people follow increasingly solitary pursuits such as video, television and radio and where club activities tend to be more segregated or the clubs themselves are either for disabled or for able-bodied.

SOCIAL INTEGRATION AFTER SCHOOL LEAVING

It seems clear that the position of older adolescents does not change significantly. Indeed, if there is a trend, it seems that social contact generally becomes *less* frequent, particularly for the more severely handicapped, and that opportunities to mix with able-bodied peers, far from increasing, become less easy. The work of Thomas et al referred to above also suggests that, for disabled young adults, friendships—even when they do exist—are often not at a level where important confidences can be exchanged. Leaving school occurs at a time when the peer group begins to alter to accommodate heterosexual couple relationships. Work, too, has a social component, but surveys show that there is a high number of disabled teenagers who are unable to find work. Lack of work means lack of opportunity to meet people in a work setting as well as a probable limit on funds to afford alternative social activity.

FACTORS INFLUENCING DIFFICULTIES IN SOCIAL INTEGRATION

There is clearly no simple causal relationship between aspects of a child's disability and the ability to integrate socially. However, some attempt to identify the main components of a complex interactional process is warranted.

Attitudes and opportunities

Research interviews into the area of social integration are supported by the overwhelming impression gained both from clinical interviews with disabled children and young people, and from ordinary, informal social conversation with them. The conclusion to be drawn from all these contacts is that the primary problem lies in the way in which disabled children are responded to and in the restricted opportunities and choices that they have when compared with their able-bodied peers. What disabled youngsters define as the problem seems entirely consistent with the way in which research findings can be interpreted. In particular, the striking contrast between reasonable friendships at school and the all too frequent lack of friends outside school points towards difficulties of opportunity as a more common explanation than personal inability to get on with other people.

Type of school

In recent years there have been important changes in the policies governing the school placement of physically handicapped children. The 1981 Education Act was generally strongly influenced by arguments in favour of integration into mainstream schools wherever possible. The act also involved the significant change that decisions about placement are now no longer based as much upon considerations about physical status as upon assessment of educational need and the duty to ensure that parents are involved as much as possible. While the implications of much of this are positive, the 1988 Education Reform Act has more recently become law in this country and has given rise to considerable concern in many quarters about the effects of the new legislation on the facilities for all children wi· h special educational needs—and whether or not it will increase parental choice for disabled children or in fact restrict it even further.

It is certainly the case that type of school affects social integration and aspirations. Handicapped children are emphatic that they do not want their friendships or opportunities for social contact to be restricted solely to other disabled people. It follows that their social needs and wishes are more readily met if they can attend mainstream school, and there is now fairly clear evidence that handicapped youngsters at mainstream school are more able to maintain social contact outside school than those at special schools.

While this finding is significant, it is important to point out that social integration is still a problem for one third or more of those at mainstream schools; and that for this group the sense of isolation and loneliness may be particularly intense in a way that is not the case for those at special residential schools where (in term-time) loneliness is not a common problem. Secondly most, if not all, special schools encourage part-time attendance wherever possible at local schools and attempt to foster other opportunities for social contact with the able-bodied. Thirdly full-time special schooling will continue to be both necessary and advisable for significant numbers of handicapped children and young people. The issue for some children and adolescents may indeed be which type of school is better; for others the issue will be how to ensure that, whatever the type of school, as much as possible is done to resolve problems of social integration.

Nature of physical handicap

Various studies have documented the association between problems in social relationships and aspects of the handicapping condition. It has been shown, for instance, that the prospects for social integration are greater for those whose handicaps do not involve impaired mobility. This is not at all surprising. The author's own study (Dorner 1975) found a highly significant correlation between problems of mobility and social isolation; other studies have come to similar conclusions.

Somewhat less obvious are the effects of 'hidden' disabilities, particularly urinary incontinence, the social aspect of which becomes increasingly problematic with age. Worry about other children discovering about incontinence and the presence of urinary appliances can become socially handicapping even when good social control of the incontinence has been achieved. In a substantial proportion of youngsters, fear of discovery leads to withdrawal from social contact (Anderson & Clarke 1982, Carr et al 1984, Dorner 1976). This can occur where mobility is not a handicapping factor; there is general agreement from research that the problem is particularly acute for boys and this presumably relates to their concerns about their masculinity (see below).

While mobility and incontinence have been shown to be the features most commonly affecting social relationships, it is worth highlighting the socially handicapping consequences of speech disorders, e.g. in cerebral palsy, and of learning difficulties.

Family relationships

Up to this point, discussion has proceeded as if a disabled youngster's social relationships occur independently of the family context. Clearly this is not the case. One of the major functions of the family is to foster social contact and integration. Most families strive energetically to ensure that the handicapped member of the family is indeed integrated as much as possible into their social activities. This is true not only of parents but also of siblings, especially older brothers and sisters, and of members of the extended family. At the same time it must be acknowledged that some parents are themselves affected by the problems of managing the day-to-day demands of handicap; reduced opportunities to go out may lead the parents themselves to a restricted social life with ensuing difficulties of social integration.

EFFECTS OF SOCIAL INTEGRATION PROBLEMS

Loneliness

Social isolation must be distinguished from loneliness, the latter being essentially a subjective experience that affects individuals, at least to some extent, independently of the frequency of their social contacts. Some very isolated people may not feel lonely and the degree of contact they maintain is often a matter of choice. Handicapped young people do not appear to feel that they have such a choice. They feel strongly, and rightly, that their opportunities for social contact are very restricted. It is therefore not surprising that loneliness is a common problem for the handicapped adolescent. Indeed, loneliness is given as the most common reason for misery or unhappiness when talking to disabled youngsters.

While misery can reasonably be regarded as a common experience in adolescence, the effects of social isolation can frequently extend to depression and in some circumstances to a belief that life is not worth living. Such emotions tend to create a vicious circle since unhappiness often leads either to further withdrawal or to reduced social attractiveness in the eyes of peers, or both.

Social skills deficits

Some useful work has been undertaken in the last few years in assessing the social skills of disabled children and young people. Common problems are lack of confidence, finding it hard to keep a conversation going, making friends and, for the older age group, going out with someone to whom they are attracted (Jowett 1982). More systematic research into this area confirms that able-bodied young people also frequently acknowledge problems in their social skills but the difference lies in the *severity* with which these problems were rated. Differences in the nature of the deficits between disabled males and females were also noted (Thomas et al 1989).

Clearly it would be unwise to attribute problems of social integration as a cause of social skills difficulties. It is just as possible that these deficits are a consequence of the limited chance to practise the necessary skills *because of* the integrative difficulties. It is the author's view that the latter is the more likely explanation.

Self-esteem and the wish to 'belong'

It would be a mistake to regard the issue of social integration as being defined simply in terms of frequency of social contact with able-bodied peers, absence of feelings of loneliness, and the acquisition of reasonable social skills. Just as important is the need of the disabled youngster to know that he is esteemed and accepted as an equal rather than merely tolerated by his peers.

Articulate handicapped teenagers argue powerfully for their right to be treated 'just like anybody else'. The sense of being different and the associated frustration or helplessness at being unable to change basic social and cultural attitudes lie at the root of problems of low self-esteem commonly felt by the disabled. In fact the experience of low self-esteem, like so much else that has been discussed in this chapter, reflects the failure of people to acknowledge the interactional imbalances that society continues to create, and this is what can make it seem so unfair.

APPROACHES TO INTERVENTION

Lack of social integration continues to be a central problem for handicapped youngsters, some evidence indicating increasing difficulties into late adolescence and beyond. It has been suggested that the problem operates at a number of different levels:

• Social attitudes towards those with disability

- Limited facilities and opportunities for the disabled
- Lack of fulfilment of a legitimate need to belong to and be accepted as equal by peers
- Problems in maintaining friendships outside school
- The experience of loneliness with attendant feelings of misery or depression.

Clearly the resolution of some of these problem areas involves broad matters of social and financial policy, which cannot be addressed in a brief chapter. However, there is scope for both statutory and voluntary agencies to work together and there are signs that attempts are being made to develop and apply systematic approaches that are needs-oriented rather than service-oriented, and which recognise everyone's entitlement to choice and participation in decision-making (Brimblecombe et al 1989).

Within this general framework the opportunity arises not only for advocacy, but also for more specific interventions. There is much that can be done using problem-solving approaches, i.e. the problem is clearly defined, the possible solutions explored, the preferred option decided upon and the plan of action made and carried out. Reference has already been made (Thomas et al 1989) to the place of social skills approaches, a type of intervention that has a recognised pedigree, as has assertiveness training. Finally, individual counselling, or occasionally psychotherapy, may be helpful to particular clients; the broad benefits of family therapy as well as some of its limitations are summarised by Goodyer (1986).

Although formal psychological help is sometimes indicated, in general there appear to be considerable advantages to developing service provision in settings that are socially 'normal' rather than settings that are identified with illness or pathology, such as hospitals or clinics. Social isolation and failure of social integration are not diseases—addressing these and similar issues in places like schools or clubs is to be preferred. Certainly attempts that have been made to establish 'clinics' for disabled youngsters have been characterised by poor attendance rates.

Finally, much can be achieved by continuing to develop social interaction through clubs for the physically handicapped and able-bodied. Perhaps the best known agency organising such activities is PHAB, but both the Spastics Society and the Association for Hydrocephalus and Spina Bifida (ASBAH), to name but two, have become energetically involved in such enterprises. One of the goals of these clubs is to reduce the sense of alienation experienced by so many disabled youngsters, but they also provide an informal opportunity for them to ventilate their feelings in discussion with the sympathetic skilled staff who run these clubs. Some organisations plan residential courses which combine social activities, group discussion and formal instruction on topics relevant to social integration.

SEXUALITY AND SEX EDUCATION

It is unwise to generalise, but it is probably the case that the last 15 years have seen a noticeably greater readiness by professionals to acknowledge that disabled youngsters have entirely natural aspirations to develop close personal and sexual relationships with other people. It is probably also the case that there continue to be significant unmet needs in this area and that the quality of the education—and the advice and counselling, where this is sought—varies considerably from locality to locality.

Sexual experience

Any professional interested in developing a programme of sex education for handicapped adolescents needs to be aware of the broader problems of social integration that have been summarised earlier in this chapter. Problems of loneliness and low self-esteem, a sense of not being accepted, lack of certain social skills, and most importantly lack of opportunity to meet people of the same age are bound to hinder the formation of hetero-sexual relationships.

Anderson & Clarke (1982) interviewed 15–16-year-olds with spina bifida or cerebral palsy and found that 80% had little or nothing to do with the opposite sex, compared with only 27% of able-bodied controls. Their study also revealed that only 14% of the disabled group had ever had a 'steady' boyfriend or girlfriend by that age, compared with 45% of controls.

The author's earlier study (Dorner 1977) suggests a similar picture. In his study, only seven out of 63 teenagers with spina bifida were going out with a member of the opposite sex at the time of interview. This study further suggested that there were particular difficulties for boys with dis-ability in forming close friendships with girls, and confirmed that these problems were, understandably, especially acute where the disability involved urinary incontinence. Concerns of this sort had far reaching psy-chological consequences in a number of cases; counselling must identify the special worries that incontinence gives rise to.

It will be seen that the opportunities to learn about sex at first hand are limited for those with disability. This covers the whole range of first-hand experience from dating to sexual intercourse. Anderson & Clarke (1982) found that only a quarter of the handicapped group had ever been out with someone of the opposite sex compared with three times as many controls. Further, it was much less likely that kissing or petting had occurred in the relationship. In Dorner's 1977 study, there was a noticeable lack of physical intimacy and, out of 46 teenagers with spina bifida, only one ex-perience (a disastrous one leading to a suicide attempt) of sexual inter-course was acknowledged. It should be pointed out that this information was obtained on the basis of an extended, single research interview and the number of those having experience of sexual intercourse may well have been underestimated. Certainly, in clinical work, as far as older disabled adolescents are concerned, there appears to be greater readiness to 'admit to' experience of intercourse.

Both the studies just referred to emphasise that the wish to establish an intimate relationship with a member of the opposite sex is very common and that there is a strong preference that boy- or girlfriends should be able-bodied. This further underlines the link between heterosexual and the broader social aspirations of disabled youngsters; any sex education programme has to respect the strength of their wish to be just like anyone else. It means that sex education and counselling must find a constructive means of accepting apparently unrealistic aspirations, since they are a legitimate part of the plans for the future that most young people make and are best discovered to be unrealistic rather than prematurely shattered. It also means that counselling must provide an opportunity for feelings of distress and anger to be adequately expressed.

It will be noted that the research that has been quoted is restricted to heterosexual contacts and activity, though Thomas et al (1989) refer briefly to the difficulties of obtaining information on homosexual interest and activity when writing about the needs of disabled young adults.

Child sexual abuse is a further, vital area that has not yet been systematically explored as far as disabled youngsters are concerned. Both from talking to other professionals and from first-hand clinical experience, there are some disabled children who are only now beginning to disclose that they have been abused—sometimes by their disabled peers, and in some cases by 'care' staff. The fact that their disability has in some cases meant that they have been physically powerless when the abuse has taken place has added to the anguish and fear generated by the experience. An encouraging development in this country is the recent formation of a Disability and Abuse Working Party to report to BASPCAN (British Association for the Study and Prevention of Child Abuse and Neglect) but much clearly needs to be done educationally and therapeutically.

Sexual information and knowledge

The unwelcome barrier between the handicapped and the able-bodied reduces and alters the former's knowledge of sex. Schofield's study (1968) showed that most able-bodied teenagers derived most of their information about sex from their peers (62% of boys and 44% of girls). This is clearly not the case for handicapped teenagers, most of whom learn about sex either from their parents, or at school or other residential institution.

The way in which the nature of the handicap affects placement affects the way in which teenagers learn about sex, since handicapped adolescents attending mainstream schools are more likely to learn about sex from their peers. This may be a welcome normalising consequence of greater educational integration. The main point, however, is that handicapped teenagers' sexual knowledge is likely to be different from that of the able-bodied, because their source is different. It is true that this may protect them from some of the anxiety-arousing adolescent mythology about sex (the dire effects of masturbation, for example), but it is also true that they are at a time of life when it is generally acknowledged that much learning must take place away from parents, rather than through the personal viewpoints or indeed prejudices of parents or other adults such as teachers or nurses.

Certainly, in talking to handicapped teenagers, one finds that a good deal of their own sex education has been of the birds and bees variety, or euphemistic in some other way. Further there has often been an assumption that the whole area of sexuality is of theoretical relevance only, especially for those with severe disability, because the opportunity for actual sexual experience will not arise.

Although adolescents with physical handicap are indeed relatively very inexperienced, the picture for adults is not the same and research and clinical experience reveal reasonable numbers of severely disabled young people able to establish sexually intimate relationships. One important practical issue here is the need to ensure that a handicapped young person has adequate knowledge not only of conception but also of contraception. Many disabled teenagers have only the vaguest knowledge about the latter and do not necessarily know what the implications of particular contraceptive methods are for their medical or physical problems. Finally, like everyone, disabled young people need to know about AIDS and sexually transmitted diseases.

So far, the dangers of viewing sexuality as an issue separate from social aspects of handicap have been underlined. This is also true of the specific question of sexual information. There are some conditions, such as those involving damage to the spinal cord, which directly affect sexual function. While sex education for such directly affected groups needs to take account of their condition, experience suggests that many disabled youngsters have major worries about their condition even when there is no physiological or neurological reason. Conversely, a number of those who do have spinal lesions claim to have sexual function and sensation that does not seem entirely consistent with the nature and level of their lesion!

Lack of systematic knowledge about their condition in general continues to be a striking finding in research into the problems of handicapped teenagers, and implies lack of specific knowledge about whether or not sexual performance will also be impaired. Worries about genetic transmission are also common and are often based on limited or misunderstood information. Typically, disabled young people either overestimate or underestimate the genetic risks involved.

CONCLUSIONS

Any programme of sex education for the young disabled has to take account of their overall psychological and social predicament, particularly their legitimate feelings of wanting to be the equals of their able-bodied peers and the resultant apathy, despair or anger when this cannot happen. The flexible use of group discussion which includes sympathetic able-bodied teenagers is helpful in generating discussion about personal relationships in which more specific counselling and discussion about sexual relationships can occur. Both the Spastics Society and the Association for Spina Bifida and Hydrocephalus are increasingly active in facilitating counselling and education around these concerns (Young ASBAH Series 1983). On an individual basis some special schools are also attempting to develop their sex education and counselling systems.

There is a need for general information, not purely sexual information. Few disabled teenagers know enough about their condition to know how their sexual activities may or may not be affected. Lack of opportunity and anxiety may prevent them from trying to find out. Some of this information can be given on a group basis but there is also a need for individual advice and counselling to be made available to take account of the private anxieties that many teenagers are bound to have and the particular nature of the disability and its severity. As in all skilled counselling the pace and content of sessions must be negotiated in a way that is acceptable to the client, not set by the counsellor.

The language of sex education is also crucial. Except in the case of people with very severe learning difficulties, the language of sex already exists. It has a vernacular and expressive vocabulary which young people understand much more readily than the multisyllabic expressions of professionals. Short words are more likely to be understood than long ones!

Personal attitudes to sex education held by the adults in the disabled teenager's network are important (Cole et al 1973). Any sex education programme may well demand that parents, educators, doctors, nurses and others will have to face their own prejudices, anxieties, and untested assumptions about sexuality.

Where teenagers live at home or are in frequent contact with their parents, the parents, too, will need the chance to express their concerns and review their attitudes and expectations. In the same way, good staff communication and open discussion are an essential ingredient of successful sex education programmes where they are school or institution based. The Family Planning Association and SPOD (Association to Aid Sexual and Personal Relationships of the Disabled) may be able to offer specialist advice, and the latter agency provides some books and advisory leaflets (e.g. Davies 1985).

REFERENCES

Anderson E, Clarke L 1982 Disability in adolescence. Methuen, London
ASBAH/SPOD 1983 Sex education for young people with spina bifida or cerebral palsy. Published by ASBAH with the cooperation of The Spastics Society and SPOD

Brimblecombe F 1987 The voice of disabled young people. Children and Society 1: 58–70

Brimblecombe F, Hoghughi M, Tripp J 1989 A new covenant with adolescents in crisis. Children and Society 3: 168–180

Carr J, Halliwell M, Pearson A 1984 The relationship of disability and school type to everyday life. Zeitschrift für Kinderchirurgie 39(11): 135–137

Cole T, Chilgren R, Rosenberg P 1973 A new programme of sex education and counselling for spinal cord injured adults and health care professionals. Paraplegia 2: 111–124

Davies M 1985 Sex education for young people with a physical disability. SPOD

Dorner S 1975 The relationship of physical handicap to stress in families with an adolescent with spina bifida. Developmental Medicine and Child Neurology 17: 765–776

Dorner S 1976 Adolescents with spina bifida: how they see their situation. Archives of Disease in Childhood 51: 439–444

Dorner S 1977 Sexual interest and activity in adolescents with spina bifida. Journal of Child Psychology and Psychiatry 18: 229–236

Goodyer I 1986 Family therapy and the handicapped child. Developmental Medicine and Child Neurology 28: 247–250

Jowett S 1982 Young disabled people: their further education, training and employment. NFER–Nelson, Windsor

Lonton A P, Cole M S J, Mercer J 1986 The integration of spina bifida children: Are their needs being met? Zeitschrift für Kinderchirurgie 41(1): 45–47

Madge N, Fassam M 1982 Ask the children. Batsford Academic and Educational, London

Schofield M 1968 The sexual behaviour of young people. Penguin, Harmondsworth

Thomas A P, Bax M C O, Smyth D P L 1989 The health and social needs of young adults with physical disability. MacKeith Press, Oxford

32. Transition into adulthood

P. Madden

WHAT IS ADULTHOOD?

When I was little it was still the standard cliché for a lad to say he wanted to be an engine driver when he grew up. Clearly, most of my contemporaries did not become one—reflecting both the changes in the market place (there aren't so many engines!) and the fact that our ideas change as we get older. Even if we stay within a particular career area, we will almost certainly change jobs several times, and have to constantly adapt our practice. It is also true today that many people would challenge such a declaration as inherently sexist—why couldn't girls become engine drivers too?

I use this small example to illustrate the complexities of what we mean by 'being grown up', by 'adulthood'. There is of course no magic answer to the question, but the more we share and make explicit our often implicit, comfortable and half-formed notions, the less likely we are to unwittingly impose inappropriate expectations, assumptions and attitudes on others. The clearer we are about our aims, the more likely we will be to find the means to achieve them. This is a particular responsibility for professionals and carers who act as 'midwives' to young people with physical disability in their journey to adulthood. There are so many subtle and not so subtle ways in which, often for the best of motives, people continue to speak for those with disability, especially if they are young, projecting their own views rather than helping the development of parental choice.

So what can we say about 'being grown-up'? Perhaps the first and most important statement is that it is both personal and yet also cultural. Every individual has a uniqueness that both exists and should be encouraged, and yet at the same time every individual is placed in a particular context, of family, friends, neighbourhood and so on. Thus any definition of adulthood, of being grown up, is both internally defined—who am I to myself?—and externally defined—what do others think of me? The challenge and the skill lies in how to manage the dynamic tension between the two.

Secondly, this is made all the more difficult in that in complex industrialised societies the very process of growing up is obscure. There is no single 'rite de passage'. To take three immediate examples (and there are many more), the ages at which a young person can marry, drive a car and vote are all different. Adolescence is a misty threshold. Nor does it stop there. Whilst whatever disagreements there may be about the age of adulthood, there would be little disagreement that it would have happened by the time a person is in their mid-20s; nevertheless adulthood itself is not a static condition—we may marry, become parents; we grow older; change our jobs. Adulthood itself is constantly changing.

Thirdly, adolescence can be a very painful process. Remarkably perhaps, the vast majority of young people become adults without extreme or protracted trauma and conflict. Nevertheless it is a challenging time for all concerned. Parents need to be able to let go and yet be available. Sometimes it is they who push the young person out of the nest, not because they are uncaring, but to force them to fly. Adolescents need to be able both to take the space offered to them, and to claim their own. Growing up always involves some torn flesh.

Challenging though all this process is for young people who do not have a disability, it is very often even more difficult for those who have. This is where the classic distinction applies between 'disability'—the innate condition, and 'handicap'—the burden which is imposed by others. Within families parents may have adopted a pattern of caring that does not easily adjust to the demands for increased independence. The disabled young person may have become used to everything being done for him or her. Also, whilst different disabilities have different stabilities and severities, a certain level of protectiveness and special caring is likely to be appropriate in adulthood as well as childhood, but there is always the danger of this becoming the inappropriate standard response.

Of course, not all families who have within them a young person with physical disability have these or similar problems. However, even where they do not, the resources made available and the attitudes demonstrated by society at large are also crucial. A young person with disability may want to live independently. That person's family may also wish it, but appropriate accommodation may simply not exist. Also, even when it is benign rather than indifferent, society's attitude is still often mawkishly sentimental, still in the vein of 'Does he take sugar?'. Too many people with disability still say that they feel condemned to permanent childhood.

So, given all these complexities and difficulties, what are the standards that should be set in helping young people with physical disability achieve adulthood?

STANDARDS FOR SERVICES

Fundamentally, the standards should be the same as for everyone else. This is the essence of Wolfensberger's (1975) notion of normalisation, which has primarily been applied to the field of mental handicap/learning difficulties, but is equally applicable to physical disability. It does not mean that 'everyone else' achieves these standards—it means that there should be no categoric difference between the culturally approved aspirations of wider society, nor of the culturally approved means of achieving them, and the aspirations and means that apply to people with a disability.

Acceptance by society is not therefore a gift, but a right: to be afforded the same opportunities, and, crucially, responsibilities as others. To re-apply Virginia Woolf's phrase about women, it is the right to the 'liberty of experiences'.

Having accepted the appropriateness of such standards, how do we make them more explicit? In the field of mental handicap/learning difficulties, which again could equally be applied to physical disability, one of the most fashionable definitions is that of the 'Five Service Accomplishments' developed by O'Brien (1989) in the US. These require services to achieve the following outcomes for service users:

1. *Sharing* the same places as ordinary citizens for living, work, social and leisure activities
2. *Making choices* and having experiences which inform choice amongst a variety of options in all areas of life
3. *Gaining a positive reputation* through having positive social roles such as householder, neighbour, friend, worker, etc.
4. *Developing skills* which increase people's independence and social competence
5. *Having valued friends* and positive relationships with ordinary community members.

It is not necessary to swallow this particular subdivision wholesale. Nor, even if it is accepted, is it sufficient. Without them becoming over-elaborate, more precise definitions are still needed of how to measure whether these standards have been achieved.

However, though it is only one way of looking at things, O'Brien's scheme emphasises three crucial features of successful services:

1. Means cannot be divorced from ends—the only way to share is to have and receive, the only way to develop choice is to practise choice, and so on.

2. Conversely, all achievements are interrelated and reinforcing. This applies to any combination of the five accomplishments, or of any other framework. People grow, grow up, organically not sequentially.

3. Particular issues and challenges have to be constantly related to the whole person—no area can develop in isolation.

Not only do we need to have standards, and standards that are sufficiently appropriate, comprehensive and explicit, we also need to have standards that can respond to changing circumstances. This means the changing circumstances not only of each individual person, but also of society at large. Consider the following statements:

a. The nature of employment is changing—there is an increasing demand for hi-tech skills, in the service industries; there are changes in the pattern of employment—earlier retirement, more job sharing, and so on

b. The number of young people available for work is substantially less than 10 years ago because of changes in the birth rate

c. There is a substantial increase in the last 20 years of the number of single parents

d. A substantial minority of families still live in considerable poverty

e. There are major changes in the organisation of health, education and social services—the closure of long stay hospitals, the move to community care, to contracted services, to a national, standard curriculum.

These statements are hardly a comprehensive analysis of social change. One by one they will also become outdated. However, even as they stand they are vitally relevant to the provision of a successful transition for young people with physical disability. Some are positive, some are negative. The persistence of poverty, for instance, means the persistence of a poverty of lifestyle, of actual as opposed to theoretical choices.

Single parenthood too increases pressure and the need for respite, and at the same time can paradoxically increase interdependence between parent and offspring.

The changes in the structure of health and other services can bring new opportunities but also can mean disruption and financial uncertainty.

The change in the nature of employment and the fall in the number of young people available for work can greatly increase the chances of real work for real pay for many young people with disability, both because jobs can be less physically demanding than hitherto and also because of employers having to adapt to find the labour force they need.

How these and other changes interplay will vary from person to location to particular disability. However, they will also vary according to the values and perceptions of the services for the physically disabled, and their readiness to not simply react but also go out and influence a change themselves. Services need therefore to see themselves as not only 'whole person' oriented, but 'whole society' oriented.

There is no magic way or time to do so. There are always difficulties. As the man said when asked how to get to Cork by the tourist, 'I wouldn't start from here'. The pace of change also never seems to slow. In that sense services can always appear 'in crisis', and this can paralyse. However, the Chinese character for crisis has always seemed particularly appropriate: it is drawn representing 'danger', but also 'opportunity'.

The ultimate test is, of course, not how these services themselves adapt to change, but how they equip the young person with disability, to quote Darwin, 'to adapt and survive'; to assume what Bronfrennbrenner (1980) has called a 'developmental trajectory', i.e. an *internalised* ability to assume a lasting change in how that young person perceives and deals with his/her environment, and in a way that assumes a momentum of its own.

To summarise this more prosaically, we need a system of transitional services which (a) has clear standards and objectives, (b) is not inappropriately different, (c) is whole person oriented, (d) is continuous and (e) is responsive to wider societal change. This can be expressed diagrammatically as in Figure 32.1.

THE CURRENT STATE OF SERVICES

How do our existing services measure up to such a vision? The answer has to be that they do so very poorly. This will obviously be modified according to the nature of the disability. Some conditions such as cerebral palsy, or visual or aural impairment have well established systems of services largely based on voluntary bodies such as the Spastics Society. Such services can sometimes be accused of being complacent and segregated,

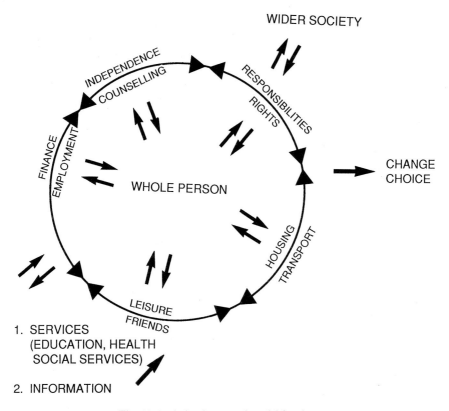

Fig. 32.1 A developmental model for change.

and are certainly not sufficient, but at least they exist, whereas young people who suffer from rarer, less numerous or 'established' conditions are much more isolated.

Notwithstanding the modifications, services can generally be considered: (1) impoverished, (2) unimaginative, and (3) fragmented.

They are *impoverished* in the sense that for many young people services such as day centres simply do not exist, never mind their quality.

They are *unimaginative* in the sense that even where they do exist they can be static and self-limiting. To stay with the example of day services, the recent Social Services Inspectorate report (1989) on day services for people with a mental handicap criticised them for having no sense of purpose, no clear policy frameworks, poor monitoring systems and little consumer participation. Many are also age inappropriate, lumping together people from 16 to 65 whose needs and energies are often vastly different. Many also have little sense of movement, of expectation that people may wish to develop and move away.

The report may have been about mental handicap, but the criticisms apply equally to day and occupation centres for people with physical disability.

Lastly, they are *fragmented* because there is often no clear system of responsibility for the delivery and coordination of services, no proper process of handover. Thus many young people and their families can find themselves without particular services, or receive them spasmodically, or from people who are not knowledgeable of their condition and/or their circumstances, or, alternatively find themselves having to attempt to become de facto case managers of a bewildering excess of different professionals—doctors, nurses, teachers, social workers—who do not seem to be aware of, or wish to communicate with, each other. Yet the need for coherence is clear. Brimblecombe (1989) cites a typical example which is worth quoting in full:

A young man of 19, physically disabled by spina bifida, suffered severe paralysis of his legs, and incontinence. His priority need was for a job; after training as an accountancy clerk he had been unemployed for 12 months. He had applied for a job in a city distant from his family home and had provisionally been offered it. In order to accept the job, he had to find suitably adapted accommodation conveniently close to the place of work, appropriate transport to take him to work and back (his wheelchair was adequate for indoor purposes but only of limited outdoor use), appropriate carer support (someone to attend to his personal needs in new accommodation), which would allow him to live away from the parental home, and the necessary finance to make the whole proposition viable. It was clear that appropriate health care would need to be continued (he suffered from recurrent urinary infections as a result of his incontinence) and if he was to progress in his work he would need further training in accountancy and computers. His social life, in a city where he was unknown, would involve making friends and having access to recreational facilities and entertainment—he very much hoped his adapted flat would be conveniently close to a public house since he enjoyed playing darts and drinking beer. He also mentioned some personal problems including his severe depression during the last year and his need for sexual counselling.

The problem is not peculiar to this country. The OECD report (1986) on transitional services showed that the problem was widespread throughout Western Europe, but this of course does not make it acceptable.

AN OPERATIONAL MODEL

So what is to be done? Perhaps the most hopeful development of the last few years has been the 1986 Disabled Persons (Services, Representation and Consultation) Act, in particular Sections 5 and 6, which are specifically focused on planning transitional services for school leavers who have disability. These sections, which are now fully legally operative, require education departments to seek the opinion of social services departments as to whether young people who are 'statemented' (i.e. have 'special educational needs') under the 1981 Education Act, are disabled within the 'adult' definition of disability contained within the 1948 National Assistance Act.

Whilst there are likely to be some variations as to precisely which young people will be referred—what of those with moderate learning difficulty, for example?— nevertheless clearly all young people with physical disability who are statemented will be. The referral will take place at the time of the annual review after the young person's 14th birthday.

The key phrase that social services departments will be mindful of in the 1948 Act definition of disability is 'permanent and substantial'. Whilst again there will no doubt be variations of opinion which may need to be clarified by precedent, it is equally also true that the vast majority of young people with physical disability who are referred will be deemed as 'adult disabled'.

Having received the deemed opinion from social services departments, education departments are then required to keep such young people 'under review', and, at least 8 months before the young person is due to leave school, must inform the social services departments of the school leaving date. Social services departments must then assess such young persons', and their families', range of needs within 5 months of being notified of the leaving date. That assessment should then be regularly reviewed.

Obviously, the operation of Sections 5 and 6 will need to 'bed in'. They are not a panacea—particularly since the government has not earmarked any more resources, and an assessment of need is not a guarantee of it being met. Nor should we assume that the existence of prescribed procedures mean that they will always be adhered to, or guarantee success— child protection tragedies have taught us that. But child protection procedures have also taught us that the existence of procedures can often ensure minimum standards where otherwise disparate or warring professionals would not meet constructively. Indeed, the existence of prescribed procedures in any area of work is now likely to be a necessary condition for the preservation or creation of resources at a time of so many competing demands.

The procedures could also do with being fleshed out. For instance, they neither acknowledge nor attempt to make more specific the crucial role played by health services, who anyway have their own internal problems of providing coherent transfer at the time when the young person leaves child orientated services and has to adjust to those provided by adults. Primary health care is often in the hands of the school doctor, especially where this is a boarding school, and where paediatric and other specialist care might have been based in the district of the child's school rather than the district to which they return after school age on transfer. The family doctor might know very little about either the young person or the wider implications of their condition, since the medical record card might still be with the school doctor; and even on leaving school, full records may not be transferred, or include a clear plan of positive medical care. Also, many young people with disability, and their families, are themselves often uncertain about the type of help they would receive from the family doctor, despite the GP's key role in providing local specialist help, and so they can often stay largely strangers to each other.

Nor do the Sections 5 and 6 procedures themselves guarantee appropriate consumer involvement, either by the young person and/or his/her family. It is possible for departments to play a private game of paper ping-pong.

Nevertheless, whilst the letter of the Act may be narrow, the spirit is wide, and its very existence increases the chances of good creative transitional planning.

What would a model of such planning look like? It could be called Individual Transitional Planning. The essence of this model already exists, to some real effect, in the guise of the system of Individual Programme Planning that is now widespread in the field of mental handicap learning difficulties, and it would be:

- *At least annual,* from the time of the first education statement review around the young person's 14th birthday
- *In active partnership* with the young person and parents or carers, providing them with a *single* reference point
- *Flexible* in location and timing
- *Limited in size* to prevent it becoming daunting, and not unnecessarily or without prior agreement including professionals who were not known to the young person and family unless they wished this
- *Multidisciplinary* with expected regular representation from education and careers departments, social services and health, as well as others as appropriate
- *Based on the young person's wishes, strengths and needs,* i.e. emphasising the forward looking positives with
- *A standard format* to ensure key issues were addressed and not forgotten
- *Whole person oriented* so that the range of areas in which appropriate and wished-for adulthood could be achieved was examined, producing

• *A clear, achievable, concise plan of action with a named person(s)* responsible for the initiation, administration, implementation and review of the plan.

Such a system would not stop when the young person left full-time education, but would be the basis for a continuing Individual Care Plan.

The responsibility for the coordination of this system should lie with the education department until the young person leaves full time education, and thereafter with the social services department. This is not to argue for 'supremacy', but simply to ensure it happens. Nor is transitional planning about passing the buck: it is about passing the baton.

An individual system of planning does not of course obviate the need for strategic planning. The spirit of the Disabled Persons Act requires the establishment of a regular method of planning between senior members of education, social services and health to review corporate issues and make policy and resource initiatives. These could include:

1. *The joint promotion of active disability policies,* akin to equal opportunities and anti-racist policies; and, in particular, a pro-active target of employing people with disability, thus providing both a direct service and a good example.

2. *Establishing joint training initiatives,* both pre- and post-qualification, and also with the young people and their parents or carers as well as multi-professionally.

3. *Making programmes and curricula* in schools, day centres and elsewhere *more complementary,* and encouraging staff interchange.

4. *Collecting information* from Individual Transitional Plans to provide adequate data about priority patterns of need.

5. *Asking consumers what they think of services,* both by meeting with representative bodies, but also by regular market research, (something non-commercial organisations are notoriously bad at)—and then acting on it!

ADVOCACY, BROKERAGE AND CONSUMER EMPOWERMENT

Some argue that a proper system of transitional planning will never come fully alive if it is left to one of the provider agencies, since by definition its staff will be one or more of the following:

a. Too cosily narrow in perspective
b. Inherently reluctant to be seriously self-critical
c. Likely to encourage inappropriate dependence
d. Too caught up in the gate-keeping role
e. Anxious not to bite the hand that pays them.

In this country, for example, the Honeylands Centre in Exeter accordingly appointed (with support from Action Research for Crippling Disease) a full-time Resource and Development Officer who is not identified with any single discipline. This officer works across all boundaries of both statutory and voluntary service provision, establishing a convenant with a young person with disability, whereby that person's needs and wishes are identified and ways are agreed to work together to advocate and present the case to the relevant authorities so that those needs are acceptably met.

Denmark has a similar system, where an independent person called a 'curator' is appointed to oversee the path of a young person with disability into independence. More radically, the Canadians have begun to establish a system of 'service brokerage', whereby adults with disability appoint independent brokers to purchase personal, flexible services on their behalf from provider agencies.

Certainly the notion of separating out purchasers from providers has become a key feature of both health and social service reforms, as has, in the White Paper on Community Care, the 'idea of personal packages' of care which are negotiated with the client/consumer.

My personal feeling is that the case is overstated. Services are not magically cheaper or necessarily less complex or quicker to organise simply because they are 'purchased'. At the same time, despite my earlier criticisms of the range and quality of services (criticisms which still stand), there have nevertheless been genuine examples of service providers changing the systems to meet the individual rather than the individual having to act, as it were, like a chameleon to fit the fixed colours of a static context.

Also, a system which assumes the narrowness and inability of agencies to change may self-fulfillingly produce the very pattern of defensive rigidity it wished to avoid.

Great strides have been made by innovative staff of all disciplines to be less rigid, less demarcative and more humble—to admit they are struggling sensitively rather than 'knowing' the answers, and to accept that the key people in a transitional planning system should depend on 'consumer chemistry' and particular needs, i.e. who gets on best with the person, who has the skills needed, rather than whose profession or agency habitually controlled the resources or practised the skills.

Advocacy and brokerage are of course not the only means of consumer involvement. I have also mentioned the importance of the style, timing and location of planning, formal representation and market research. Other ways come to mind: the establishment and proper use of student councils in the later years in schools, or in centres, or a national youth-oriented magazine equivalent to the very successful *Who Cares* for young people in care.

There is no single magic, comprehensive answer. It is primarily a question of attitude, of willingness to appreciate the significance and validity of the concept and to try out ways to put it into effect.

Consumer empowerment is fundamentally a 'good thing' for three reasons. The first is that in the most fundamental sense they are the 'reason' for the services—without them there would be no professionals to get paid. Therefore the services are first and foremost 'theirs' before they are anyone elses.

The second reason refers back to the basic model of standards and practice (Fig. 32.1). It is only in the doing that the skills are learnt. The Americans have an apt phrase: 'pre-' means never'.

The third reason is that the services provided (which are anyway in extremely scarce supply and therefore cannot afford to be wasted) are more likely to be accurate and appropriate if they are checked out with those they are provided for. No-one tells me whether I need a fridge more than a holiday. No-one should presume day centres are more important than employment opportunities.

It is likely that genuine attempts at increasing consumer involvement will be slower, less convenient, sometimes angrier and usually much more challenging than professionally taking unilateral decisions; but it is also likely to be worth the investment in creative discomfort.

One of the difficulties that is often presented is that it is difficult to know who is the consumer, at both the wider societal and individual family level. Thus it can be stated that an individual group should not be listened to because it is not representative, and a parent should not be listened to because the young person should be speaking for him/herself. Yet surely this is a false problem—we do not refuse to recognise our political parties because they do not speak for everyone, or because they have dominant leaders.

Deaf single-mindedness is hardly unheard of in managers in professional agencies!

The groups that do exist are at least representative of themselves, or else they would wither, and usually there are few alternative voices.

Equally it is arrogant to assume that parents are not speaking for or with the agreement of their offspring. Most families do agree on most major issues let alone that parents have their own rights because of, so often, their unique knowledge, their passionate commitment and the fact that they are still usually the most continuous carer. Indeed, for young people with dual handicap, i.e. physical disability and severe intellectual impairment, the parent may indeed have to continue to wear the mantle or primary responsibility for much longer.

Of course parents may be overprotective or unimaginative—but that criticism can be equally applied to professionals. Often indeed it can be individual parents who can be the most assertive and imaginative, and who can make most things happen.

This is certainly the case in the United States, where there is now a substantial network of what are called Parent Training Centres. These were set up with federal funding because it became clear that despite ritual homage to the idea of partnership by professionals, many parents with children who have special needs were lacking knowledge and were isolated. The centres exist specifically to empower parents to be more effective partners in the provision of the right services for their children. They are primarily staffed by parents who themselves have children with special needs. The parents are paid a salary in recognition of how impossible it is to do it consistently on a voluntary basis. Each centre is a unique constellation of people and skills, and each state has different issues, but all work across all disabilities, and together they provide an impressive and energetic range of services, from counselling to lobbying to information to matching volunteers to training, often on a joint learn-together basis with professionals. This systematic empowerment has done much to raise the overall standards of services, a view that research shows the professionals also feel—however bumpy the ride sometimes.

Parent Training Centres were initially established to push issues to do with special education, but right from the start the centres have inevitably and rightly looked at wider whole life issues that impinge upon educational attainment. Also, their children grow up, and the focus of need changes to what will happen after school, and so centres are increasingly focusing their attention on adult services.

The evidence suggests that they most emphatically are not achieving their objectives by 'presuming to know what is best', but by careful dialogue and discussion with their young adults, and are impressively capable of encouraging independence.

None of this is to deny the need to continually increase the ways in which young people with disability can learn to speak for themselves. It is simply to say that the distinction between the parent voice and the young person's voice is often far more arbitrary than that between the professionals and the young person.

Information

However, whatever the precise methods of consumer empowerment, they cannot thrive without information. Knowledge is power. This means a commitment by professionals to the maximum sharing of information and decision making in individual planning. It also means the organised and systematic provision of information to young people with disability about what is going on, in a form that, whilst certainly not patronisingly trendy, is sufficiently modern to be accessible and attractive, and is concerned with issues that young people particularly care about such as sexual problems, leisure, how to find a place to live, as well as the latest developments and ideas about specific conditions.

Indeed the provision of up-to-date information about services is not only a need of young people with disability. It is a need of their parents, and of professionals themselves, so vast is the area to be covered, and so rapid the rate and complexity of change, whether it be in the way services are organised, or, say, the particular entitlement to benefit.

In fact it could be argued that one of the most significant contributions health, social services and education agencies could make to transitional services would be to jointly finance a particular local disability pressure group or voluntary body, an equivalent of a Parent Training Centre, its own joint enterprise, or better still all three, to regularly make available up to date information for both consumers and professionals, so that people are reasonably aware of the new questions and 'answers', and—if they don't know themselves—whom they can contact to find out.

Such knowledge can either mean making use of resources and ideas already available, or marshalling arguments about the extent of needs or how they can be met.

Independent living

Certainly there are many areas of clearly established but unmet need. I have already used the terms impoverished and unimaginative, and cited some examples. There are other key areas. One of these is the need for independent living. Most young people with disability continue to live at home. The responsibility for their care, which is all too often a mutually implosive burden, lies with their parents. Studies have continually shown that the most consistent priority need for carers is adequate, sensitive, available, appropriate respite care. Yet, whilst it would be wrong to assume that it is an innate need of every young person, whether or not disabled, to live independently, it is certainly a clear need for very many, and in that sense the answer is not more respite, but more permanent independence. The models already exist—particularly in Sweden but also (in scattered form) in the UK—where young people become tenants of specially adapted, usually housing association, accommodation, with a network of health and social services staff, together often with trained volunteers from the Community Service Volunteers scheme, who provide appropriate 'live in' or peripatetic domiciliary back-up.

Employment and further education

Another need is proper employment. Certainly this is the dominant theme of Parent Training Centres as young people become adult—how to get a job? This in part reflects the extreme importance of employment as a means of adult validity in the US, but the difference is only a matter of degree. Employment is vitally important in this country too. It is usually only well-paid TV pundits who speculate on the post-employment era. It is important both as an achievement, an end in itself, and also, because it pays, as a means to express existence, to have meaningful choice. Yet, according to the 1989 figure from the Department of Employment, nearly 80% of all disabled people who are of working age are unemployed, compared to a national average of 6%.

Many would argue that making day centres more age-appropriate and dynamic is lambing the mutton—it is the wrong meat in the first place. They would say that the system of Supported Employment (Madden 1988) which has been extensively developed in the US for people with severe intellectual impairment, is equally appropriate for people with physical disability, and clearly demonstrates the essential employability of anyone with a disability. Supported Employment is based on the idea of people with disability obtaining, with the help of specially trained 'job coaches', 'real' jobs for which they are paid, proportionately to output, the same wages as everyone else. The keys to its success are a sensitive matching of the individual to the culture of the firm, an appropriate compartmentalisation of the tasks, the regular support of the job coaches, benefit flexibility, and success breeding success. The system is subsidised but no more expensive than traditional services, and often less so. Also many of the people who are thus employed stay longer, have better sickness records, and usually earn considerably more than if they were on benefit—all clear counters to arguments about exploitation.

Nor are the innovations solely confined to abroad. Creative careers officers and disablement resettlement officers have made imaginative individual placements. The further education units, particularly the work of David Hutchinson at North Notts College, have shown how young people with disability can take advantage of further education opportunities.

The time is clearly right for a root and branch change in the UK, too. Mention has already been made about the relative shortfall of young people available for employment. There is general concern about the poor take–up of further education and continuing education, particularly amongst working class young people. 'Relevance' and 'work oriented' are key terms, whether in the introduction of the national curriculum, the replacement of the training agency by the employer-led enterprise councils, or the establishment of a comprehensive system of national vocational qualification. The Confederation of British Industry (CBI) has called for a voucher system enabling young people to 'buy' an appropriate package of further education.

Assuming there are resources behind this rhetoric, then it is vital that young people with disability are seen as part of these developments, both for their own sake and for the contribution they can make. It is important therefore that they are not, as is now potentially provided for, 'exempted' from the expectations of the national curriculum—despite the best intentions this can condemn them to second class citizenship.

It is also important that sharp local teeth are put into the national toothless fangs of the Education Reform Act's expectation that colleges of higher education must simply 'have regard to' the needs of young people with disability. It is crucial that young people with disability do not lose out financially—that any voucher or existing system takes proper note of their extra expenses for accommodation, transport and so on; that starting a job, and then perhaps losing it, does not affect entitlement to benefit.

CONCLUSIONS

There are other areas of need and potential—the use of leisure, advice about sexuality, and so on. There is so much to be done. Perhaps it is time for a new charter for young people with disability, equivalent to the Barnardo's 'If You Let Me' campaign for young people with intellectual impairment, and designed to push services into qualitative progress.

But all progress is valid, however incremental. Indeed it is often a series of apparently unconnected incremental changes that suddenly synthesise and produce the next qualitative progress rather than vice versa. It is vital that professionals, parents and young people with disability themselves find shared ground and positive challenges.

Certainly, neither progress nor deterioration in services is inevitable— only change is.

Oscar Wilde said the price of democracy was eternal vigilance. The history of the improvement of disability services is the history of expectations, and so perhaps the price of progress in transitional services is eternal expectation.

REFERENCES

Brimblecombe F, Hoghugi M, Tripp J 1989 A new covenant with adolescents in crisis. Children and Society vol 3 (2)
Bronfrennbrenner A 1980 The ecology of human development. Harvard University Press, Cambridge, Mass.
Madden P 1988 Real work, real pay. Community Care (16.4.88)
O'Brien J 1989 Design for accomplishment responsive systems associates. Georgia, USA
OECD 1986 Towards a unified concept of transition. Available from The Further Education Unit, London
Social Services Inspectorate 1989 Inspection of day services for people with a mental handicap. DSS Health Publicity Unit
Wolfensberger W 1975 Programme analysis service systems (PASS 3). National Institute of Mental Retardation, Canada

33. Enabling independence in daily living

M. Jones

WORKING TOWARDS INDEPENDENCE

Children with physical disabilities experience similar difficulties to those presented by adults with physical disabilities. It can be helpful to refer to the same information systems, such as the Disabled Living Foundation or Naidex. Contact with local occupational therapists from the health authority and social services is recommended to ensure that the child is fully assessed and that local services are provided.

The drive to become as independent as possible must be nurtured throughout childhood and the child needs to have positive experiences on which to build. Thus it is advisable to avoid situations where the child is unlikely to succeed. This should not, however, discourage the introduction of new situations and experiences, as this is part of the learning process. Even where physical limitations prevent total independence, the child should be encouraged to make choices, give directions and to start to take responsibility for him/herself and for the task.

It is often possible to achieve a high level of physical independence (with or without aids and equipment) but at great cost in terms of time and fatigue. A balance must be sought where the child still has time and energy for play and schoolwork. For instance, it may be unrealistic to expect a child who has severe difficulties to fulfil a complex dressing programme before school each day, but a smaller part of the programme could be practised daily, with a greater time commitment at weekends and school holidays.

Undressing, particularly nightclothes, is an easier task to practise than dressing and can be timed to be part of the daily routine rather than a chore. The child may gain a great deal from assisting with dressing: for instance, understanding the sequence; paying attention to the task; recognising the clothes and where they go; learning about colour, temperature; and developing visual motor skills and body awareness.

Adapting the environment

Decisions about major adaptations to the child's environment should be delayed until the prognosis is clear, although minor work such as reor-

553

ganising furniture to allow floor space or to provide a stimulating position where the immobile child can see family activity can be suggested very early on. Where it becomes obvious that the child will be dependent on a wheel-chair for mobility outdoors, modifications such as levelling paths and ramping steps can be considered. Mobility using a trolley or chariot should be established early. Provision of aids for mobility at an early age will not preclude development of independent mobility later.

If the child's level of disability indicates that independent mobility in-doors will not be achieved, or will require more space than is available in order to be mobile, decisions must be made about whether to adapt the interior of the home or extend the home to provide special accommodation.

These decisions must be made in conjunction with the local social services occupational therapists, since funding may be available to pay for all or part of any adaptation or extension to the home.

Dressing

Allow the child and helper to experiment in order to find the position that provides greatest stability or greatest reach while dressing. This may be on the bed, floor or chair, standing, leaning or kneeling. A firm mattress may provide a sufficiently stable base for the less disabled child to sit on to dress if the feet are supported; otherwise, transfer onto a low chair (feet flat on the floor), to the floor or to the wheelchair. Help the child to choose easy, fashionable, loose-fitting clothes that can stretch and which do not have complex fastenings. They should be easy to organise with easily located arm and neck holes.

Small adaptations to clothing—such as tape loops attached inside the waistbands of trousers or pants to assist the use of a dressing stick or wall mounted hook—can be valuable. Extending waistband fastenings through loops can simplify going to the toilet by allowing loosening of waistbands instead of releasing. Lengthened fly openings and zipped trouser seams can help with the management of urinary devices and putting trousers over orthoses. The presence of lower limb orthoses and spinal jackets will com-plicate the dressing process. Care must be taken to ensure that fastenings are velcro and easily accessible. To avoid frustration, aspects of independ-ent dressing may have to be shelved for a short while following the intro-duction of new orthoses. Velcro concealed under buttons or replacing press studs and rings/loops on zips can enable a child to cope with school uni-form. Velcro fastenings on shoes can be valuable although they may have a tendency to loosen more quickly than buckles or laces.

Techniques such as backward chaining, where the helper assists to the last stage of the process, leaving the child to complete the task, can be very successful. The helper then expects the child to complete a larger final part of the task each time until the child achieves the whole task.

The practice of dressing the weaker or less mobile side first and undressing that side last is often appropriate, although an open mind must be kept, as the child may well find his or her own solution. Much can be achieved with the assistance of a helper—the continuing need for assistance should not rule out opportunities for assisted dressing practice.

Where reach is very restricted, a dressing stick with a double hook to help with fastenings, or a rubber end to hold clothes, may be sufficient aid although the precise length and bend of the stick will be critical. Wall-mounted hooks, bars or a dressing stand can be useful where there is limited reach or very stiff joints. Adjustments and location of these items is again critical to enable maximum use.

Toilet

Early potty training is an important aspect of the child's development. It is one of the earliest steps towards independence; in order to succeed, the child must feel comfortable and safe. Many infants with physical handicaps will manage to sit on standard nursery potties and chairs, although adaptation to these items may be necessary (Fig. 33.1a and b). As the dependent child grows up, the helper must be aware of the increasing need for privacy and dignity in order to develop self-respect. As weight increases, a hoist may be needed to assist the helper with transfer.

For larger children a choice can be made from the range of child-sized toilet seats and commodes. Frequently a standard infant or junior sized toilet in school can be used in conjunction with grab bars to provide sufficient support (Fig. 33.2). Where the full-sized family toilet is used, adaptations must be easily removable and not bulky. Examples include the Taylor Chailey (Fig. 33.3a), the Chailey moulded seat (Fig. 33.3b), the

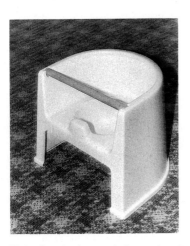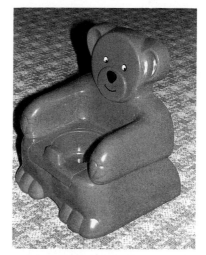

Fig. 33.1   Standard potty chairs can be adapted if necessary.

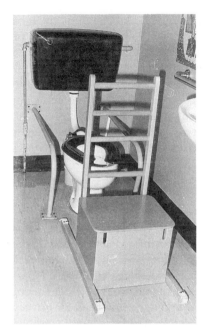

Fig. 33.2 A ladderback chair to grasp may provide enough security if feet are supported.

a

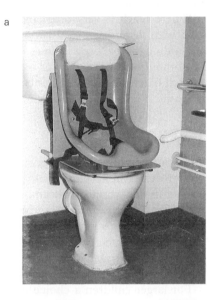

b

c

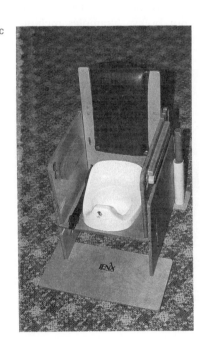

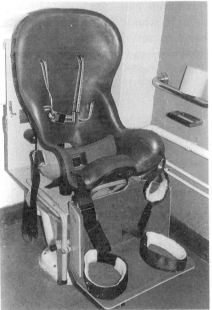

Fig. 33.3 Specialised toilets can provide an appropriate level of support and padding. **a.** Taylor Chailey. **b.** Chailey (personally moulded). **c.** Jenx.

Jenx potty seat (Fig. 33.3c), and the Everest and Jennings child's toilet seat. Grab bars fixed either side of the toilet, or a drop-down horizontal bar in front (Fig. 33.4), can give confidence to a child who lacks stability—particularly if used with a step and toilet seat insert.

Space for sideways transfer from a wheelchair is frequently lacking, and re-design may be necessary to enable manoeuvrability and independence generally.

A double wall hook or dressing stick, used in conjunction with a drop-down rail, may be required near the toilet in order to manage pants especially if orthoses are worn.

A changing table with a backrest, used in conjunction with a mirror, may allow the child to learn self-catheterisation. This must be situated in a private place with no danger of interruption. An abduction splint may be needed to help the child maintain the position.

Attention must be paid to the exact position of the basin, flush, toilet paper and lightswitch if independence is to be achieved.

For boys, aim in urination can be a problem. If the child is sitting to urinate, a Chailey urine deflector or a urinal can be useful. If the boy stands and has problems with reach or aim, a loop or channel on a stick (a 'willy wand') can be guided by short upper limbs or mouth.

Techniques for cleansing can include the use of wiping aids and the learning of techniques such as the use of trunk flexion to increase reach, or wedging the paper onto a clip on the seat.

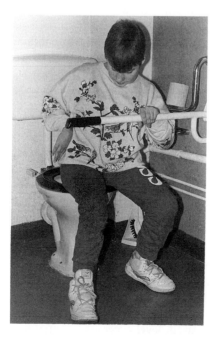

Fig. 33.4 A drop-down horizontal bar can allow the stability necessary for self-cleaning.

Try to teach girls to wipe from 'front to back' in order to reduce the risk of urinary tract infection. A horizontal drop-down grab bar in front of the child can be used to lean over and provide stability while wiping the bottom—this technique can be valuable for a child with lower limb orthoses. Always ensure that the rail will lock away in the upright position; some models can drop down again, knocking the child. A non-slip surface on the floor in front of the toilet can prevent feet slipping while getting on and off the toilet. A Closomat toilet can be considered where other attempts at independence on the toilet have been unsuccessful. However, a trial is advised as the Closomat may well soak lower limb orthoses or spray too powerfully for the child.

Bathroom

The extent of the child's physical handicap will dictate how independent he or she is able to be, particularly in the bathroom. However, the range of equipment designed for adults can often be used for children (see Disabled Living Foundation Centre publications).

For a child who is dependent on help while bathing, assistance for the parents may be required. Use of the Chailey swimming aid can be a simple means of maintaining the face clear of the water while the child lies in the bottom of the bath—preferably on a non-slip mat. Stooping to lift a slippery child from the bottom of the bath can be avoided by the use of a Shallowbath insert to reduce the depth of the bath, or a lifter such as the Bealift (Fig. 33.5a and b). Postural support in the bath can be achieved by a range of bath seats, although some of these maintain the child in too high a position, necessitating the use of a great deal of warm water before the water level reaches the child.

A start towards independence may involve the use of a bath board in combination with a bath seat. Sideways transfers can be made from a chair onto the bath board and the bath seat will reduce the depth ready for transfer out. The Shallowbath can be valuable for early independence: transfers can be made sideways (or from the end if the bathroom allows). Beware when assisting a chubby child to use a Shallowbath: a tidal wave can be created that results in wet feet for the helper!

A great drawback of the bath aids described above is that they are bulky, causing problems in storing at home and in portability when on holiday. Grab rails attached above the bath can assist in transfers and confidence.

Bathing versus showering can present a dilemma to parents. Points to bear in mind include: the child's preference; the effect of the shower/bath on postural tone; space available and family needs; hygiene, continence and the need for a good soak; danger/presence of pressure sores.

If a shower is to be used, level access is essential for easy use by a wheel-chair user or an ambulant child with a physical handicap, to avoid the need

a

b

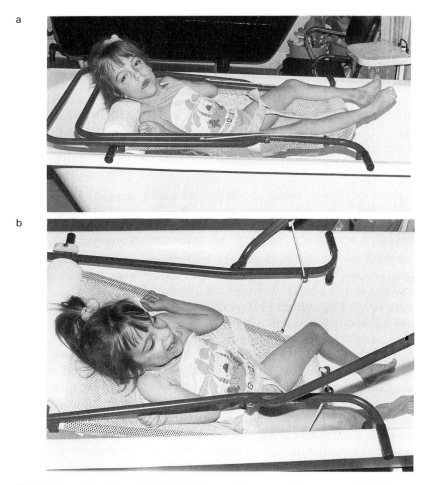

Fig. 33.5a and b.   A portable bath aid that provides postural support, and which lowers and lifts the child into and out of the bath.

to negotiate a step. There are a range of child and adult sized shower chairs; some are self-propelling. The cost of shower chairs is high and a trial should be requested from the company before a decision is made. Knee access under the washbasin, possibly used in conjunction with lever taps, can assist where reach is a problem.

Toothbrush handles can be bent or built up to assist grip and reach, or toothbrushes can be wall-mounted and the child's head movement utilised to make a brushing action. Holding the toothbrush with the added support of a wrist-strap is an alternative. For children with low motivation or poor hand coordination, an electric toothbrush can be an inspiration.

Hair washing is often best learnt under the shower. Shampoo can be dispensed via a standard lever soap dispenser mounted on the wall. A long-handled, short-bristled hairbrush can be used during shampooing to help lather if reach is too short. Short hair is easier to manage although individual preference often overrules practical issues.

Hairbrushes and combs can be attached to long handles or to the wall. Built-up handles can assist the child who lacks sustained grasp. Bent handles can help a child to reach the back of the head.

A hand strap can be attached to provide extra stability for an electric razor. Alternatively, mount it on the wall or select a model which is easier to grip.

Bedroom

A child with a physical handicap will benefit from provision of a spacious bedroom with easy access to the bathroom. In addition to accommodating the child's special equipment (orthoses, walking aid, wheelchair, etc.) some thought must be given to bedroom furniture. Where possible, accessible clothes and toy storage is desirable. An appropriate lightswitch within easy reach when the child is in bed, and an alarm switch for a non-vocal child should be considered. Environmental control systems are occasionally provided by the Department of Health and can incorporate other functions such as TV and radio control and curtain opening and closing.

When positioning, handling and therapy have maintained the child in a symmetrical posture during the day, care should be taken to ensure that the good effect is not lost at night when postural support and control ceases. Night sleeping wedges can be made to maintain symmetry, hip abduction or side-lying (see Fig. 33.13, p. 569). These must be well padded and introduced gradually to ensure that they can be tolerated. Side-lying can be assisted by placing the bed in such a way that all stimulating items such as a window, door or posters can only be seen when the child lies in the desired position. The same technique can be used to encourage head turning to a particular side.

Bed sides or a firmly tucked in sheet over a duvet may be needed if the child cannot maintain a position and moves constantly, tending to become uncovered or falling out of bed. Ensure that there is no danger of arms and legs becoming trapped in the cot/bed sides.

Eating and drinking

Eating together is an important part of family life and although it may be difficult to include the child who needs to be fed, the child's social development will be enhanced. Including the child at mealtimes will be easier if the child is supported in a good sitting position and if all family members are familiar with the techniques so that the task can be shared from meal to meal.

There is a wide range of special eating and drinking equipment for children and adults (Figs. 33.6–9), available commercially.

When assessing a child with regard to eating and drinking it is essential to obtain the optimum sitting posture (see Ch. 25) and table height. A speech therapist will be able to advise on techniques to promote good oral function and may also contribute to evaluating a good position for feeding.

Suitability of materials used in the manufacture of cutlery should be considered whilst assessing feeding difficulties. Many children with highly sensitive mouths (e.g. children with cerebral palsy) will not be able to tolerate metal. Horn spoons have now been largely superceded by

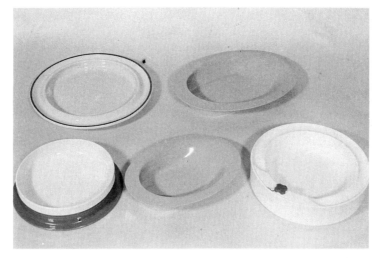

Fig. 33.6 Dishes are available to facilitate scooping and to keep food warm.

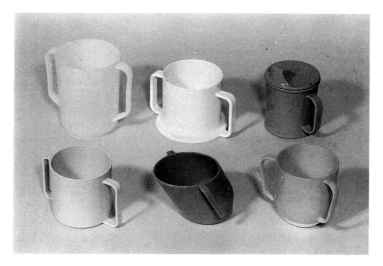

Fig. 33.7 Two-handled mugs can encourage symmetry.

a

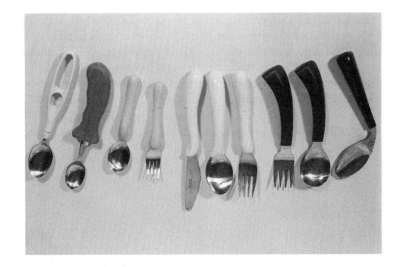

b

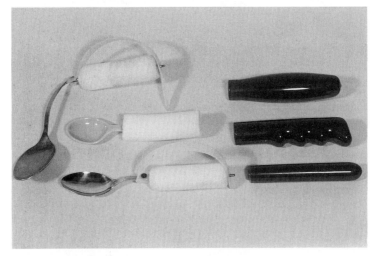

Fig. 33.8a and b. Cutlery with adapted grips to assist grasp.

polycarbonate spoons, which are equally warm to the touch but do not splinter or shatter when bitten. Choose a spoon that is the correct size for the child, with a shallow bowl so that the food will be easy to position in the mouth or easy for the child to take off the spoon, e.g. the Crystallon spoon from the Spastics Society.

Very simple modifications to cutlery can often have good results; for example, a slight bend in the handle close to the bowl of the spoon may be all that is required for a child who has difficulty rotating his hand to present the spoon to his mouth—but ensure that the bent spoon can still scoop food from the dish. Foam padding or chubby grips can stabilise a spoon within a hand, and a strap around the back of the fingers can save a

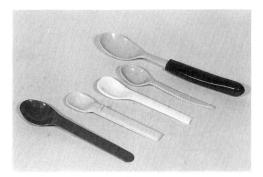

Fig. 33.9 Polyethylene or polycarbonate spoons are advised for hypersensitive mouths.

spoon or fork being dropped accidentally. Consider the use of non-slip matting, plates with rims or scooper ends, keep-warm plates for slow eaters and, of course, suitability of the food being presented (see Chs 1 and 7).

Where range of arm and shoulder movement, or reach generally, is the presenting problem, adapting spoons or forks to minimise movements required is often possible.

When only head movement is available a feeding aid can occasionally be a solution (Fig. 33.10). However, very refined head control, trunk stability and balance, as well as good perceptual skills combined with practice and determination are necessary. Use of a feeding aid can be very tiring so may not necessarily be used for all meals.

Spouted beakers for drinking may not be considered the best option since they can tend to reinforce primitive suckling. Beakers with two handles (large enough for hands), only partly filled with drink, may better enable success especially if the child learns to stabilise on the elbows. A slanted cup or one with a cutaway opposite the nose can also be helpful as it enables the child's head to be kept in the vertical position and avoids tipping the head back. Slanted beakers are also useful if the helper is giving the drink, since they give a clear view of the quantity being given and allow controlled small sips to be attempted.

Some children, particularly those with restricted movement and power, (for example those with Duchenne muscular dystrophy or spinal muscular atrophy) may prefer to use a drinking straw. Mugs can be obtained with a hole through the lid to direct a straw, or a pen clip can be used to clip a straw to the side of the beaker. Flexible straws are recommended. Where power suck is restricted, a Pat Saunders valved straw will keep the liquid within the straw, thus eliminating some of the effort.

Kitchen

All children need the opportunity to be in the kitchen while meals are prepared and cleared away. A table or worktop of suitable height, with

a

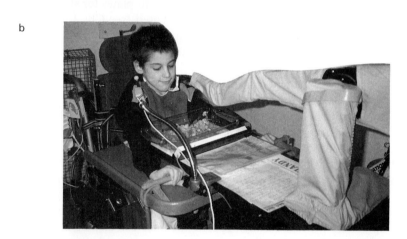

b

c

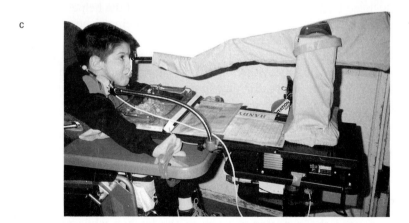

Fig. 33.10a, b and c.   Child feeding himself with the Handy 1 Robotic Feeding Aid.

knee space underneath, can allow the child to help with meal preparation. If a wheelchair is used, sufficient space for turning may be a problem. Some children may prefer to stand or to use a clicker walker or flexistand while working.

As the child's future physical abilities become clear, often at around 10–12 years old, it is appropriate to consider further kitchen adaptations/extension/equipment to meet the needs and allow some independence. Reference to Design for People with Disabilities will now be useful (Goldsmith 1984).

Car/transport

Babies and small children can generally be accommodated in the reclining type of baby car seats now available. The seats may require additional padding and support for the child but care must be taken not to alter the safety aspects, i.e. type of harness fitted.

Backward facing seats for the very young infants can be most valuable for a baby with poor head control. Older children may manage with an ordinary booster seat and harness, Britax Handicapped child's car seat, or other types of seat such as the Hansa Booster (Possum). If parents/carers comment on difficulty in lifting the child in and out of fixed seats, a swivel car seat may need to be considered.

For a child who needs postural support in sitting, some specialised seating systems (such as the Adaptaseat) can be used in a car in conjunction with an adult seatbelt, although they are not safety seats. The need to lift seat and child into the car (either together or separately) still presents a problem. A roomy estate car—to give space for carrying a wheelchair—is advisable.

There is a range of vehicles with high roofs and ramps so that the wheelchair and occupant can be wheeled straight in. Care must be taken to ensure that the roof is high enough and the wheelchair is sufficiently sturdy and stable to be used for this purpose. Windows should be at a suitable height for the wheelchair occupant, allowing travel to be an enjoyable and stimulating experience. Check also that clamps are available to hold the chair in place.

Many standard cars can be fitted with hoists, either to assist transfers or to help with packing away the folded wheelchair. The Car Chair adaptation consists of a wheelchair combined with a hoist, which locates in the driving or front passenger position in place of a regular car seat. Details of this and other car adaptations can be obtained from the Mobility Roadshow or the Disabled Living Foundation (see references).

On public transport a 'buggy major' may be required if the family are to use a bus, and this item is often available from the Disablement Services Centre in addition to the child's wheelchair. Rail travel with a wheelchair is possible but it is advisable to contact stations first to ensure that access is available and that time and help will be allowed for loading and unloading.

School

If it is planned for the child to attend a local school rather than a special school, a visit should be made in advance to check that the environment is suitable. Ideally the visit should be planned to include the child, parents, therapists, teacher and a representative from the department of education who will be responsible for any work that is recommended.

Where possible, adaptations should be designed to meet the needs of other children and adults with physical handicaps.

Privacy in the school toilet is vital for children who are coping with incontinence, catheterisation, orthoses or prostheses. Space may be required in the toilet for sideways transfers from a wheelchair and also for a plinth for managing incontinence. This may need to be at a suitable height for a helper, or an adjustable height variety may be required. Storage may be required for clean dressings: this is frequently a problem when looking at adapting school toilets.

Consideration should be given to ease of mobility within school generally, and proximity to all communal rooms, especially toilets. The amount and frequency of movement between classrooms, width of corridors and doorways must also be borne in mind, as well as the question—how will the child cope at playtime?

Extra space in the classroom for the child's equipment should also be considered. In class, methods for recording work done may need to be devised. Pencils and pens can be adapted with special grips to enhance grasp. Even when writing is laborious, it is worthwhile to encourage some level of skill (Fig. 33.11).

Alternatives may need to be considered when quantity and speed of output becomes a problem. A computer or electronic typewriter may suffice. Portability and other functions of a computer must be borne in mind when reaching a decision. A switch system may be required but utilisation of the same switches (or type of switch) for powered driving and

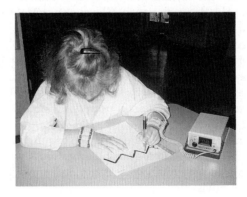

Fig. 33.11   Weighted bracelets can occasionally be useful in ataxia.

computer work may either simplify or complicate the child's introduction to switches, so careful assessment is required. Consideration must be given to which part of the body is to operate the switch and how complex the switch should be. Whether head, chin, hand or foot switches are proposed, it is advisable to observe the effect of the switch use on the child's postural stability (see Ch. 25). A page turner can also be utilised, controlled by the child's usual switch.

Correct positioning is vital whether handwriting or keyboard work is being undertaken. The best height for both table and chair must be ascertained. Consideration should also be given to comfort and whether extra postural support should be provided while the child is concentrating on the task. Adjustable heights for tables and computer trolleys are desirable, and adaptations can be devised to assist with function (Fig. 33.12). Prone standers and standing frames can permit a change of position and improve hand function and head control.

To assist with stabilisation of paper, experimentation with non-slip matting under a clipboard or a metal writing board with magnetic strips resting on the paper can be helpful. When a metal writing board is used, rulers and technical drawing equipment can be fitted with magnetised strips to maintain position. Rulers can also be weighted to keep them in place.

Angled bookrests and writing desks can assist the child with a visual perceptual problem and, additionally can be advantageous where hand coordination is affected.

There are many types of scissors available—some sprung, others with training handles to enable help to be given. When the use of standard scissors is not possible, scissors can be mounted on a plate for lever action use. Alternative ways of cutting can be explored, e.g. electric scissors, cutters and shielded guillotine.

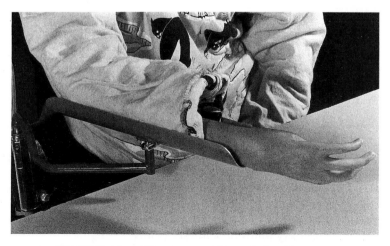

Fig. 33.12   A mobile arm support for use in the classroom.

Selecting the optimum position within the classroom should also be considered, taking into account any sensory losses and problems with head control or attention span.

Positioning for activity

All children benefit from experiencing many positions during the day. The able-bodied child constantly changes position and level, e.g. chair to floor to standing. Physically handicapped children should benefit from the same range of experiences.

The prone position can help the child to weightbear symmetrically, and to develop extension and control of head and limbs. It can also provide a position for play on the floor.

For a child of low physical ability, side-lying can provide a stable posture in which hands can come together in front of the face. Standing is known to inhibit spasticity, encourage circulation, urinary tract function and stability of hip joints, and help prevent osteoporosis; standing can frequently be achieved through the use of a prone stander or flexistand. Additional benefits gained from the standing position include being the equivalent height of peers, and having a normal orientation to the environment (see. Ch. 25).

Commercial companies are now producing a wide variety of positioning equipment, and reference to the Disabled Living Foundation publications or to the Naidex exhibition is advised.

Adaptations to positioning equipment are frequently necessary—extra straps or support blocks can be tried, extra padding is often indicated and grab bars may be required for trays to enable the child to stabilise his posture (see Chs 7 and 25).

SOURCES OF FUNDING AND PRACTICAL BACK-UP

A detailed knowledge of the resources available in the locality is valuable for obtaining individual items of equipment, or adaptation of a standard piece. The following notes give ideas on the types or organisations which may be found locally:

1. *Local occupational therapists* based either in the local authority social services department or the local hospital. Therapists often have access to technical support for individual work and will also advise on design or selection of a piece of equipment. A referral to an occupational therapist employed by social services will include an assessment (possibly jointly with the treating therapist), advice on possible techniques, equipment or alterations for the client and information on routes for funding the work, such as local authority funds or statutory grants.

2. *Rehabilitation Engineering Movement Advisory Panels (REMAP):* panels

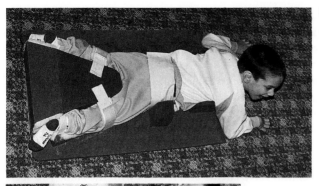

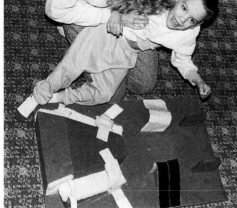

Fig. 33.13a and b. A night wedge can help the child to maintain symmetry and reduce spasm.

of experts, often from industry, working in a voluntary capacity with clinical advisors utilising their skills in solving individual problems presented to the panel.

3. *Chailey Heritage Rehabilitation Engineering Unit* manufactures one-off aids designed in conjunction with clinical input.

4. *Local carpenters.* People with specific skills can be contacted through local papers or radio. The client/customer will be expected to finance the work unless local charitable funds can be identified.

5. *Local trusts and charities.* Many towns and villages have trusts specifically aimed at helping certain categories of local people. Trusts are frequently seeking suitable recipients.

6. *Organisations linked to diagnostic groups.* Many diagnostic groups have their own national and local organisations and can frequently be a source of both information and practical support.

7. *Specific fundraising efforts.* Local organisations, pubs and schools might consider fundraising for a 'good cause', but care needs to be taken that the beneficiary (and family) can cope with the publicity that will surround the effort and that sufficient funds are also raised to cover the future maintenance costs of the item. Advice may be required to ensure the suitability of the item to be purchased.

8. *The Family Fund.* This organisation (see Appendix for address) will often consider a grant for children under 16 years of age. Grants may be made for items not generally available through social services or the National Health Service.

9. *Local health authorities.* Some health authorities have supplies of equipment such as standard commodes and hoists for short-term loan. Health Authority paediatric occupational therapists and physiotherapists occasionally carry a small stock of children's equipment for short-term loan. Wheelchairs and prostheses are available from local health authority Disablement Services Centres.

10. *Local day centres* may have clients and leaders with the skills you seek. However, some funding may be required.

11. *The Disabled Living Foundation* have a wide range of equipment for the individual to try. They also publish a wide range of information.

12. *Naidex exhibitions* of assistive devices and equipment are held in a different venue each year and in London.

13. *Mobility Roadshow.* An annual exhibition is held at Crowthorne, Berkshire.

REFERENCES AND FURTHER READING

Chailey Heritage (annually) Assistive devices. Rehabilitation Engineering Unit, Chailey Heritage
Dunn Klein M 1983 Pre-dressing skills. Communication Skill Builders and Winslow Press
Dunn Klein M 1987 Pre-scissor skills. Communication Skill Builders and Winslow Press
Finnie N 1968 Handling the young CP child at home. Heinemann, London
Goldsmith S 1963 Designing for the disabled. RIBA, London
Jay P 1985 Help yourselves: a handbook for hemiplegics and their families. RADAR, London
Harpin P 1981 With a little help. Muscular Dystrophy Group of Great Britain, London
Holgate L 1985 Hydrocephalus: learning aid development. ASBAH, London
Mandelstam M 1990 How to get equipment for disability. Jessica Kingsley Publishers and Kogan Page for the Disabled Living Foundation, London
National Toy Libraries Association 1989 Positions for play. Play Matters, London
Ouvry C 1987 Educating children with profound handicaps. British Institute of Mental Handicap, Kidderminster
RADAR 1988 Directory for disabled people.
RADAR 1988 Motoring and mobility for disabled people.
Sassoon R 1991 Helping your handwriting. (Teacher's guide). Arnold Wheaton
Warner J 1981 Helping the handicapped child with early feeding. Winslow Press

Publications from the following organisations are recommended for further reading:

Disabled Living Foundation, London
Health Publications Unit, HMSO, London
Mencap, London
National Children's Bureau, London
Oxfordshire Health Authority ('Equipment for disabled people' series)
Spastics Society, London

Appendix
Select list of useful organisations

The following organisations are only a few of the many who offer information, advice and counselling. In addition, the following book will be a useful source reference:

Directory for disabled people, compiled (and regularly updated) by A. Darnbrough and D. Kinrade, and published by Woodhead-Faulkner, Cambridge.

United Kingdom

Association For All Speech Impaired Children (AFASIC)
347 Central Markets, Smithfield
London EC1A 9NH   071-236 6487

Association to Aid Sexual and Personal Relationships of
Disabled People (SPOD)
286 Camden Road
London N7 OBJ   071-607 8851

Association for Spina Bifida and Hydrocephalus (ASBAH)
ASBAH House, 42 Park Road
Peterborough, Cambridgeshire PE1 2UQ   0733 555988

British Colostomy Association
15 Station Road
Reading, Berkshire RG1 1LG   0734 391537

British Epilepsy Association
Anstey House, 40 Hanover Square
Leeds LS3 1BE   0532 439393

British Sports Association for the Disabled
Hayward House, Barnard Crescent
Aylesbury, Buckinghamshire HP21 9PP   0296 27889

The Compassionate Friends
6 Denmark Street
Bristol BS1 5DQ   0272 292778

The Family Fund
Joseph Rowntree Memorial Trust
Beverley House, Skipton Road
PO Box 50
York YO1 1UY

Friedreich's Ataxia Group
Copse Edge, Thursley Road, Elstead
Godalming, Surrey GU8 6DJ   0252 702864

Headway
200 Mansfield Road
Nottingham NG1 3HX   0602 622382

ICAN
Allen Graham House, 198 City Road
London EC1V 2PH   071-608 2462

Ileostomy Association of Great Britain and Ireland
Amblehurst House, Black Scotch Lane
Mansfield, Nottinghamshire NG18 4PF   0623 28099

The International Cerebral Palsy Society
5a Netherhall Gardens
London NW3 5RN   071-794 9761

Lady Hoare Trust for Physically Disabled Children
37 Oakwood, Bepton Road, Midhurst
West Sussex GU29 9QS   073081 3696

Medic-Alert Foundation
17 Bridge Wharf, 156 Caledonian Road
London N1 9UU   071-833 3034

Muscular Dystrophy Group of Great Britain
Nattrass House, 35 Macaulay Road
London SW4 0QP   071-720 8055

Naidex Conventions Ltd
90 Calverley Road
Tunbridge Wells TN1 2UN

National Bureau for Students with Disabilities (SKILL)
336 Brixton Road
London SW9 7AA   071-274 0565

The National Deaf Children's Society
45 Hereford Road
London W2 5AH   071-229 9272

National Toy Libraries Association
68 Churchway
London NW1 1LT   071-387 9592

Physically Handicapped and Able Bodied (PHAB)
12–14 London Road, Croydon
Surrey CR0 2TA   081-667 9443

Rehabilitation Engineering Movement Advisory Panels
  (REMAP)
25 Mortimer Street
London W1N 8AB   071-637 5400

Riding for the Disabled Association
Avenue Road, National Agricultural Centre
Kenilworth, Warwickshire CV8 2LY   0203 696510

Royal Association for Disability and Rehabilitation
  (RADAR)
25 Mortimer Street
London W1N 8AB   071-637 5400

Royal National Institute for the Blind
224–228 Great Portland Street
London W1N 6AA   071–388 1266

Royal National Institute for the Deaf
105 Gower Street
London WC1E 6AH   071-387 8033

Scottish Council for Spastics
22 Corstorphine Road
Edinburgh EH12 6DD   031 337 9876

Scottish Council on Disability
5 Shandwick Place
Edinburgh EH2 4RG   031 229 8632

Scottish Spina Bifida Association
190 Queensferry Road
Edinburgh EH4 2BN   031 332 0743

Scottish Spinal Cord Injury Association
Unit 22, 100 Elderpark Street
Glasgow G51 3TR   041 440 0960

Scottish Sports Association for the Disabled
Fife Sports Institute, Viewfield Road
Glenrothes, Fife KY6 2RA   0592 771700

Sense
311 Gray's Inn Road
London WC1X 8PT

Spastics Society
12 Park Crescent
London W1N 4EQ   071-636 5020

Spinal Injuries Association
76 St James Lane
London N10 3DF   081-444 2121

Voluntary Council for Handicapped Children
National Children's Bureau, 8 Wakley Street
London EC1V 7QE   071-278 9441

Western Cerebral Palsy Centre
Bobath Centre, 5 Netherhall Gardens
London NW3 5RN   071-435 3895

Australia

New South Wales

Independent Living Centre
600 Victoria Road, Ryde
Sydney, New South Wales 2112   02-808 2322

Muscular Dystrophy Association of New South Wales
c/o Mr E. Parmenter, Executive Officer
GPO Box 9932, Sydney, New South Wales 2001   02-267 6622

Nadow Training Program, Training Centre for Disabled
27 Atchinson Street, St Leonards
Sydney, New South Wales   02-436 0303

New South Wales Society for Crippled Children
30 Cowper Street, Parramatta
Sydney, New South Wales 2150   02-893 1000

New South Wales Sports Council for the Disabled
PO Box 135, Flemington Markets
Sydney, New South Wales 2129   02-763 0155

Paraquad Association
33–35 Burlington Road, Homebush
Sydney, New South Wales 2140   02-764 4166

Spastics Centre of New South Wales
189 Allambie Road, Allambie Heights
Sydney, New South Wales   02-451 9022

Spina Bifida Association of New South Wales
PO Box 15, Carlingford
Sydney, New South Wales 2118   02-893 1000

Technical Aid to the Disabled (TAD)
227 Morrison Road, Ryde
Sydney, New South Wales 2112

Wheelchair Sports Association of New South Wales
Ralph Place, Mount Druitt
Sydney, New South Wales   02-675 2617

Victoria

Yooralla Society
52 Thistlewaite Street
Melbourne, Victoria   03-699 2066

Queensland

Spina Bifida Association of Queensland
387 Old Cleveland Road
Cooparoo, Queensland   07-394 3822

Australian National Organisations

Australian Council for Rehabilitation of the Disabled
   (ACROD)
PO Box 60, Curtin, Canberra 2605   06-282 4333

The Children's Growth Foundation
PO Box 459, Maroubra
Sydney, New South Wales 2035

Limbkids (Limb Deficiency)
c/o Mrs Diane Bell, 14 Faul Street
Aspley, Queensland 4034   07-263 1513

The Little People's Association of Australia
The Summit Road
Port Macquarie, New South Wales 2444   06-582 0574

Osteogenesis Imperfecta Society of New South Wales
PO Box 401, Epping
Sydney, New South Wales 2121

Spinal Muscular Atrophy Association
c/o Mrs Caroline Maltby, 67 Donaldson Street
Mackay, Queensland 4740

New Zealand

Mrs W. Gregory, Spina Bifida Association
PO Box 19281
Evondale, Auckland

Mrs L. Thurston, Spina Bifida Group
PO Box 354
Rotorua

New Zealand Crippled Children's Society
PO Box 6349
Te-Aro, Wellington

Canada

Advocacy Resource Centre for the Handicapped
40 Orchard View Boulevard, Suite 255
Toronto, Ontario M4R 1B9

Autism Society Canada
20 College Street, Suite 2
Toronto, Ontario M5G 1K2   416-924 4189

Canadian Association for Community Living
Kinsmen Building, York University Campus
4700 Keele Street, Downsview, Ontario M3J 1P3   416-661 9611

Canadian Association of the Deaf
271 Spadina Road, Suite 311
Toronto, Ontario M5R 2V3   416-928 1350

Canadian Cerebral Palsy Association
880 Wellington Street, Suite 612
City Centre, Ottawa, Ontario K1R 6K7   613-235 2144

Canadian Cleft Lip and Palate Family Association
180 Dundas Street West, Suite 1508
Toronto, Ontario M5G 1X8   416-598 2311

Canadian Co-ordinating Council on Deafness
116 Lisgar Street, Suite 203
Ottawa, Ontario K2P OC2   613-737 7499

Canadian Council of the Blind
220 Dundas Street, Suite 510
London, Ontario N6A 1H3   519-433 3946

Canadian Down Syndrome Society
5232 4th Street SW
Calgary, Alberta T2V OZ4   403-253 5835

Canadian Hearing Society
271 Spadina Road
Toronto, Ontario M5R 2V3   416-964 9595

Canadian Hemophilia Society
1450 City Councillors Street, Suite 840
Montreal, Quebec H3A 2E6   514-848 0503

Canadian Institute of Child Health
17 York Street, Suite 105
Ottawa, Ontario K1N 5S7   613-238 8425

Canadian National Institute for the Blind
1931 Bayview Avenue
Toronto, Ontario M4G 4C8   416-480 7580

Canadian Paediatric Society
c/o Children's Hospital of Eastern Ontario
401 Smyth Road
Ottawa, Ontario K1H 8L1   613-737 2728

Canadian Rett Syndrome Association
260 Adelaide Street East, PO Box 97
Toronto, Ontario M5A 1N0   416-226 0559

Disability Information Services of Canada
839 5th Avenue SW, Suite 610
Calgary, Alberta T2P 3C8   403-270 8100

Easter Seal Communication Institute
24 Ferrand Drive
Don Mills, Ontario M3C 3N2

Muscular Dystrophy Association of Canada
150 Eglinton Avenue East, Suite 400
Toronto, Ontario M4P 1E8   416-488 0030

Spina Bifida Association of Canada
633 Wellington Crescent
Winnipeg, Manitoba R3M 0A8   204-452 7580

Glossary

acheiria Absence of a hand

achondroplasia A type of short-limbed dwarfism

adactylia Absence of fingers

agonist muscles Muscles producing movement around a joint

amblyopia Absence of vision or poor vision not caused by any discoverable lesion in the eye

amelia Absence of a limb

amino-acid An organic acid in which one or more of the hydrogen ions are replaced by NH_2; any one of the hydrolytic products of protein breakdown, some of which are indispensable to growth in higher animals

antagonist muscles The muscles which oppose the agonists to provide stability arond a joint

anterior horn cells The nerve cells present in the anterior horn of the spinal cord which connect with the motor nerves forming the lower motor neurone

antibody Specific constituent of serum proteins which develop in response to an antigen as part of the defence mechanism of the body

anti-emetics Drugs which inhibit nausea and vomiting

antigen Any substance which, after introduction into the body, is capable of producing an antibody and thus inducing immunity

apnoea Absence of breathing

apodia Absence of a foot

arthrodesis Surgical fixation of bone by the artificial production of bony union

arthrogryposis Curved stiff joints

ataxia Incoordination of muscular action caused by damage to the cerebellum or its nervous pathways

athetosis Slow, writhing involuntary movements of the limbs and trunk caused by damage to the basal ganglia

autosomal recessive inheritance A trait whose expression is dependent upon the homozygous state, i.e. inheritance of the gene occurs from both parents

autosome One of the pairs of chromosomes numbered 1–22; a chromosome other than an X or Y

579

bioengineer   A person who combines engineering and life sciences in the study of biological processes

biofeedback   Devices developed to assist control of body function by giving a recognisable signal of a particular function, e.g. head control

biopsy   Removal of a small piece of tissue for examination under the microscope in order to make a diagnosis

bulbar signs   Neurological signs caused by damage to the cranial nerves arising in the medulla causing swallowing and speaking difficulties

caudate nucleus   Part of the corpus striatum of the basal ganglion, so called because it has a long tail, the other parts being the putamen and globus pallidus

choroid plexus   The highly vascular tissue derived from ependymal cells projecting frond-like into the cavities of the cerebral ventricles and producing cerebrospinal fluid (CSF)

complement   A protein which takes part in the reaction between antigens and antibodies

concussion   A state of unconsciousness or impaired consciousness usually caused by mechanical force applied to the skull, not causing disruption of tissue and usually followed by amnesia

congenital   A disorder present at birth, not necessarily inherited

contusion   A bruise from a blow by a blunt instrument inflicted without breaking the integument (skin)

craniosynostosis   Premature fusion of the cranial sutures

creatine phosphokinase   An enzyme normally present in muscle which leaks into the serum in muscular dystrophy and other muscle disorders

cystogram   A radiograph of the bladder

detrusor   The main muscle of the bladder

detrusor sphincter dyssynergia   Failure of coordination between detrusor muscle contraction and sphincter relaxation during bladder emptying

diplegia   Paralysis of symmetrical parts. *Spastic diplegia*: spastic paralysis more marked in the legs, but also affecting the arms

dopa   Dopamine, one of the biogenic amine neurotransmitters

dorsiflexion   Upward movement of the foot from 90 to 45 degrees

dysarthria   Impaired articulation arising from neuromuscular conditions affecting muscle tone and the action of the muscles used in articulation

dysmelia   An imperfect or faulty limb

dysmorphic   A structural abnormality resulting from a primary defect in the morphogenesis of a structure: it can range from an altered fingerprint pattern to complex congenital heart disease

dysphasia   Incomplete language function caused by impairment of the dominant cerebral hemisphere serving the special intellectual functions concerned with the use of language

dysphonia   Impairment of voice production caused by damage to the larynx or the control of voice

dyspraxia Impairment of motor performance

dysraphism Imperfect closure of the neural tube causing a defect of the spinal cord or its surrounding structures

electrocochleography A test of hearing which records the effect of stimulating the 8th cranial nerve (cochlear) and measuring the cortical EEG responses over the temporal lobe of the brain

electroencephalogram (EEG) A record of cerebral action currents

electromyogram (EMG) A record of the action currents of muscle

fasciculation Visible spontaneous contractions of groups of muscle fibres — a feature seen in the tongue associated with atrophy in spinal muscular atrophy

fibrillation Localised irregular twitching of individual muscle fibres also seen in spinal muscular atrophy

fundal plication A surgical operation to repair a hiatus hernia

gamma-aminobutyricacid (GABA) An inhibitory neurotransmitter in the central nervous system

gastrocnemius and soleus The two large muscles of the calf responsible for plantarflexion

gastrostomy An artificial opening from the stomach to the abdominal wall to allow tube feeding to be carried out

gelastic seizures Seizures associated with pathological laughter

hallux valgus Deviation of the great toe towards the others

hamartoma A tumour of embryonic tissue

hemiplegia Paralysis of the arm and leg on the same side of the body caused by an upper motor neurone lesion

hiatus hernia Protrusion of the upper part of the stomach through the oesophageal opening of the diaphragm into the chest

hypercapnia A raised level of carbon dioxide in the blood caused by respiratory failure

incidence The number of new cases of a disorder occurring during a certain time period in a defined population at risk

infarction Death of tissue caused by interruption of end-arterial blood supply

kernicterus Damage to the basal ganglia caused by high level of circulating bilirubin in jaundice of the newborn

kinaesthesia The sense by which movements of the body, weight, position or resistance are perceived by stimulation of specific receptor muscles, tendons or joints

kinetics The study of moving bodies and the forces that act to produce the motion

kyphosis Backward curvature of the spine (hump-back)

laceration A tear or rupture

lordosis Forward curvature of the spine

lower motor neurone The motor nerve supply arising from the anterior horn cell in the spinal cord and terminating in the skeletal muscle

malleolus Part of a bone shaped like a hammer, e.g. at the ankle, medial and lateral malleoli

Milwaukee brace A spinal brace designed to exert distractive force between the pelvis and the head, incorporating a neck extension which takes weight through the occiput and chin

myelination The process of development of the lipid and protein sheath around nerve axons which acts as electrical insulaton and speeds nerve conduction

myelogram A radiograph which outlines the spinal cord and its connections by injection of a radio-opaque dye or air

neural tube The tube of cells in embryological development from which the brain and spinal cord develop

neuropathic bladder Abnormality of the bladder caused by abnormality of its nerve supply

nystagmus Lateral oscillations of the eyes

ocular motor dyspraxia Difficulty in moving the eyes voluntarily in the desired direction when random and reflex movements are intact

oesophageal reflux The return of acid stomach contents into the oesophagus

optic fundus The view of the optic nerve and retina obtained through the pupil with an ophthalmoscope

optokinetic nystagmus Short lateral oscillations of the eyes in response to a series of moving images passing before them. An example is the nystagmus seen when an individual looks out of a moving train. It is a brainstem reflex

orthosis A splint for a disabled part of the body

osteotomy Division of bone or removal of a section of bone

paraplegia Paralysis of the lower half of the body

paraxial hemimelia Absence of one forearm or leg bone; the name of the deficient bone is used as a prefix

periventricular leukomalacia Damage to nervous tissue in the region around the cerebral ventricles at boundary zones between blood vessel territories. In the early stages there is softening of brain tissue, later white spots develop due to fat-laden cells, and finally there may be gliotic scars and cystic areas

pes cavus A foot with very high arches

phocomelia A short flipper-like arm or leg

phonological Concerning the voice

plantarflexion Downward movement of the foot from 90 to 180 degrees

prevalence The number of cases of a disorder present during a certain time period or at a single point in time

proprioception The awareness of position in space and relationship of one part of the body to the rest

prosthesis An artificial substitute for a part of the body which is absent or has been surgically removed

quadriceps The large muscle on the front of the thigh made up of four parts

quadriplegia Paralysis of all four limbs of equal severity

radial club hand deformity Absence of the radius with acute deviation of the hand to the radial side of the wrist

recessive trait A characteristic which only manifests itself in persons who are homozygous for the mutant gene concerned, i.e. who have received a double dose of the gene

rehabilitation engineering The branch of bioengineering associated with treatment of the disabled

renogram Radioactive isotope studies to show individual kidney function

rhizotomy Cutting of nerve roots

saccades or saccadic movements Rapid successive movements of the eyes from one point of fixation to another. All voluntary eye movements (except when following a moving object, when smooth pursuit movements occur) take the form of saccades

scoliosis Lateral curvature of the spine

siblings Brothers and sisters who collectively form a sibship

subluxation Partial dislocation of a joint

subtalar joint The joint below the ankle joint between the talus and the calcaneus

syndrome A recognisable collection of abnormal features or symptoms

syringomyelia Dilatation of the central canal of the spinal cord causing pressure on the neural tissue

talipes Club foot

talipes calcaneus Bent upwards at the heel, i.e. dorsiflexed

talipes equinus (horse-like deformity) On the toes, i.e. the foot is plantar flexed

talipes valgus Turned outwards

talipes varus Turned inwards

tendo calcaneus The large tendon at the back of the heel joining the soleus (calf) muscle to the calcaneum (heel bone); often called the Achilles tendon

tenodesis Fixation of a joint by fixation of tendons passing about the joint

tenotomy Division of a tendon

tibialis anterior A muscle situated at the front of the leg responsible for maintaining balance at the ankle and initiating the arch of the foot

transverse terminal hemimelia (peromelia) Absence of the distal segment of a limb in its entirety

Trendelenburg lurch A waddling gait due to paralysis of the gluteal muscles

trisomy The presence of a triple dose of a single chromosome such as the three No. 21 chromosomes in trisomy-21—Down syndrome

upper motor neurone A nerve cell originating in the motor area of the cerebral cortex and terminating in the motor nuclei of the cranial nerves or in the central grey column of the spinal cord

ureter The duct conveying the urine from the renal pelvis to the bladder

urethra The channel through which the urine is excreted from the bladder

urodynamic studies Studies taken during bladder filling and emptying to demonstrate bladder function

vesical Relating to the bladder

visually evoked responses (VER) A test of vision measuring the cortical EEG response to a visual stimulus

X-linked inheritance A specific pattern of inheritance associated with transmission of abnormality via the X chromosome. The disorder is present in males and transmitted by females

Index